Contents

PART 4 Uncommon Endocrine Disorders

PART 5 Therapeutics and Endocrine Tests

Contributors

Ross Bond BVMS PhD DVD DipECVD MRCVS
Dermatology Unit, Royal Veterinary College, Hawkshead Lane, North Mymms, Hatfield, Herts AL9 7TA, UK

Scott A. Brown VMD PhD DipACVIM
Department of Physiology, University of Georgia College of Veterinary Medicine, 1 Agriculture Drive, Athens, GA 30602, USA

Audrey K. Cook BVM&S DipACVIM MRCVS
Veterinary Internal Medicine, 316 Winston Salem Avenue, 501 Virginia Beach, VA 23451, USA

Richard M. Dixon BVMS CertVR MRCVS
Department of Veterinary Clinical Studies, University of Glasgow Veterinary School, Bearsden Road, Bearsden, Glasgow G61 1QH, UK

Joan Duncan BVMS PhD CertVR MRCVS
Grange Laboratories, Grange House, Sandbeck Way, Wetherby, West Yorkshire LS22 4DN, UK

John K. Dunn MA BVM&S MVetSc DSAM DipECVIM MRCVS
Department of Clinical Veterinary Medicine, University of Cambridge, Madingley Road, Cambridge CB3 0ES, UK

Jonathan Elliott MA VetMB PhD CertSAC MRCVS
Department of Veterinary Basic Sciences, Royal Veterinary College, Royal College Street, London NW1 0TU, UK

Gary England BVetMed PhD DVetMed CertVA DVR DVRep DipACT FRCVS
Royal Veterinary College, Hawkshead Lane, North Mymms, Hatfield, Herts AL9 7TA, UK

Peter A. Graham BVMS PhD CertVR MRCVS
Endocrine Section, Animal Health Diagnostic Laboratory, Michigan State University, PO Box 30076, Lansing, MI 48909-7576, USA

Amanda J. Hawthorne BSc PhD
Waltham Centre for Pet Nutrition, Freeby Lane, Waltham-on-the-Wolds, Melton Mowbray, Leics LE14 4RT, UK

Michael E. Herrtage MA BVSc DVR DVD DSAM DipECVDI DipECVIM MRCVS
Department of Clinical Veterinary Medicine, University of Cambridge, Madingley Road, Cambridge CB3 0ES, UK

Boyd R. Jones BVSc FACVSc MRCVS
Department of Small Animal Clinical Studies, University College Dublin, Ballsbridge, Dublin 4, Republic of Ireland

Elizabeth McNiel DVM MS DipACVIM
Department of Radiological Health Sciences, College of Veterinary Medicine and Biomedical Sciences, Colorado State University, Fort Collins, CO 80523, USA

Carmel T. Mooney MVB MPhil PhD MRCVS
Department of Small Animal Clinical Studies, University College Dublin, Ballsbridge, Dublin 4, Republic of Ireland

Ray F. Nachreiner DVM PhD
Endocrine Section, Animal Health Diagnostic Laboratory, Michigan State University, PO Box 30076, Lansing, MI 48909-7576, USA

Elizabeth J. Norman BVSc MACVSc MRCVS
Department of Veterinary Clinical Studies, University of Glasgow Veterinary School, Bearsden Road, Bearsden, Glasgow G61 1QH, UK

David L. Panciera DVM MS DipACVIM
Alameda East Veterinary Hospital, 9870 East Alameda Avenue, Denver, CO 80231, USA

Mark E. Peterson DVM DipACVIM
The Animal Medical Center, 510 East 62nd Street, New York, NY 10021, USA

Kent R. Refsal DVM PhD
Endocrine Section, Animal Health Diagnostic Laboratory, Michigan State University, PO Box 30076, Lansing, MI 48909-7576, USA

Kenneth W. Simpson BVM&S PhD DipACVIM MRCVS
College of Veterinary Medicine, Cornell University, Ithaca, NY 14853, USA

Jörg Steiner medvet Drmedvet DipACVIM DipECVIM-CA
Gastrointestinal Laboratory, Department of Small Animal Medicine and Surgery, Texas A&M University, College Station, TX 778483-4474, USA

Andrew G. Torrance MA VetMB PhD DipACVIM DipECVIM-CA MRCVS
Bloxham Veterinary Laboratories, George Street, Teignmouth, Devon TQ14 8AH, UK

David C. Twedt DVM DipACVIM
Department of Clinical Sciences, College of Veterinary Medicine and Biomedical Sciences, Colorado State University, Fort Collins, CO 80521, USA

Timothy D.G. Watson BVM&S PhD MRCVS
Waltham Centre for Pet Nutrition, Freeby Lane, Waltham-on-the-Wolds, Melton Mowbray, Leics LE14 4RT, UK

Foreword

The rapid advancement in the knowledge of small animal endocrinopathies has led to a need for a complete revision of the highly successful first edition of the *Manual of Small Animal Endocrinology*. New authors, truly international experts in their own fields, have been recruited from all over the world. This has resulted in an expanded volume with greater emphasis being placed on the clinical case. Full colour photographs and easily read tables complement previously unreported disorders and improvements in diagnostic techniques,

The first part of the book has a diagnostic approach to endocrinological clinical syndromes which should be of major benefit to the busy practitioner. Section two deals with the major endocrinopathies followed by the less common disorders and finally with the all important treatment and testing regimens.

The editors are to be congratulated on producing a book which will maintain both the interest and the skills of the veterinary surgeon in general practice

David F. Wadsworth
BSAVA President 1997-98

Preface

Small animal endocrinology has advanced rapidly over the last few years with the recognition of previously unreported disorders, improvements in diagnostic tests including development of in-house techniques, and the emergence of novel options and refinements for treatment. This edition of the *Manual of Small Animal Endocrinology* is, therefore, not simply an update or revision of that published in 1990. It is a new manual offering the practitioner a concise source of readily accessible, up-to-date, information presented in a format reflecting the relative importance of the different endocrine disorders currently encountered in practice.

The structure of the text breaks with tradition to provide a fresh approach to endocrinology in practice. Instead of a sequential list of endocrine organs and abnormalities, a new format has been selected that divides the subject into five relevant sections. The first section deals with the diagnostic approach to common endocrine problems and provides useful advice on the systematic investigation of patients in the practice situation. The second section presents detailed descriptions of the major endocrinopathies encountered in practice, while sections three and four deal with more complex and uncommon disorders, respectively. The final section provides an easy reference to therapeutics and endocrine tests including dynamic test protocols.

Throughout the book, information of greatest clinical relevance is emphasised, including presenting features, diagnostic testing and treatment. Where applicable, separate descriptions of disorders are presented for dogs and cats. Algorithms, tables and figures appear frequently and provide the practitioner with readily accessible material ensuring that this manual will be a well-thumbed addition to the practice library.

Clinical endocrinology is a fascinating subject requiring in-depth knowledge not only of internal medicine but also of physiology, clinical pathology, anatomy and surgery. This manual provides the most comprehensive information available today in a format designed specifically for the busy small animal practitioner.

Andrew G. Torrance
Carmel T. Mooney
February 1998

PART ONE

The Clinical Approach to Endocrine Problems

CHAPTER ONE

The Dog with Polydipsia and Polyuria

John K. Dunn

INTRODUCTION

Polydipsia is defined as a fluid intake >100 ml/kg/24 hours. In dogs, polyuria is defined as the formation and excretion of large volumes of urine (>50 ml/kg/24 hours). Polyuria is frequently accompanied by pollakiuria (increased frequency of urination) and nocturia (a voluntary desire to urinate at night). The converse, however, is not always the case, i.e. pollakiuria and nocturia are not always indicative of polyuria and may be caused by numerous inflammatory, neoplastic and functional disorders of the lower urinary tract which compromise the normal function and filling capacity of the bladder.

Water is taken into the body by ingestion and is produced in the body by the oxidation of carbohydrate, fat, and protein. Daily fluid intake must compensate for water that is lost in faeces and urine and by evaporation from the skin and respiratory tract. A healthy dog drinks approximately 50–60 ml/kg/24 hours of water, depending on the moisture content of its diet, and normal urine output varies between 20 and 40 ml/kg/24 hours. Thirst and the renal control of salt and water excretion are the two main mechanisms for balancing water intake with water loss. The physiology of normal water balance is described in more detail in Chapter 18.

PATHOPHYSIOLOGY

Most disorders of water balance that cause polydipsia and polyuria are the result of impaired ability of the kidneys to conserve water. In most cases, polydipsia represents a compensatory mechanism to maintain total body fluids within normal limits. Less frequently polydipsia is primary and compensatory polyuria occurs in response to the excess water load.

Conditions causing water diuresis
Water diuresis may be associated with impaired synthesis or secretion of vasopressin (antidiuretic hormone, ADH) from the neurohypophysis (central diabetes insipidus, CDI) or an inability of distal renal tubules and collecting ducts to respond to ADH (nephrogenic diabetes insipidus, NDI).

Central diabetes insipidus is a rare condition caused by a complete or partial deficiency of ADH. Most cases are classified as idiopathic although CDI may occur as a sequel to head trauma or in association with pituitary or hypothalamic tumours. A complete deficiency of ADH is characterised by

Pyelonephritis
Chronic renal failure
Hypercalcaemia
Hypokalaemia
Pyometra
Hyperadrenocorticism
Hepatic failure
Hyperthyroidism

Table 1.1: *Disorders associated with impaired responsiveness of renal tubules and collecting ducts to antidiuretic hormone (acquired nephrogenic diabetes insipidus).*

hyposthenuria i.e. the production of urine with low specific gravity (usually <1.005). With a partial deficiency of ADH, urine may be minimally concentrated i.e. urine specific gravity may be within the isosthenuric range (1.008–1.012). Certain drugs, most notably glucocorticoids, inhibit the release of ADH. Most cases of NDI are acquired and occur secondary to numerous metabolic disorders (Table 1.1). Primary NDI is an extremely rare congenital renal abnormality.

Water diuresis also occurs in cases of primary (psychogenic) polydipsia where the excessive intake of water over a prolonged period results in renal medullary washout. The net result with any of these conditions is the production of a large volume of dilute solute-free urine. The investigation of persistent hyposthenuria is discussed in more detail in Chapter 18.

Conditions causing solute diuresis
A large amount of solute, e.g. glucose, urea or sodium in the glomerular filtrate overwhelms the reabsorptive capacity of proximal tubular epithelial cells and results in the obligatory excretion of water. Conditions where solute or osmotic diuresis contribute to polyuria include diabetes mellitus, primary renal glycosuria and chronic renal failure, and the diuresis that occurs following relief of urethral obstruction (postobstructive diuresis).

Renal medullary washout
In response to ADH, water is reabsorbed along concentration gradients established in the renal medulla. Renal medullary hypertonicity is maintained by the efflux of high levels of sodium, chloride and urea from the loop of Henle and collecting ducts. Loss of this osmotic gradient,

HISTORY CHECK LIST

Consider breed, age and sex of animal; sexually intact or neutered? Quantify water intake in ml/kg/24 hours	• Endotoxaemia e.g. pyometra • Uraemia (chronic renal failure) • Ketoacidosis (diabetes mellitus) • Hypoadrenocorticism • Hypercalcaemia
Urination Abnormal volume, colour or smell? Nocturia? Incontinent? Frequency?	**Behavioural changes or central nervous system signs?** • Hepatic encephalopathy • Expanding pituitary tumour
Diet Moisture content? Recent changes?	**Exercise intolerance/muscle weakness?** • Hyperadrenocorticism
Appetite normal or polyphagic? • Primary polydipsia • Diabetes insipidus • Diabetes mellitus • Hyperadrenocorticism	**Reproductive abnormalities?** Recent oestrus? Vaginal discharge? Recent administration of oestrogens? Loss of libido?
Inappetent or anorexic? • Pyometra • Chronic renal failure • Liver disease • Diabetes mellitus (ketoacidosis) • Hypoadrenocorticism • Hypercalcaemia	**Environmental changes or trauma?** • Primary polydipsia • Secondary diabetes insipidus
General health Weight loss? Lethargic or depressed? Vomiting or diarrhoea? *(continues)*	**Recent or current drug administration?** • Frusemide • Mannitol • Dextrose • Intravenous fluids (crystalloids) • Anticonvulsant drugs (primidone, phenobarbitol, phenytoin) • Glucocorticoids

CLINICAL EXAMINATION CHECK LIST

Record body weight Assess hydration status	**Peripheral lymphadenopathy?** • Multicentric lymphosarcoma (check for hypercalcaemia)
Palpate abdomen	
Kidneys enlarged or painful? • Glomerulonephritis • Renal lymphosarcoma • Pyelonephritis	**Palpable thyroid mass?** Hyperthyroidism is rare in dogs and when present is usually due to a thyroid carcinoma
Kidneys small and misshapen? • Chronic interstitial nephritis • Congenital renal dysplasia	**External genitalia** Vaginal discharge (open-cervix pyometra)? Testicular atrophy (hyperadrenocorticism)?
Liver enlarged? • Diabetes mellitus • Hyperadrenocorticism • Chronic active hepatitis • Hepatic neoplasia	**Eyes** Cataract formation (diabetes mellitus)?
	Skin changes? Endocrine alopecia, thin, non-elastic skin, comedone formation and pendulous abdomen suggestive of hyperadrenocorticism
Uterus distended? • Closed cervix-pyometra	**Bradycardia?** • Hypoadrenocorticism • Hypercalcaemia
Pendulous abdomen? • Hyperadrenocorticism	

Table 1.2: *Investigation of polydipsia and polyuria in the dog: history and clinical examination check lists.*

for example due to chronic sodium wasting in dogs with hypoadrenocorticism, results in submaximal concentration of urine even in the presence of adequate ADH.

In many cases the pathophysiological mechanism of polyuria is multifactorial. For example the polyuria and polydipsia associated with chronic liver disease may be due partly to decreased conversion of ammonia to urea (and a resultant loss of medullary hypertonicity), and partly to other mechanisms such as decreased release of ADH caused by increased levels of circulating cortisol. The polyuria associated with primary polydipsia can be attributed to the effects of renal medullary washout and overhydration resulting in a relative lack of ADH.

DIAGNOSTIC APPROACH

History

The causes of polydipsia and polyuria in the dog are numerous. An accurate history is often extremely informative and may help to rule out some of the more common differential diagnoses. Consideration should be given to the general health of the animal, diet, environmental factors, reproductive history, and recent or current drug administration. These aspects are summarised in Table 1.2.

Primary *versus* secondary polydipsia

Primary or psychogenic polydipsia (compulsive water drinking) is an uncommon disorder characterised by a marked increase in water intake. Water consumption exceeds the body's requirements, resulting in overhydration and compensatory (secondary) polyuria. The aetiology is uncertain; it may represent a behavioural abnormality triggered by an environmental or emotional stimulus. Less frequently, primary polydipsia is associated with lesions involving the hypothalamic thirst centre. The ability to concentrate urine is retained although frequently this may be impaired due to the effects of renal medullary washout. The condition requires differentiation from CDI and NDI. The diagnosis and management of primary polydipsia is discussed more fully in Chapter 18.

With most polydipsic conditions, excessive drinking represents a compensatory secondary response to an obligatory polyuria. Although an observant owner may notice their dog is drinking more, it is often the polyuria, particularly if the animal is unable to retain large volumes of urine overnight, that provides the stimulus for veterinary consultation.

Polyuria, nocturia and urinary incontinence

Nocturia must in the first instance be distinguished from true urinary incontinence. Typically, urinary incontinence associated with sphincter mechanism incompetence (oestrogen-responsive incontinence) occurs in medium and large breed dogs and is characterised by the passive leakage of urine when the dog is either lying down resting or sleeping. The problem is most frequently observed in overweight, middle-aged bitches that have been spayed. Nocturia and urinary incontinence may be initiated or exacerbated in any dog that is polyuric.

Breed, age and sex

Some polyuric/polydipsic conditions occur more frequently in certain breeds of dog; for example, Miniature Poodles are predisposed to hyperadrenocorticism and diabetes mellitus, Dobermann Pinschers to chronic active hepatitis, and Lhaso Apsos and Shih Tzus to familial renal dysplasia. Pyometra is more common in middle-aged bitches, i.e. 8–10 years old. Primary polydipsia occurs more frequently in young, hyperexcitable, large breed dogs.

Verify and quantify the polydipsia

The volume of water drunk should be quantified at an early stage. In most cases this can be simply done by asking the owner to measure water intake at home for at least 3 consecutive days. Accurate measurement of water intake may be difficult in polydipsic dogs which persist in drinking from a range of sources, e.g. puddles and toilets or even their own urine. Similar difficulties may be encountered in multipet households, and hospitalisation may be necessary to assess an individual animal's water intake.

Dogs with diabetes insipidus or primary polydipsia are usually severely polydipsic, i.e. there may be a 4–6-fold increase in water consumption. Frequently, simply hospitalising a dog with primary polydipsia may significantly reduce its water intake, presumably by removing or altering the precipitating emotional or stress factor.

Appetite and diet

When assessing water intake, the nature and composition of the diet should be taken into account. Dogs fed a complete dry cereal-based diet invariably drink more water than those fed a meat-based diet. Low protein diets may also result in renal medullary washout and primary polyuria.

Many systemic diseases which cause polydipsia also affect appetite.

General health

The presence of non-specific clinical signs such as anorexia, lethargy, depression, and weight loss is of limited diagnostic value. Signs which relate directly to the underlying disease process responsible for the polydipsia and polyuria are generally more informative.

Vomiting, with or without diarrhoea, may occur with pyometra (endotoxaemia), chronic renal failure (uraemia), hepatic failure, hypoadrenocorticism, hypercalcaemia, and diabetes mellitus (ketoacidosis).

Hepatic encephalopathy (due to portosystemic shunts or acquired chronic liver disease) and large expanding pituitary neoplasms in dogs with pituitary-dependent hyperadrenocorticism may result in a variety of behavioural abnormalities and central nervous system (CNS) signs, e.g. ataxia, central blindness, seizures, mental stupor, head pressing, and aimless wandering. In addition, dogs with hyperadrenocorticism become exercise intolerant due to progressive generalised muscle weakness.

Reproductive history

Pyometra is typically a disorder of middle-aged bitches, clinical signs usually occurring during or immediately

Condition	Clinical signs other than poly-dipsia and polyuria	Haematology/ Biochemistry	Urinalysis	Radiology	Additional diagnostic tests	Mechanism of polydipsia and polyuria
Chronic renal insufficiency/failure due to:						
Chronic interstitial nephritis (CIN)	Weight loss, anorexia, depression, vomiting, 'rubber jaw', ± melaena	Non-regenerative anaemia, lymphopenia, ↑ urea, creatinine, and phosphate	Isosthenuria, ± casts, ± protein	Kidneys small, ± signs of secondary renal hyperpara-thyroidism		Decrease in number of functional nephrons, osmotic diuresis, decreased renal medullary hypertonicity
Glomerulonephro-pathy/nephrotic syndrome: Renal amyloidosis Renal lymphoma Glomerulonephritis	As for CIN ± peripheral oedema, occasionally ascites	As for CIN ± ↑ cholesterol, hypoalbuminaemia	Significant proteinuria	± enlarged kidneys, ± signs of secondary renal hyperpara-thyroidism	Urine protein: creatinine ratio, renal ultrasonography, and biopsy	As for CIN
Pyelonephritis	As for CIN ± pyrexia, sublumbar pain	As for CIN + neutrophilia ± left shift	White blood cells (WBCs), protein, bacteria, and casts	Kidney size variable (may be markedly enlarged)	Intravenous urography, urine culture, renal ultrasonography	As for CIN, destruction of countercurrent mechanism in renal medulla
Chronic liver disease: Portosystemic shunts Chronic active hepatitis (CAH) Fibrosis and cirrhosis Neoplasia	Vomiting, diarrhoea, weight loss, ± jaundice, ± ascites, ± CNS signs	Mild non-regenerative anaemia, hypoproteinaemia (↓ albumin), ↓ urea, ± ↑ ALT, ALP and ɣ-GT, ± ↓ glucose, ± ↑ bilirubin, ↑ pre- and post-prandial bile acids	Variable urine specific gravity, biurate crystals (especially portosytemic shunts), ± ↑ bilirubin	Liver size ↓ (portosystemic shunts, cirrhosis), liver size ↑ (CAH, neoplasia)	Pre- and post-prandial bile acids, ↑ blood clotting times (OSPT/APTT), ↑ plasma ammonia, liver biopsy	Decreased medullary hypertonicity, hypercortisolaemia, impaired action and release of ADH and aldosterone
Pyometra and other toxaemic states	Anorexia, depression, weight loss, vomiting, abdominal distension, vaginal discharge (if open)	Neutrophilia with a left shift; WBC count may be normal if open, pre-renal azotaemia	WBCs, protein	Coiled soft tissue dense viscus in mid-caudal abdomen		Endotoxin-induced renal tubular insensitivity to ADH; immune-complex glomerulonephritis
Primary (psychogenic) polydipsia	Severe polydipsia and polyuria	± Low normal plasma osmolality	Hyposthenuria		Equivocal response to water deprivation and ADH indicating submaximal concentration of urine	Failure of collecting ducts to respond to ADH, medullary washout
Primary renal glycosuria	Inherited in Norwegian Elkhounds	Normal blood glucose	Glycosuria			Osmotic diuresis
Fanconi's syndrome	Inherited in Basenjis	Normal blood glucose	Glycosuria, ↑ urinary excretion of amino acids, phosphate, sodium and bicarbonate			Osmotic diuresis
Hypercalcaemia: Hypercalcaemia of malignancy Metastatic bone tumours Renal dysplasia	Weakness, depression, anorexia, muscle tremors, bradycardia, vomiting, signs associated with primary neoplasm e.g. enlarged lymph nodes	± Non-regenerative anaemia, initially ↑ calcium and ↓ phosphate; later increases in urea, creatinine and phosphate (nephrocalcinosis)	Frequently isosthenuria, casts		Identify underlying cause; may require lymph node or bone marrow aspirate/biopsy to rule out neoplasia, PTH or PTHrp measurement	Nephrocalcinosis resulting in chronic renal failure, impaired action of ADH on renal receptors
Hypokalaemia: Excessive gastro-intestinal loss Excessive renal loss e.g. diabetes mellitus, renal failure, diuretic therapy	Muscle weakness (hypokalaemic myopathy), gastric atony, paralytic ileus, cardiac arrhythmias	↓ Potassium	Non-specific		Response to potassium supplementation	Intracellular dehydration resulting in stimulation of thirst centre, failure of collecting ducts to respond to ADH, ?impaired release of ADH, medullary washout
Hyperviscosity syndromes: Polycythaemia vera Hypergammaglob-ulinaemia e.g. plasma cell myeloma	Bleeding diatheses, CNS signs or congestive heart failure	↑ Haemoglobin, total red blood cell count and packed cell volume			Serum protein electrophoresis, bone marrow aspiration	Uncertain

ADH, antidiuretic hormone; ALT, alanine aminotransferase; ALP, alkaline phosphatase; APTT, activated partial thromboplastin time; ɣ-GT, gamma-glutamyltransferase; OSPT, one-stage prothrombin time; PTH, parathyroid hormone; PTHrp, parathyroid hormone related protein.

Table 1.3: *Non-endocrine causes of polydipsia and polyuria.*

after the dioestrous phase of the oestrous cycle. Occasionally open- or closed-cervix pyometra occurs in younger animals following the administration of oestrogens for misalliance. Open-cervix pyometra is characterised by the presence of a purulent and/or sanguinous vaginal discharge approximately 4–8 weeks after oestrus.

In the bitch, hyperadrenocorticism may result in prolonged anoestrus; in males, the excessive secretion of cortisol results in testicular atrophy which in the stud dog may result in a loss of libido.

Environmental stress factors and trauma

Occasionally in dogs with pyschogenic polydipsia, it is possible to identify a stress factor preceding the onset of the polydipsia. This may take the form of some sudden alteration to the animal's immediate environment such as moving house or the arrival of a new baby. Secondary CDI caused by either a complete or partial deficiency of ADH occasionally occurs as a sequel to head trauma resulting in disruption of the pituitary stalk.

Recent or current drug administration

Many drugs can cause polydipsia and polyuria and can therefore influence urine specific gravity and urine output, e.g. the administration of frusemide, dextrose, mannitol, or intravenous crystalloid solutions results in obligatory solute diuresis and compensatory polydipsia. Other drugs such as glucocorticoids, phenytoin, primidone and phenobarbitol either inhibit the release of ADH from the pituitary gland or interfere with its action on renal tubular epithelial cells and collecting ducts.

CLINICAL EXAMINATION

The significance of various clinical abnormalities in the context of investigation of polydipsia and polyuria is summarised in Table 1.2.

Dogs with diabetes insipidus or primary (psychogenic) polydipsia are generally bright and active and show few, if any, clinical abnormalities. Other disorders may be ruled in or out on the basis of a thorough clinical examination which should include careful palpation of the abdomen, peripheral lymph nodes and external genitalia. During abdominal palpation particular attention should be paid to the size and shape of the kidneys and the size of the liver. If closed-cervix pyometra is suspected, palpation should be performed with great care to minimise the risk of perforating the distended uterus.

Ophthalmic examination for cataract formation (diabetes mellitus) and a thorough neurological examination should be performed in any animal with a history of CNS or behavioural abnormalities.

SCREENING LABORATORY TESTS

A minimum data base for the laboratory investigation of polydipsia and polyuria includes full routine haematology, a complete biochemistry screen, and urinalysis.

A biochemistry screen consisting of total plasma protein, albumin, globulin, sodium, potassium, chloride, calcium, phosphate, glucose, liver enzymes (alanine amino-transferase, aspartate aminotransferase, alkaline phosphatase, gamma-glutamyl transferase), urea and creatinine determinations is a cost effective way of identifying or ruling out many of the differential diagnoses listed in Tables 1.3 and 1.4.

Urinalysis

Urine specific gravity is dependent on particle size and molecular weight as well as the total number of solute molecules. An approximate relationship exists between the specific gravity and total concentration of urinary solute. Urine specific gravity in normal dogs varies from approximately 1.015 to 1.045.

Osmolality represents the concentration of osmotically active particles in solution and is expressed as mOsm/kg. Osmolality is directly related to osmotic pressure and is not influenced by particle size or molecular weight. Urine osmolality in the dog varies from 500 to 1200 mOsm/kg.

It has been shown that there is considerable intra- and interindividual variation in both urine specific gravity and osmolality values in healthy dogs of various ages. Urine specific gravity values as low as 1.006 and above 1.050, and osmolality values ranging from 161 to 2830 mOsm/kg have been reported in healthy dogs. Urine concentration is generally lower in the evening than in the morning and it also decreases with age.

Urine can be classified into one of four categories on the basis of urine specific gravity:

- Hyposthenuria (specific gravity 1.001–1.007); urine more dilute than plasma
- Isosthenuria (1.008–1.012); urine has similar concentration to plasma i.e. specific gravity is within the 'fixed' range typical of chronic renal failure
- Range of minimal concentration (1.013–1.029); ability to concentrate urine is submaximal
- Hypersthenuric (>1.030); urine more concentrated than plasma.

Persistent hyposthenuria is suggestive of a deficiency of ADH or lack of responsiveness to ADH; it does not however indicate abnormal tubular function since urine is actively diluted in the ascending limb of the loop of Henlé. The investigation of persistent hyposthenuria is described in Chapter 18.

In addition to urine specific gravity, urine should be examined for protein, blood, bilirubin and urobilinogen. Urine sediment should be examined microscopically for the presence of red and white blood cells, epithelial cells, bacteria, casts, and crystals. Bacteriological culture of a urine sample, preferably obtained by cystocentesis, should be considered even when urinary sediment is unremarkable.

Plasma osmolality

Normal plasma osmolality varies with the state of hydration (approximately 275–305 mOsm/kg). Dogs with

Condition	Clinical signs other than polydipsia and polyuria	Haematology/ Biochemistry	Urinalysis	Radiology	Additional diagnostic tests	Mechanism of polydipsia and polyuria
Diabetes insipidus: Central diabetes insipidus (CDI)	Severe polydipsia and polyuria, ± marginal dehydration, ± central nervous system signs, ± weight loss (restlessness), ± vomiting following excessive water intake	± slight increases in packed cell volume, plasma proteins and plasma osmolality, ± ↑ urea, creatinine, sodium, and chloride (if water depleted)	Hyposthenuria, urine osmolality 40–200 mOsm/kg		Negative response to water deprivation; positive response to ADH	Decreased secretion of ADH
Nephrogenic diabetes insipidus (see Table 1.1)	As for CDI	As for CDI	As for CDI		Negative response to water deprivation and to ADH administration	Distal tubules and collecting ducts unresponsive to ADH
Diabetes mellitus (may be associated with hyperadrenocorticism)	Obese or progressive weight loss, polyphagia, lethargy; anorexia and vomiting if ketoacidotic, hepatomegaly, dry scurfy hair coat, cataract formation	± Leucocytosis or stress haemogram, ↑ glucose, ↑ ALT/ALP, ± ↑ cholesterol, lipaemic plasma, low or normal potassium, ± pre-renal azotaemia, ↑ amylase and lipase if concurrent pancreatitis	Glycosuria,± ketonuria, urine specific gravity typically >1.030	Hepatomegaly	Plasma fructosamine, glycosylated haemoglobin	Osmotic diuresis
Hyperadreno- corticism (may be associated with diabetes mellitus)	Alopecia, hyperpig- mentation, loss of skin elasticity, calcinosis cutis, muscle weakness/ atrophy, exercise intolerance, polyphagia, hepatomegaly, pendulous abdomen, testicular atrophy	Stress haemogram (neutrophilia, lymphopenia, eosinopenia ± monocytosis), ↑ ALP and ALT, ± ↑ glucose, ± ↑ cholesterol	Variable urine specific gravity (often hyposthenuric or isosthenuric), urinary tract infections common, ± glycosuria	Hepatomegaly, bronchial/tracheal calcification, calcification along fascial planes, calcinosis cutis, osteoporosis, mineralisation of adrenal gland (neoplasia)	ACTH response test, low and high dose dexamethasone suppression tests	Excessive production of cortisol inhibits the release and interferes with the action of ADH, increase in glomerular filtration rate
Hypoadrenocorticism: Acute	Hypovolaemia, shock (collapse), dehydration, bradycardia, ± gastrointestinal haemorrhage, abdominal pain	Variable eosinophilia and lymphocytosis, mild non-regenerative anaemia (regenerative if gastrointestinal haemorrhage), pre-renal azotaemia, ↓ sodium, ↑ potassium, (sodium:potassium ratio <23:1), mild hypercalcaemia, ± ↓ glucose	Variable urine specific gravity; often isosthenuric	Microcardia, hyperlucent lung fields (decreased pulmonary perfusion), narrow posterior vena cava	ECG: with severe hyperkalaemia peaked T waves, absent P waves and bradycardia; negative response to ACTH stimulation	Renal sodium wasting results in renal medullary washout, may be due also to effects of hypovolaemia and hypercalcaemia
Chronic	Polydipsia/polyuria in 15% of cases, anorexia, weight loss, depression, muscle weakness, tremors, intermittent vomiting and diarrhoea					
Hyperthyroidism (rare; usually thyroid carcinomas)	Weight loss, polyphagia, palpable thyroid mass (if large may result in dysphagia, cough, respiratory distress, vomiting)	Non-specific		± Cardiomegaly and signs of congestive heart failure	T4 assay (only 5– 10%) of tumours are functional) ECG biopsy	Multifactorial?, impaired action of ADH, increased renal blood flow results in medullary washout, ?compulsive polydipsia
Acromegaly: Administration of progestogens May occur spontaneously during dioestrus	Excessive skin folds around head, neck and limbs, inspiratory stridor, general increase in body size, protruding mandible, increased interdental spaces,	± ↑ Glucose, ↑ ALP/ALT, ↑ phosphate (mild)	± Glycosuria	Hyperostosis of the skull, soft tissue swelling of the head, neck, limbs and oropharyngeal region	Skin biopsy (increased dermal collagen deposition); growth hormone or insulin-like growth factor assay	Excessive production of growth hormone results in insulin- resistant diabetes mellitus
Hypercalcaemia: Functional para- thyroid adenoma Hypervitaminosis D Hypoadrenocorticism	see Non-endocrine causes of hypercalcaemia (Table 1.3)	see Non-endocrine causes of hypercalcaemia (Table 1.3)	see Non-endocrine causes of hypercalcaemia (Table 1.3)	Skeletal osteoporosis (parathyroid adenomas)	PTH assay, vitamin D assay, exploratory surgery	see Non-endocrine causes of hypercalcaemia (Table 1.3)
Hypocalcaemia: Idiopathic hypo- parathyroidism Thyroid carcinoma (hypercalcitoninism)	Central nervous system signs predominate (seizures, ataxia, muscle tremors, tetany), vomiting and diarrhoea, cataract formation	↓ calcium, ↑ phosphate			PTH assay	Uncertain

ACTH, adrenocorticotropic hormone; ADH, antidiuretic hormone; ALP, alkaline phosphatase; ALT, alanine aminotransferase; ECG, electrocardiogram; PTH, parathyroid hormone.

Table 1.4: *Endocrine causes of polydipsia and polyuria.*

diabetes insipidus usually have high normal or slightly increased plasma osmolality because of the continuous loss of solute-free water in their urine. In comparison, dogs with primary polydipsia may have slightly low plasma osmolality due to water overload.

RADIOGRAPHY AND ULTRASONOGRAPHY

Abdominal radiographs are indicated in most dogs with polydipsia and polyuria to further evaluate the size and shape of the kidneys, liver, uterus and adrenal glands. When available, ultrasonographic examination complements radiography by assessing the internal structure of organs and identifying the presence of focal lesions. In skilled hands ultrasonography provides a more accurate assessment of adrenal size and shape than radiography.

SPECIFIC DIAGNOSTIC TESTS

Many causes of polydipsia and polyuria can be excluded by careful assessment of the history, clinical findings and results of the minimum data base. The differential diagnosis of polydipsia and polyuria and specific diagnostic tests are described in Tables 1.3 and 1.4.

CHAPTER TWO

The Obese Dog

Timothy D.G. Watson and Amanda J. Hawthorne

INTRODUCTION

Obesity is common in dogs and has important conse-quences for their long-term health. The observed incidence, as reported from surveys conducted in veterinary practices, ranges from 24% to 44% (Markwell and Butterwick, 1994). Certain breeds appear to be more susceptible to obesity, while others are at reduced risk (Edney and Smith, 1986). The reasons for this are unclear, although feeding behav-iours, regulation of food intake and inherent metabolic differences may play important roles. Obesity appears to be more common in middle-aged dogs (6–8 years).

Complications of obesity in dogs include traumatic and degenerative orthopaedic diseases (rupture of cruciate ligaments, hip dysplasia and elbow problems), cardiopul-monary compromise (increased risk of congestive heart failure, hypertension, respiratory embarrassment), heat and exercise intolerance, glucose intolerance, diabetes mellitus, pancreatitis, and fatty infiltration of the liver. Although a number of other consequences of obesity have been suggested, including increased risks of infection, perioperative complications, altered drug metabolism, dystocia, dermatological problems and certain neoplasias, the evidence cited for these associations is weak and open to criticism (Buffington, 1994).

CAUSES OF OBESITY

Obesity is a pathological condition characterised by the accu-mulation of adipose tissue in excess of that required for optimal body function. Excess adipose tissue is formed when energy intake chronically exceeds energy expenditure.

Typically this imbalance is attributed to overeating, under-exercising, or a combination of both factors. It has been suggested that at least 95% of canine obesity is due to simple overeating (Glickman *et al.*, 1995). Although it is possible that changes in metabolic efficiency may also contribute to obesity, such anomalies have not been well defined in dogs. Certain endocrine diseases are associated with obesity and these include hypothyroidism, hyper-adrenocorticism, hyper-insulinaemia and hypogonadism. It is unclear, however, whether the relationship of these conditions to obesity reflects overeating, under-exercising, or real changes in meta-bolic efficiency associated with the endocrinopathy. Hypothyroidism is believed to cause a reduction in resting metabolic rate; hyperadrenocorticism and hyperinsulinaemia are associated with polyphagia; hyperadrenocorticism results in increased fat storage; and hypogonadism is associated with reduced energy expenditure. Chronic administration of drugs, such as megoestrol acetate and some anticonvulsants, may be associated with polyphagia and the development of obesity.

Neutering has been identified as an important risk factor for obesity, particularly in females where neutered bitches are twice as likely to be obese as entire animals (Edney and Smith, 1986). Energy intake does not appear to be influenced by neutering, suggesting that changes in energy expenditure, in terms of exercise, or efficiency of energy utilisation are responsible for the development of obesity in neutered dogs (Glickman *et al.*, 1995). Calorie consumption of adult dogs does not appear to be related to age (Glickman *et al.*, 1995), suggesting that age-related declines in exercise or metabolic efficiency are primarily responsible for the development of obesity in middle age. It has been recently reported that the maintenance energy requirements of a group of senior dogs (>8 years of age)

Breed	Typical body weight (kg)					
	Male			**Female**		
	Mean	**Min**	**Max**	**Mean**	**Min**	**Max**
Basset Hound	28.5	23.1	32.1	25.1	23.0	30.4
Beagle	14.9	11.0	19.1	13.0	10.4	16.0
Cairn Terrier	7.8	6.3	8.6	7.2	5.3	9.3
Cavalier King Charles Spaniel	9.0	6.8	11.5	7.9	4.7	10.0
Cocker Spaniel	13.7	10.7	19.0	11.6	8.8	16.5
Labrador Retriever	38.3	26.1	44.7	31.8	26.3	40.0
Shetland Sheepdog	8.8	6.4	16.4	7.8	6.0	10.6

Table 2.1: *Breeds predisposed to obesity. Typical body weights for non-obese males and females are represented as mean, minimum (min) and maximum (max) from adult dogs weighed at Championship Shows in the UK. (D. Booles, unpublished data.)*

Failure to adjust food offered according to the individual dog's needs and activity
Giving additional calories in the form of snacks, treats, or table scraps
Encouraging appetite as a sign of good health
Using food to develop and sustain the owner–dog bond
Indulging begging behaviour
Giving food as a palliative, e.g. for when the dog is left alone
Providing inadequate exercise

Table 2.2: Owner lifestyle and behavioural characteristics that contribute to the development of obesity in dogs. (Adapted from Markwell and Butterwick, 1994.)

of mixed breeds were on average 20% lower than that of young adult dogs (<6 years of age) (Harper, 1997). Failure to compensate by reducing meal size will, therefore, result in relative overfeeding and the development of obesity.

The predisposition of certain breeds to obesity (Table 2.1) suggests a familial aetiology but no genetic factor has been identified in dogs. In reality it is difficult to separate genetic from environmental influences. However, the identification of genes and gene products that regulate energy balance in man and rodents, such as leptin and neuropeptide Y, has re-awakened interest in genetic causes of obesity. It is possible that homologous genes exist in other species, including the dog, and that defects in these genes, or the receptors with which their products interact, result in ineffective regulation of energy intake and metabolism.

Owner lifestyles and behaviours make a significant contribution to the development of obesity by resulting in overfeeding and under-exercising (Table 2.2). It is important to recognise the contribution of these various factors as long-term weight maintenance is dependent upon their modification. Feeding patterns, particularly table scraps, and choice of diet are important factors. In one US study, table scraps accounted for approximately one-third of total daily energy intake (Glickman *et al.*, 1995). Energy-dense, highly palatable dry foods have been associated with obesity in cats (Scarlett *et al.*, 1994), although no equivalent data exist for dogs. High fat diets may be problematical because fat: delivers 2.25 times the calories of equivalent weights of protein and carbohydrate; blunts diet-induced thermogenesis; and enhances palatability, thereby potentially over-riding normal mechanisms of appetite control. It has been suggested that dogs fed home-prepared diets are more likely to become obese (Mason, 1970), but this is a rare practice and an insignificant factor in the current prevalence of obesity.

RECOGNITION AND ASSESSMENT OF OBESITY

Recognition of obesity by the owner and veterinarian is the first step in successful weight management. Unfortunately there are no robust, objective criteria on which to base this recognition and monitor the effectiveness of weight loss programmes. Obesity has been arbitrarily defined as body weights in excess of 110%, 115% or 120% of the animal's ideal or optimum weight. While such definitions provide the means of convincing owners of the gravity of their dog's condition, major difficulties

lie in deciding what is the optimum weight for an individual dog, when the latter is clearly influenced by breed, gender and conformation. Information on 'ideal' body weights for pedigree dogs can be obtained from breed tables and this may assist in deciding an ideal body weight as the target for weight reduction. Typical body weights for breeds most at risk of obesity are included in Table 2.1.

Although body condition scoring is subjective, it is useful when pre-defined visible and palpable criteria are used (Edney and Smith, 1986; Laflamme, 1997) and currently represents the most reliable means of assessing obesity in a clinical situation. Body condition scoring can easily be incorporated into a physical examination and has been shown to provide accurate assessment of percentage body fat and to be reasonably repeatable within individual animals and between assessors (Laflamme, 1997). More objective means of assessing obesity, such as dual energy X-ray absorptiometry (Munday, 1994) and isotope dilution to measure total body water (Sheng and Huggins, 1979), offer great potential in obesity research but are unfortunately not practical in clinical situations.

CLINICAL INVESTIGATION

Prior to instituting a weight loss programme (Table 2.3), it is essential to check the patient for any concurrent disease that might be associated with the development of obesity, e.g. endocrine disorders, or that may complicate the long-term success of its management, e.g. cardiopulmonary or orthopaedic disease. Specifically, clinical examination and routine laboratory tests should be used to monitor for hypothyroidism, hyperadrenocorticism, hyperinsulinaemia and hypogonadism. A minimum database should include a complete blood count, chemistry panel, and urinalysis. Indications of underlying disease should then be followed up with more targeted testing procedures, as outlined elsewhere in this book.

CLINICAL MANAGEMENT OF OBESITY

An effective weight loss programme comprises energy restriction and increased energy expenditure through exercise, monitoring of weight loss, and modification of owner and dog behaviours that have contributed to excess energy intake or insufficient exercise (Table 2.4). Owner commitment is crucial for success, especially when the programme may take 6–12 months to complete, require

1	Recognition of obesity by owner and veterinarian
2	Identification and treatment of any underlying or concurrent disease
3	Controlled weight loss programme
4	Prevention of weight rebound

Table 2.3. Route to successful management of obesity in dogs.

1	Calculate energy restriction
2	Select appropriate diet
3	Modify owner/dog behaviours that contribute to overfeeding or insufficient exercise
4	Design a realistic exercise programme
5	Regularly monitor weight loss

Table 2.4: Clinical management of obesity – components of an effective weight loss programme.

significant effort in monitoring food intake and exercise patterns, and possibly involve substantial changes in the owner's lifestyle.

In dogs where obesity is complicated by the presence of hypothyroidism or hyperadrenocorticism, the primary aim should be to restore normal thyroid or adrenal function with appropriate therapies. If the obesity persists once the patient is stable, then a programme of weight loss should be instituted. Excessive weight loss may indicate inappropriate doses of replacement thyroid hormones.

Energy restriction

The aim of energy restriction is to lose weight from adipose and not lean body tissue. Loss of lean body mass is associated with very rapid rates of weight loss, which can be detrimental to the health of the patient, as well as resulting in significant weight gain once energy restriction is discontinued. Starvation is well tolerated by dogs, but results in weight loss of 4–5% per week. This is in excess of the 2% loss of body weight per week that is considered safe. It requires hospitalisation to be effective, is of questionable humanity, does not address problematic behaviours or the importance of exercise for weight maintenance, and is generally associated with rapid weight rebound.

A number of strategies are described for controlled energy restriction. These are based on daily energy requirements at either current body weight, optimum body weight, or a 15% reduction in body weight. Given the difficulties in estimating optimum body weight, the latter is preferable in that it represents a safe and achievable target. Daily energy intake may be calculated in terms of resting or maintenance energy requirements (MER) and a number of equations exist for these (Legrand-Defretin, 1994). Sixty percent energy restriction is usually applied to the optimum or target body weight, such that the patient will receive 40% of MER for that weight. If an initial target body weight of 85% of current weight is set, this means that the daily energy intake at the outset of the programme will be 34% of current requirements. Such levels of energy restriction have been shown to be well tolerated by dogs, with no adverse effects, resulting in weight loss of approximately 1% per week (Markwell and Butterwick, 1994).

The relative safety and efficacy of several energy restriction regimens has recently been assessed (Laflamme *et al.*, 1997). Adult dogs that were approximately 20% overweight were fed 100%, 75%, 60% or 50% of MER for their estimated ideal body weights for a 16-week period. All dogs fed 50% of MER achieved target weight, compared to 40%, 73% and 75% of dogs fed 100%, 75% and 60% of MER, respectively. The rate of weight loss was related to the degree of energy restriction. No adverse health effects were observed with any of the regimens. Subsequent weight maintenance was investigated in a follow-on study, where half the dogs in each group were given free access to food and the other half fed to actual energy needs (Laflamme and Kuhlman, 1995). The dogs given free access to food gained weight, which was correlated with the amount of weight previously lost, such that after a further 26 weeks there was no difference in percentage weight lost between dogs from all four treatment groups. In contrast, the dogs fed an energy-controlled diet maintained their reduced body weight.

This work highlighted the potential for weight rebound in dogs undergoing weight loss, suggesting that the magnitude of weight rebound is related to the amount of weight lost. This reinforces the need to control energy intake once an ideal or target body weight has been achieved. This said, the dogs that lost weight at approximately 1% of body weight per week experienced minimal weight gain, even when given free access to food, reinforcing the long-term efficacy of this rate of weight loss.

Dietary selection

From a nutritional standpoint, it is essential to restrict energy intake while preserving the consumption of essential macro- and micronutrients, i.e. protein, essential fatty acids, and certain vitamins and minerals. For this reason, it is unacceptable in the long term to simply reduce the amount of the dog's usual diet, which will reduce the intake of essential nutrients by as much as 70% because the nutrient profile of standard prepared petfoods is linked to the energy content. In addition, certain properties of the dog's usual diet may well have contributed to the development of obesity. To get around this problem, a number of veterinary diets are available for use in weight loss programmes. These are balanced so that, when fed according to the manufacturers' recommendation, the intake of energy is restricted and the consumption of other nutrients preserved. These products are usually accompanied by feeding recommendations that remove the inconvenience of the sometimes complex calculations used for energy restriction.

Other key characteristics of veterinary weight loss diets are a low energy density and fat content, together with a degree of palatability that encourages compliance. A low energy density means that a larger daily volume can be fed, thereby discouraging owner perception that they are 'starving' their dog and maximising the satiation potential of the diet. Energy density is reduced in such products by reducing the fat content and increasing the level of components with little or no caloric value, i.e. fibre, air or moisture. Further benefits can be achieved by dividing the daily allowance into more than one meal a day. This, in turn, may reduce the likelihood of owners feeding snacks, treats or other foods in response to begging behaviour.

Reducing the fat content is theoretically beneficial because fat is associated with lower thermic energy loss, compared with protein or carbohydrate, and supports the retention of body weight. There are a number of contradictory studies on the effects of dietary fat intake during weight loss in humans, with some showing no effect and others reporting greater weight loss or loss of body fat with low fat intakes. In a recent canine weight reduction study, a diet low in fat (and high in fibre) was associated with significantly greater loss of body fat, but not body weight, compared with a high fat diet (Borne *et al.*, 1996). This suggested that energy, rather than fat content *per se*, is the primary dietary determinant of weight loss in dogs.

Supplemental dietary fibre has been advocated because of its potential to bind water and slow gastric emptying, thereby promoting satiety. This said, there are contradictory studies on the effects of fibre on food intake in dogs (see below). There are also concerns that excessive dietary fibre may be detrimental in terms of palatability, faeces quality and volume, skin and coat condition, and the digestibility of nutrients (Bartges and Anderson, 1997).

Two studies have evaluated the effects of fibre on food intake using challenge meals to quantify hunger. In the first, normal weight Beagle dogs were fed to maintenance energy requirements diets containing low, medium and high fibre contents (Jewell and Toll, 1996). Animals fed the high fibre diet voluntarily consumed significantly fewer calories during their daily meals and ate significantly less food and calories at the challenge meal, which was fed 75 minutes after the daily meal, compared with those fed the low fibre diet. There was no significant effect of the medium fibre diet. These data indicate that high dietary fibre intakes may reduce hunger in normal weight dogs when fed for weight maintenance, which may be of potential benefit in dogs that have successfully lost weight.

The effects of dietary fibre on satiety and hunger during weight reduction in overweight dogs were investigated in the second study (Butterwick and Markwell, 1997). In contrast to the previous work, the dogs were: overweight; and fed according to recommendations for weight reduction, with daily food allowances corresponding to 45% of MER at a target body weight of 85% of starting body weight. In this study, feeding diets high in soluble or insoluble fibre had no significant effect on intake of a challenge meal, the perception of hunger, as estimated by behavioural characteristics, or body weight change. These data indicate that high fibre intakes have no significant effect on satiety, hunger or weight loss, thereby questioning the benefits of diets rich in dietary fibre for overweight dogs undergoing weight reduction.

The palatability of the product used for weight reduction is important as it encourages compliance with the regimen, which is essential for long-term success, and reduces the temptation to offer other forms of food. High dietary fibre may reduce palatability, as suggested by the reduced intake observed in dogs fed foods with a high fibre content (Jewell and Toll, 1996).

Modification of owner behaviours

Behavioural therapy is targeted at both the owner and the patient and should specify clearly defined and achievable goals. It is particularly crucial for success in cases where simple use of a restricted energy diet has failed to achieve significant weight loss. The first step in the process is an assessment of the client's problem and this requires accurate information gathering. An approach to this is to ask owners to record over a 7-day period the dog's daily food and hence energy intake, the pattern of feeding (where, when, who), availability or access to other food, and level of play and exercise. Owner recall should not be relied upon as this may underestimate energy intake and hide key behaviours. The log will help identify areas for attention and provide a baseline by which owners can appreciate the changes in lifestyle that they develop during the programme.

The aim is to provide regular meals, limit snacks and offer only low energy treats, the energy content of which is compensated for by reducing the amount of food fed at meal times. Attention should also be paid to limit begging behaviours by stimulus control modification, which entails reducing the normal cues associated with eating through feeding only at strict times and always in the same place (Norris and Beaver, 1993). Because feeding sustains the bond between owner and pet, it is desirable to substitute feeding with non-feeding behaviours that can serve the same purpose, for example play and exercise.

Exercise programme

Exercise is the only practical way of increasing energy expenditure, which occurs through the energy cost of the exercise and positive effects on diet-induced thermogenesis and resting metabolic rate. Exercise is also important because it helps offset the reduction in metabolic rate that accompanies weight loss, and promotes the maintenance of lean body mass. It has been estimated that energy expenditure can be increased by approximately 10% for every hour's increase in activity each day (Burger, 1994). Unfortunately effective exercise programmes have not been designed for dogs undergoing weight loss, and typical recommendations of 20–60 minutes of brisk walking per day may be too much for severely obese dogs. Recent studies demonstrated that for some obese human subjects walking at a slow pace on a flat surface constituted a major exercise challenge (Gately *et al.*, 1997). The level of exercise will, to a large extent, be determined by what the dog is capable of, especially if there are significant complications of obesity influencing exercise tolerance, and what is realistic for the owners to achieve within their lifestyles.

Monitoring weight loss

Regular monitoring during the weight loss programme is essential to reinforce the commitment of the owner, allowing them the opportunity to see the results of their efforts and receive recognition. This can be facilitated by daily recording of food intake and activity level, combined with weekly or bi-weekly body weights at an obesity clinic within the veterinary practice. Close monitoring becomes particularly important whenever the rate of weight loss slows and written records of food intake and exercise can help identify the reasons for this.

Once the target weight has been achieved, the dog should be placed on a dietary regimen that encourages weight maintenance. If the dog is still considered over-weight at the initial target weight, then further cycles of weight loss can be progressed until an optimal condition is achieved.

Prevention of weight rebound

Many of the components of a weight reduction pro-gramme are essential to the long-term maintenance of weight loss. Exercise and continual attention to feeding practices are critical, especially control of energy intake. Feeding foods with a relatively lower energy density designed for avoidance of obesity may help at this stage.

PHARMACOLOGICAL MANAGEMENT OF WEIGHT LOSS

Drugs for the management of obesity fall into two broad categories: appetite suppressants and thermogenic aids. Appetite suppressants generally work through activation of β-adrenergic and/or dopamine receptors, or serotonin neurotransmission, and may be associated with stimula-tion of the central nervous and cardiovascular systems. Of these agents, only fenfluramine has been evaluated for use in dogs, with disappointing results (Bromson and Parker, 1975). Thermogenic agents, which have α- and/or β-adrenergic activity, act to increase energy expenditure. Although yohimbine, an α_2-agonist, has undergone pre-liminary evaluation in dogs (Galitzky et al., 1991) there are no data on its clinical efficacy and current research in humans is focused on β_3-agonists because of their selec-tive effects.

Dehydroepiandrosterone (DHEA) sulphate has been shown to produce moderate, but significant weight loss in dogs without a reduction in food intake (Kurzman et al., 1990). The mode of action of DHEA is uncertain and long term studies of safety and efficacy are required before the drug becomes acceptable in clinical practice. Preliminary evidence of enhanced weight loss in overweight dogs on energy restriction has been presented (MacEwen and Kurzman, 1991).

Anti-obesity agents should be considered only as an adjunct to energy restriction, behavioural modification and exercise in a weight loss programme. It should be remembered that the last three factors are essential for long-term success.

SUMMARY

Obesity is a common condition of dogs which, through detrimental consequences for long-term health, warrants effective management. Having recognised that a dog is obese, efforts should be made to identify whether there are concurrent endocrine diseases prior to instituting a weight loss programme. Effective weight loss can be achieved through implementation of appropriate energy reduction and exercise programmes, supported by modification of owner and pet behaviours that have previously contributed to excessive energy intake.

ACKNOWLEDGEMENTS
The authors gratefully acknowledge the contributions of their colleagues Richard Butterwick and Derek Booles in the preparation of the manuscript.

REFERENCES

Bartges J and Anderson WH (1997) Dietary fiber. *Veterinary Clinical Nutrition* **4**, 25–28

Borne AT, Wolfsheimer KJ, Truett AA, Kiene J, Wojciechowski T, Davenport DJ, Ford RB and West DB (1996) Differential metabolic effects of energy restriction in dogs using diets varying in fat and fibre content. *Obesity Research* **4**, 337–345

Bromson L and Parker CHL (1975) Effect of fenfluramine on overweight spayed bitches. *Veterinary Record* **96**, 202–203

Buffington CAT (1994) Management of obesity – the clinical nutritionist's experience. *International Journal of Obesity* **18** (Supplement 1), S29–S35

Burger IH (1994) Energy needs of companion animals: matching food intakes to requirements throughout the life cycle. *Journal of Nutrition* **124**, S2584–S2593

Butterwick RF and Markwell PJ (1997) Effect of amount and type of dietary fiber on food intake in energy-restricted dogs. *American Journal of Veterinary Research* **58**, 272–276

Edney ATB and Smith PM (1986) Study of obesity in dogs visiting veterinary practices in the United Kingdom. *Veterinary Record* **118**, 391–396

Galitzky J, Vermorel M, Lafontan M, Montastuc P and Berlan M (1991) Thermogenic and lipolytic effect of yohimbine in the dog. *British Journal of Pharmacology* **104**, 514–518

Gately PJ, Cooke CB, Barth JH and Butterley RJ (1997). Exercise tolerance in a sample of morbidly obese subjects. *International Journal of Obesity* **21** (Supplement 2), S129

Glickman LT, Sonnenschein EG, Glickman NW, Donoghue S and Goldschmidt MH (1995) Pattern of diet and obesity in female adult pet dogs. *Veterinary Clinical Nutrition* **2**, 9–13

Harper J. (1997). The energy requirements of senior dogs. *Waltham Focus* **7** (2), 32

Jewell DE and Toll PW (1996) Effects of fiber on food intake in dogs. *Veterinary Clinical Nutrition* **3**, 115–118

Kurzman ID, MacEwen EG and Haffa ALM (1990) Reduction in body weight and cholesterol in spontaneously obese dogs by dehydro-epiandrosterone. *International Journal of Obesity* **14**, 95–104

Laflamme DP (1997) Development and validation of a body condition scoring system for dogs. *Canine Practice* **22**, 10–15

Laflamme DP and Kuhlman G (1995) The effects of weight loss regimen on subsequent weight maintenance in dogs. *Nutrition Research* **15**, 1019–1028

Laflamme DP, Kuhlman G and Lawler DF (1997) Evaluation of weight loss protocols for dogs. *Journal of the American Animal Hospital Association* **33**, 253–259

Legrand-Defretin V (1994) Energy requirements of cats and dogs – what goes wrong? *International Journal of Obesity* **18** (Supplement 1), S8–S13

MacEwen EG and Kurzman ID (1991) Obesity in the dog: role of the adrenal steroid dehydroepiandrosterone (DHEA). *Journal of Nutrition* **121**, S51–S55

Markwell PJ and Butterwick RF (1994) Obesity. In: *The Waltham Book of Clinical Nutrition of the Dog and Cat*, ed. JM Wills and KW Simpson, pp.131–148. Elsevier Science, Oxford

Mason E (1970) Obesity in pet dogs. *Veterinary Record* **86**, 612–616

Munday HS (1994) Assessment of body composition in cats and dogs. *International Journal of Obesity* **18** (Supplement 1), S14–S21

Norris MP and Beaver BV (1993) Application of behaviour therapy techniques to the treatment of obesity in companion animals.

Journal of the American Veterinary Medical Association **202,** 728–730

Scarlett JM, Donoghue S, Saidla J and Wills J (1994) Overweight cats: prevalence and risk factors. *International Journal of Obesity* **18**

(Supplement 1), S22–S28

Sheng H-P and Huggins RA (1979). A review of body composition studies with emphasis on total body water and fat. *American Journal of Clinical Nutrition* **32,** 630–647

CHAPTER THREE

The Dog with Symmetrical Alopecia

Ross Bond

INTRODUCTION

Dog owners usually recognise abnormalities of their pet's hair coat early in the course of a disease. Alopecia (absence of hair in an area where it is normally present) or hypotrichosis (partial hair loss) may present no risk to the patient and may be nothing more than a cosmetic problem, albeit one which may cause the owner considerable distress. Alternatively, alopecia may be a manifestation of an internal disease that has potentially serious consequences. A methodical approach and accurate diagnosis are prerequisites for successful management of cases presenting with alopecia. The purpose of this chapter is to present an overview of the biology of hair growth and the mechanisms by which alopecia may develop, and to suggest an approach to the diagnosis of symmetrical alopecia in the dog, with emphasis on cutaneous endocrine disorders and their impersonators.

ANATOMY AND PHYSIOLOGY

Dogs generally possess a dense hair coat which covers the entire skin surface, with the exception of the nasal planum, footpads, lips, teats and anus. The length, thickness, density and colour of the hair coat varies between individuals and, especially, between different breeds. Dogs exhibit compound hair follicle grouping whereby a primary hair and 2–15 secondary hairs emerge from the same pore. There are 100–600 hair follicle ostia per square centimetre (Kristensen, 1975). Hair has important thermoregulatory, protective and sensory functions.

In hair-bearing animals, a cyclical pattern of hair shedding, followed by new growth and replacement has evolved. The growing, or 'anagen', phase is characterised by the production of a hair shaft. Stem cells located in the hair matrix (Figure 3.1) give rise to a population of epidermal cells which terminally differentiate and keratinise, forming the hair shaft and inner root sheath. Anagen usually accounts for 80–90% of the duration of the hair growth cycle. The cessation of active hair growth heralds the onset of 'catagen', a short transitional phase during which the inferior portion of the hair follicle undergoes regression. The 'telogen', or resting, phase is characterised by a period of apparent inactivity during which the fully grown hair remains anchored in the follicle by an expanded and keratinised base known as a 'club'. The hair shaft is normally retained in the follicle during catagen or telogen unless removed by vigorous grooming. Shedding of the hair occurs only after the next anagen phase has progressed such that a new hair shaft enters the follicular canal. In the dog, the hair growth cycle in each body region is asynchronous and hairs are replaced in a mosaic pattern.

The hair growth cycle reflects the intrinsic rhythmic activity of the follicle which results from local regulatory processes that are poorly understood. Dermal papilla cells (Figure 3.1), a permanent and stable population of specialised fibroblasts which interact with the follicular epidermis during embryonic development and throughout adult life, are thought to provide potent factors which stimulate both epidermal proliferation and follicle morphogenesis (Jahoda and Oliver, 1990). Systemic factors are also important, and several hormonal systems influence follicular activity. Hormones probably provide the link between environmental factors such as photoperiod and ambient temperature, and seasonal changes in follicular activity (Ebling *et al.*, 1991). Gonadal, thyroidal, adrenocortical, pituitary and pineal hormones have all been shown to influence the hair growth cycle in many species. For example, thyroxine (T4) accelerates the rate of hair growth and reduces the duration of telogen, whereas corticosteroids generally inhibit follicular activity (Ebling *et al.*, 1991).

PATHOPHYSIOLOGY

Dunstan (1995) has described an approach to diseases of hair follicles based on pathophysiological processes and

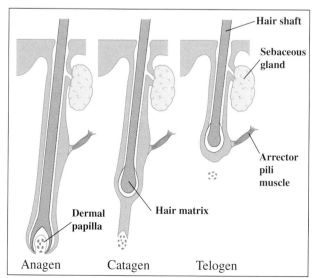

Figure 3.1: Anatomy of the hair follicle at different stages of the hair growth cycle.

Labels in figure: Hair shaft, Sebaceous gland, Arrector pili muscle, Hair matrix, Dermal papilla, Anagen, Catagen, Telogen

which provides a useful framework for consideration of the possible causes of alopecia. Diseases characterised by alopecia can be divided into *scarring* (or potentially scarring) and *non-scarring* disorders. In scarring alopecia, there is destruction or distortion of the follicle such that hair regrowth is not possible, usually as a consequence of an inflammatory process. A common example would be deep pyoderma secondary to demodicosis. By contrast, non-scarring alopecias generally result from either structural or growth cycle abnormalities of the follicle without inflammation, and can be classified into four subtypes (Table 3.1). Of these, atrophic follicular diseases associated with endocrinopathies are the most common cause of symmetrical alopecia in the dog. Follicular dysplasias, diseases characterised by incompletely or abnormally formed hair follicles and hair shafts, are less common but the clinical picture may closely resemble that of an endocrinopathy. Some authors use the term 'follicular dystrophy' to describe these diseases (Gross *et al.*, 1992; Yager and Wilcock, 1994; Dunstan, 1995), which implies a disorder of structure and function caused by abnormal nutrition of the tissues.

DIAGNOSTIC APPROACH

Alopecia may be a feature of myriad skin diseases, including, for example, parasitic, allergic, endocrine and neoplastic conditions. The list of differential diagnoses in dogs with symmetrical alopecia accompanied by marked pruritus and cutaneous inflammation is often lengthy, and a detailed discussion of the approach to this presentation is beyond the scope of this chapter. However, symmetrical alopecia without historical or clinical evidence of cutaneous inflammation is also a relatively common presentation, and the presence of symmetrical skin lesions usually implies a systemically mediated disease. Acquired, bilaterally symmetrical, non-pruritic alopecia, with easily epilated hairs and variable disturbances of skin and hair pigmentation, is the classical presentation of atrophic hair follicle diseases associated with hormonal disorders. However, it is important to consider a number of 'endocrine impersonators', such as colour dilution alopecia and follicular dysplasias, when faced with this presentation. The diagnostic approach to symmetrical alopecia is initially based upon a consideration of the historical and clinical features. Further tests required to establish a definitive diagnosis in such cases, are selected based on the historical and clinical findings (see Figure 3.2).

History

A general medical and dermatological history is required in all cases of skin disease; however, there are a number of points of particular relevance in cases of symmetrical alopecia.

Breed

Breed predilections have been reported for many of the acquired endocrine diseases and are of importance in follicular dysplasias (Tables 3.2 and 3.3). Follicular

Subtypes	Mechanism	Examples
Atrophic alopecias	Abnormal hair cycle leading to shortened anagen and prolonged telogen (follicles are 'asleep')	Hypothyroidism, hyperadrenocorticism
Follicular dystrophies	Disorder of morphogens or structural proteins causing malformation of shaft or follicle such that hair growth is impossible	Congenital alopecia in Chinese Crested Dogs
Matrix cell–melanocyte abnormalities	Abnormal dispersal of melanosomes and, or, disruption of matrix cells	Colour dilution alopecia, black hair follicular dysplasia
Traumatic alopecias	Hair removed in pruritic or psychogenic disease	Alopecia in allergic skin diseases

Table 3.1: *Types of non-scarring alopecia in the dog according to the classification of Dunstan (1995).*

A CASE STUDY

A 6-year-old, neutered female, black Cocker Spaniel was presented in August with a 4-month history of progressive, non-pruritic symmetrical alopecia of the flanks. The dog was in good health otherwise. Physical examination showed only alopecia without inflammation. Remaining hairs could be easily epilated in affected areas. There were no other special features indicative of endocrine or systemic disease but a previous biopsy taken by another veterinary surgeon showed atrophic changes, with telogen hairs predominating. This was interpreted by the pathologist as being consistent with an endocrine disease; dystrophic/dysplastic changes were not observed. There was no response to thyroid supplementation over 1 month. This treatment was stopped by the owner and a further opinion was sought.

History and clinical examination confirmed no pruritus or inflammation. The age of onset excluded a congenital disorder. The dog was black all over, and a relationship to coat colour could not be determined. Parasites were not found on skin scrapings. Haemogram and biochemical profiles were normal. The thyroid stimulation test and low-dose dexamethasone suppression test were normal. While awaiting the results of the laboratory tests, hair regrowth was evident, and complete regrowth was observed within 2 months.

These findings are most consistent with seasonal flank alopecia. In this case, the alopecia developed during the next spring and regrew again in the autumn, confirming this diagnosis. No treatment was given.

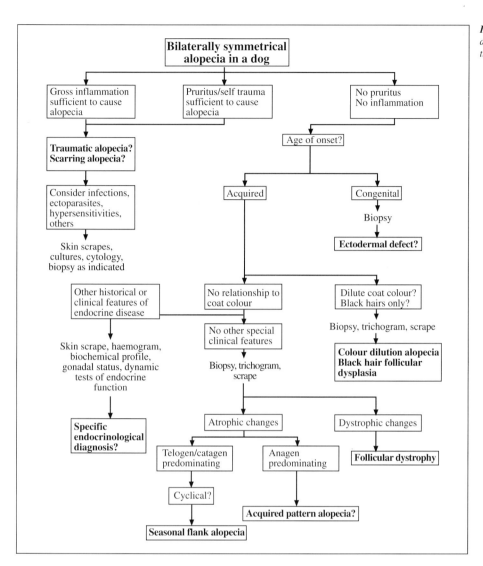

Figure 3.2: *Suggested approach to the diagnosis of symmetrical alopecia in the dog.*

dysplasias have been recognised in Curly Coat Retrievers, Irish Water Spaniels, Portuguese Water Dogs, Siberian Huskies, Dobermann Pinschers and other breeds (Miller, 1990b; Gross *et al.*, 1992; Miller and Scott, 1995; Scott *et al.*, 1995b). Acquired pattern alopecia is most often seen in Dachshunds (Table 3.3).

Age of onset
The age of the dog at onset of alopecia can be helpful. For example, congenital ectodermal defects causing alopecia from birth are occasionally encountered (Foil, 1990; Ihrke *et al.*, 1993). Symmetrical, non-inflammatory alopecia acquired during the first year of life is suggestive of some follicular dystrophies, matrix cell/melanocyte abnormalities, or congenital endocrine diseases such as congenital hypothyroidism or pituitary dwarfism. The most common acquired endocrine diseases, hypothyroidism and hyper-adrenocorticism, are usually seen in middle aged or elderly dogs.

Pruritus
A history of moderate or severe pruritus in a dog with symmetrical alopecia may indicate a traumatic aetiology or a scarring (inflammatory) disease. However, dogs with basically non-inflammatory diseases such as endocrinopathies may also be pruritic if the disease is complicated by a secondary microbial infection, most often staphylococcal pyoderma. If the distribution and severity of the pyoderma lesions do not correlate with the degree of alopecia, then the clinician should suspect an atrophic or dystrophic follicular disease underlying the skin infection. Re-evaluation after antimicrobial therapy may be helpful in such cases.

Signs of internal disease
In endocrine diseases such as hypothyroidism and hyperadrenocorticism, there may be historical features indicating abnormalities of other organ systems. For example, the owners of dogs with hyperadrenocorticism often report polyuria, polydipsia and polyphagia. In hypothyroidism, the owner may describe signs that reflect the slowing of cellular metabolism, such as lethargy and weight gain.

Recent stressful events
Telogen effluvium (telogen defluxion), a transient disorder of excessive hair shedding which results from a synchronous cessation of anagen, usually follows pregnancy,

Disease	Underlying pathology	Breed predilection	Age of onset	Clinical signs (other than skin)	Special dermatological features
Hypothyroidism	Lymphocytic thyroiditis or idiopathic atrophy	Various, large breeds	6–10 years	Lethargy/exercise intolerance, weight gain, bradycardia, corneal lipid deposits	Cool, puffy, thickened skin (uncommon)
Hyperadrenocorticism (spontaneous)	Pituitary or adrenal neoplasia	Various, Boxers, Poodles, Dachshunds, terriers	6–12 years	Abdominal enlargement, hepatomegaly, muscle wasting, testicular atrophy	Calcinosis cutis, thin skin, prominent superficial vessels
Adrenal sex hormone imbalance/'Growth hormone-responsive dermatosis'	Abnormal adrenocortical steroidogenesis due to adrenal enzyme deficiencies?	Pomeranians, Keeshond, Poodle, Chow Chow	1–3 years	None	Hair regrowth at sites of biopsy or other trauma to the skin
Sertoli cell tumour (male)	Functional testicular neoplasia	Not reported	Adult	Testicular mass, retained testis, prostatomegaly, attractiveness to male dogs, gynaecomastia, pendulous prepuce	None
Hyperoestrogenism (female)	Ovarian 'cysts' or functional neoplasia	Not reported	Adult	Enlarged nipples and vulva, irregular or prolonged oestrus, or prior oestrogen therapy?	None

Table 3.2: Atrophic hair follicle diseases of dogs associated with endocrinopathies that commonly present with symmetrical alopecia. The information is intended only as a guide, as in some cases the features may be absent.

Disease	Underlying pathology	Breed predilection	Age of onset	Clinical signs (other than skin)	Main diagnostic features
Telogen effluvium	Synchronous cessation of anagen, followed by shedding and regrowth	None	Variable	Often none. Previous systemic disease or physiological stress	Rapid spontaneous resolution, stressful event 1–3 months previously
Seasonal flank alopecia	Unknown. Related to photoperiod? Mediated via pineal gland — melatonin?	Boxers, Dobermanns, Airedale Terriers, Schnauzers	1–12 years (usually between 2 and 6 years)	None	Cyclical or seasonal course, exclude other diseases
Oestrogen-responsive dermatosis	Unknown	Not reported	Adult	Infantile vulva? Urinary incontinence?	Exclude other diseases, response to therapy (care)
Testosterone-responsive dermatosis	Unknown	Not reported	Adult	None	Exclude other diseases, response to therapy (care)
Acquired pattern alopecia (pattern baldness)	Unknown	Dachshund, Manchester Terrier, Boston Terrier, Whippet	6–12 months	None	Histopathology: miniaturisation of hair follicles

Table 3.3: Atrophic hair follicle diseases of unknown or non-hormonal aetiology that may present as symmetrical alopecia. The information is intended only as a guide, as in some cases the features may be absent.

lactation, severe illness or a similar stressful event which occurred 1–3 months previously.

Seasonal or cyclical episodes

Seasonal or cyclical episodes of non-inflammatory symmetrical truncal alopecia followed by spontaneous hair regrowth is a typical feature of seasonal flank alopecia (Miller and Dunstan, 1993; Curtis, 1995), and also occurs in occasional cases of follicular dystrophies, such as that seen in the Portuguese Water Dog (Miller and Scott, 1995).

Reproductive history

Male dogs with oestrogen-producing testicular tumours may have a history of signs suggesting feminisation (attractiveness to male dogs, gynaecomastia, pendulous prepuce). In female dogs, anoestrus and infertility may be reported in hypothyroid bitches, and prolonged oestrus has been reported in bitches with ovarian disorders and hyperoestrogenism (Davidson and Feldman, 1995).

Drug administration

The clinician should also enquire about previous drug administration; for example, long-term glucocorticoid therapy may cause iatrogenic hyperglucocorticoidism, and oestrogens and cytotoxic drugs such as cyclophosphamide may also interfere with hair growth. The response, or lack of response, to previous therapy may also be helpful; for example, failure of hair regrowth after 3–5 months of supplementation with T4 at an appropriate dose suggests that hypothyroidism is unlikely.

Clinical signs

A general physical examination may reveal clinical signs in other systems that may be related to the skin disease, particularly in dogs with hypothyroidism, hyperadrenocorticism and abnormalities of the reproductive system (Tables 3.2 and 3.3). Although it is important to appreciate that clinical signs may be confined to the skin in some dogs with these diseases, additional physical findings can be very helpful in listing differential diagnoses in order of priority, enabling further tests to be performed in a rational order. The reader is referred to other chapters in this book for comprehensive accounts of endocrine diseases of the dog.

Physical examination of the skin should allow the clinician to determine whether the alopecia results from a scarring or non-scarring alopecia. Scarring alopecias may show a predominance of lesions such as erythema, papules, pustules, furuncles and crusts. Alopecia without cutaneous inflammation suggests either an atrophic disease, a follicular dystrophy, or matrix cell/melanocyte abnormalities. Colour dilution alopecia (Figure 3.3) should be strongly suspected if the dog has a dilute coat colour (e.g. blue Dobermanns), and black hair follicular dysplasia should be considered if the alopecia is confined to black (or dark) haired areas; these two diseases usually develop during the first year of life (Carlotti, 1990; Miller, 1990a).

Dogs with symmetrical alopecia should be carefully evaluated for additional skin lesions. Comedones (blackheads), which are dilated hair follicles plugged with keratin and sebaceous debris, commonly develop in endocrine disease but may also be seen in demodicosis and in primary defects of keratinisation affecting the upper portion of the hair follicle. Thinning of the skin with prominent subcutaneous vessels occurs in hyperadrenocorticism, whereas dogs with hypothyroidism may have thickened skin due to increased deposition of dermal mucin (myxoedema). In hyperadrenocorticism, the deposition of calcium salts along dermal collagen fibres may result in calcinosis cutis; lesions consist of yellow or white papules, nodules and plaques which feel firm and gritty when palpated.

Intense hyperpigmentation of the alopecic areas is most commonly seen in dogs with seasonal flank alopecia and adrenal sex hormone imbalances/growth hormone (GH)-responsive dermatosis (Table 3.3). This poorly defined disorder is principally recognised in 'plush-coated' breeds such as the Pomeranian, Miniature Poodle, Chow Chow, Keeshond and Samoyed. Alopecia is often first observed between 1 and 3 years of age. Both male and female, neutered and entire, dogs are affected. Symmetrical alopecia affects the trunk, caudal thighs, perineum or neck, and changes in coat colour and coat quality may also be seen (Figure 3.4). Hair regrowth is often observed at sites of trauma, such as skin biopsy sites.

A lightening of the coat colour (leucotrichia) is not uncommon in dogs with hyperadrenocorticism.

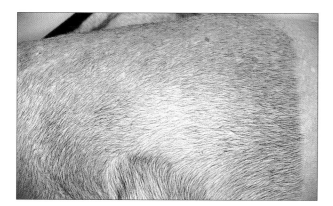

Figure 3.3: Diffuse truncal hypotrichosis in a Dobermann with colour dilution alopecia.

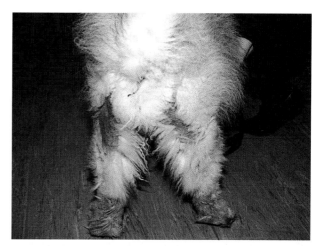

Figure 3.4: Bilaterally symmetrical alopecia with intense hyperpigmentation on the caudal aspect of the thighs in a 3 year old Chow Chow with growth hormone-responsive dermatosis.

Disease	Haemogram	Blood biochemical profile	Urinalysis	Hormone assays
Hypothyroidism	Normocytic, normochromic, non-regenerative anaemia	Hypercholesterolaemia, hypertriglyceridaemia, elevated ALT (mild), elevated ALP (mild)	Normal	Low serum thyroxine concentrations pre- and post-TSH or TRH stimulation. Low basal thyroxine and high TSH concentrations
Hyperadrenocorticism	Mature neutrophilia, eosinopenia, lymphopenia	Elevated ALP (often very high), elevated ALT, elevated cholesterol, elevated glucose	SG <1.015, UTI	Inadequate suppression of cortisol levels after low-dose of dexamethasone. Excessive cortisol levels in response to ACTH stimulation
Hyperoestrogenism	Non-regenerative anaemia, thrombocytopenia, myeloid hyperplasia or hypoplasia	Normal	Normal	Elevated basal oestradiol
Adrenal sex hormone imbalance – 'Growth hormone-responsive dermatosis'	Normal	Normal	Normal	High concentrations of adrenal progestogens (or androgens) in response to ACTH stimulation

Table 3.4: *Results of laboratory tests in dogs with symmetrical alopecia caused by endocrinopathies. The information is intended only as a guide, as in some cases the features may be absent.*
ACTH, adrenocorticotropic hormone; ALT, alanine aminotransferase; ALP, alkaline phosphatase; SG, specific gravity; TRH, thyrotropin releasing hormone; TSH, thyroid stimulating hormone; UTI, urinary tract infection

Changes in coat colour and coat quality are also seen in many of the follicular dysplasias (Gross *et al.*, 1992). The presence of miniaturised ('vellus') hairs is a key feature in acquired pattern alopecia (Table 3.3), a rare disease usually seen in Dachshunds, which presents with symmetrical non-inflammatory alopecia of the pinnae and/or the ventrum (Scott *et al.*, 1995b).

Laboratory investigation
Laboratory tests are required for the definitive diagnosis of most cases of symmetrical alopecia.

Skin scrapings and plucked hairs
The microscopic examination of skin scrapings for demodicid mites is probably warranted in all cases of alopecia in the dog. In dogs with non-inflammatory symmetrical alopecia, the microscopic examinations of plucked hairs (trichograms) and skin biopsy specimens may be of value. Dystrophic diseases and melanocytic disorders are often characterised by the production of hairs with structural abnormalities which can be detected on microscopy; for example, large melanin clumps with hair shaft distortion and fracture may be seen in colour dilution alopecia and black hair follicular dysplasia (Miller, 1990a; Hargis *et al.*, 1991). Alternatively, the presence of large numbers of easily epilated, club hairs suggests arrest of the hair growth cycle in the telogen phase, as seen in endocrine diseases.

Skin biopsy
Skin biopsy is required for the diagnosis of follicular dystrophies and matrix cell/melanocyte abnormalities. Biopsies are also indicated in cases where the diagnosis cannot be readily confirmed by other means. As a general rule, multiple biopsy specimens should be obtained from the most alopecic areas (Gross *et al.*, 1992); samples from marginal areas may be confusing because growing hairs may still be present. However, in alopecia areata, a rare disease associated with a lymphocytic cellular infiltrate which is centred around the hair matrix and dermal papilla, the key histopathological feature may be observed only in specimens obtained from the periphery of the lesion. Few of the atrophic diseases can be diagnosed definitively by the histopathological examination of skin alone; other clinical or laboratory data are usually required. Features suggesting one particular form of endocrine disease may be present in occasional specimens, and the findings may allow the 'endocrine impersonators' to be excluded. The histopathological changes in hair follicle diseases can be subtle and it may be preferable to submit biopsy specimens to a veterinary pathologist with a special interest in skin disease. The reader is referred to dermatopathology texts for a more detailed discussion of this area (Gross *et al.*, 1992; Yager and Wilcock, 1994).

Biochemistry
Blood for haematology and biochemistry, and urine samples, should be obtained for routine analyses in dogs suspected of having endocrine diseases. The biochemical profile should include measurements of total protein, albumin, alkaline phosphatase, alanine aminotransferase, bilirubin, calcium, phosphate, urea, creatinine, cholesterol and glucose. Urinalysis should include a chemistry strip, sediment examination, measurement of specific gravity and possibly bacterial culture. The laboratory findings may support a diagnosis of a particular endocrine disease, and specific hormone assays can then be performed as indicated (Table 3.4).

Hormone assays
Specific assays for many of the relevant hormones are

available from commercial laboratories. In general, dynamic tests of endocrine function are preferred because basal hormone concentrations may fluctuate widely in response to both physiological and pathological factors (Scott *et al.*, 1995a).

Tests designed to assess thyroid and pituitary/adrenal function are mandatory in dogs with clinical signs and laboratory test results suggestive of hypothyroidism and hyperadrenocorticism; these tests are described in chapters 10 and 14. Thyroid and pituitary/adrenal function should also be routinely assessed in dogs that have atrophic follicular diseases, without other historical, clinical and laboratory features of endocrine diseases because the more typical features of hypothyroidism and hyperadrenocorticism do not occur in all cases. Basal oestradiol concentrations are elevated in some dogs with hyperoestrogenism.

A protocol for the assessment of adrenal hormones before and after adrenocorticotropic hormone (ACTH) stimulation has been described for use in dogs suspected of having adrenal sex hormone imbalances, once hypothyroidism and hyperadrenocorticism have been excluded by specific tests (Schmeitzel *et al.*, 1995). However, the pathogenesis of this disease, or group of diseases, is not clear. Some dogs regrow hair after castration or supplementation with methyltestosterone. Others respond to GH supplementation, but in one study of Pomeranians, dynamic tests of GH function showed no differences in blood concentrations in both healthy and affected groups (Schmeitzel and Lothrop, 1990). The authors hypothesised that an abnormality of adrenal steroid synthesis related to a partial deficiency of an enzyme, 21-hydroxylase, might explain the elevated pro-gesterone and androgen concentrations which were observed before and/or after ACTH stimulation in these dogs. This theory will remain unproven until an assay for canine 21-hydroxylase is available. Furthermore, Dunstan (1995) has proposed that this clinical presentation might reflect a localised abnormality of hair follicle metabolism rather than a systemic defect, wherein a number of different treatments or insults can stimulate hair follicles to restart their normal growth cycle. This is clearly an area which requires further research. Normal values for 17-hydroxyprogesterone before and after ACTH stimulation have been established by a UK-based laboratory. In the USA, a wider array of hormones can be evaluated but this is expensive.

TREATMENT

Specific therapy is available for most of the endocrinopathies but is not possible in dogs with follicular dystrophies or matrix cell/melanocyte abnormalities. In general, the treatment of dogs with symmetrical alopecia by hormonal supplementation without a specific indication based on laboratory testing is to be discouraged. The therapy for hypothyroidism and hyperadrenocorticism is described in Chapters 14 and 10.

Dogs with adrenal sex hormone imbalances may respond to castration, methyltestosterone, lysodren or GH

(Schmeitzel *et al.*, 1995). Castration of the intact male dog may be the first treatment of choice. In neutered male dogs, methyltestosterone supplementation at 1 mg/kg orally every other day (maximum dose 30 mg) for 3 months, followed by weekly maintenance therapy, may be attempted. However, behavioural changes, seborrhoea oleosa and hepatic disease are potential adverse effects (Schmeitzel *et al.*, 1995). Lysodren is often effective in the treatment of adrenal sex hormone imbalances; an initial dose of 15–25 mg/kg daily for 5 days is followed by maintenance doses of 15–25 mg/kg every 7–14 days (Schmeitzel and Parker, 1993; Schmeitzel *et al.*, 1995). These dogs should be carefully monitored for signs of hypocortisolaemia, hyperkalaemia and hyponatraemia, particularly during initial therapy. Hair regrowth is often evident within 4–12 weeks. Although some dogs respond favourably to GH supplementation, this hormone is potentially diabetogenic and is expensive.

A response to trial therapy is required to establish diagnoses of both oestrogen-responsive and testosterone-responsive dermatosis. Supplementation with these hormones is potentially hazardous, and they should only be used in cases where other more common endocrine diseases have been definitively excluded. Some owners prefer to accept the alopecia once the clinician has explained the potential adverse effects of supplementation with these hormones. Dogs with gonadal neoplasia without evidence of metastases should be neutered. Therapy is not currently available for seasonal flank alopecia; however, in an unpublished study, Paradis (1995) reported that the next predicted episode of alopecia was prevented by melatonin supplementation in all nine dogs treated. There is no rationale for supplementation with thyroid, reproductive and GH in seasonal flank alopecia (Curtis *et al.*, 1996).

Only palliative therapy is available for dogs with follicular dystrophies and matrix cell/melanocyte abnormalities. Any secondary pyoderma should be treated with an antibacterial agent effective against *Staphylococcus intermedius* such as lincomycin or cephalexin. Topical therapy with shampoos may be helpful in dogs with scaling disorders, and as adjunctive therapy in superficial pyoderma.

CONCLUSION

Endocrinopathies, especially hypothyroidism, hyperadrenocorticism, and reproductive hormone imbalances, commonly present with non-inflammatory symmetrical alopecia. However, other atrophic and dystrophic hair follicle diseases can impersonate hormonal disorders. A careful review of the historical and clinical features, followed by additional laboratory tests, is required to establish a diagnosis in these cases. The prognosis for hair regrowth in symmetrical alopecia caused by endocrine disorders is often good with specific therapy, whereas permanent alopecia can be expected in most dogs with follicular dystrophies or matrix cell/melanocyte abnormalities. Therapeutic trials with hormones are not indicated unless the case has been fully evaluated.

REFERENCES

Carlotti DN (1990) Canine hereditary black hair follicular dysplasia and colour mutant alopecia: clinical and histopathological aspects. In: *Advances in Veterinary Dermatology*, vol 1. ed. C von Tscharner and REW Halliwell, pp. 43–46. Baillière Tindall, London

Curtis CF (1995) Clinical features of canine idiopathic cyclical flank alopecia. *Veterinary Dermatology Newsletter* **17**, 53–54

Curtis CF, Evans H and Lloyd DH (1996) Investigation of the reproductive and growth hormone status of dogs affected by idiopathic recurrent flank alopecia. *Journal of Small Animal Practice* **37**, 417–422

Davidson AP and Feldman EC (1995) Ovarian and oestrus cycle abnormalities in the bitch. In: *Textbook of Veterinary Internal Medicine, 4th edn*, ed. SJ Ettinger and EC Feldman, pp. 1607–1613. WB Saunders, Philadelphia

Dunstan RW (1995) A pathomechanistic approach to diseases of the hair follicle. *Veterinary Dermatology Newsletter* **17**, 37–41

Ebling FJG, Hale PA and Randall VA (1991) Hormones and hair growth. In: *Physiology, Biochemistry, and Molecular Biology of the Skin*, ed. LA Goldsmith, pp. 660–696. Oxford University Press, New York

Foil CS (1990) The skin. In: *Veterinary Pediatrics*, ed. JM Hoskins, pp. 364–369. WB Saunders, Philadelphia

Gross TL, Ihrke PJ and Walder EJ (1992) *Veterinary Dermatopathology: A Macroscopic and Microscopic Evaluation of Canine and Feline Skin Disease*. Mosby Year Book, St Louis

Hargis AM, Brignac MM, Kareem Al-Bagdadi FA, Muggli F and Mundell A (1991) Black hair follicular dysplasia in black and white Saluki dogs: differentiation from colour mutant alopecia in the Doberman Pinscher by microscopic examination of hairs. *Veterinary Dermatology* **2**, 69–83

Ihrke PJ, Mueller RS and Stannard AA (1993) Generalized congenital hypotrichosis in a female Rottweiler. *Veterinary Dermatology* **4**, 65–69

Jahoda CAB and Oliver RF (1990) The dermal papilla and the growth of hair. In: *Hair and Hair Diseases*, ed. CE Orfanos and R Happle, pp. 19–44. Springer-Verlag, Berlin

Kristensen S (1975) A study of skin diseases in dogs and cats. I. Histology of the hairy skin of dogs and cats. *Nordisk Veterinaermedicin* **27**, 593–603

Miller MA and Dunstan RW (1993) Seasonal flank alopecia in Boxers and Airedale terriers: 24 cases (1985–1992). *Journal of the American Veterinary Medical Association* **203**, 1567–1572

Miller WH (1990a) Colour dilution alopecia in Doberman Pinschers with blue or fawn coat colours: a study on the incidence and histopathology of this disorder. *Veterinary Dermatology* **1**, 113–122

Miller WH (1990b) Follicular dysplasia in adult black and red Doberman Pinschers. *Veterinary Dermatology* **1**, 181–187

Miller WH and Scott DW (1995) Follicular dysplasia of the Portuguese Water Dog. *Veterinary Dermatology* **6**, 67–74

Paradis, M (1995) Canine recurrent flank alopecia: treatment with melatonin. *Proceedings of the American College of Veterinary Dermatology Annual Meeting, Santa Fe, 1995*, p.49

Schmeitzel LP and Lothrop CD (1990) Hormonal abnormalities in Pomeranians with normal coat and in Pomeranians with growth hormone-responsive dermatosis. *Journal of the American Veterinary Medical Association* **197**, 1333–1341

Schmeitzel LP, Lothrop CD and Rosenkrantz WS (1995) Congenital adrenal hyperplasia-like syndrome. In: *Kirk's Current Veterinary Therapy XII*, ed. JD Bonagura, pp. 600–604. WB Saunders, Philadelphia

Schmeitzel LP and Parker W (1993) Growth hormone and sex hormone alopecia. In: *Advances in Veterinary Dermatology*, Vol. 2, ed. PJ Ihrke *et al.*, pp. 451–454. Pergamon Press, Oxford

Scott DW, Miller WH and Griffin CE (1995a) Endocrine and metabolic disease. In: *Muller and Kirk's Small Animal Dermatology*, ed. DW Scott *et al.*, pp. 627–719. WB Saunders, Philadelphia

Scott DW, Miller WH and Griffin CE (1995b) Acquired alopecia. In: *Muller and Kirk's Small Animal Dermatology*, ed. DW Scott *et al.*, pp. 720–735. WB Saunders, Philadelphia

Yager JA and Wilcock BP (1994) Atrophic dermatoses. In: *Colour Atlas and Text of Surgical Pathology in the Dog and Cat. Dermatopathology and Skin Tumors*, pp. 217–237. Wolfe Publishing, London

CHAPTER FOUR

The Uncontrollable Diabetic

Peter A. Graham

INTRODUCTION

Most diabetic dogs and cats can be stabilised and managed without difficulty but there are occasional individuals, or phases of an individual's therapy, which may be described as 'difficult to regulate' or 'uncontrollable'. The point at which a diabetic animal is described as uncontrollable may depend on the expectations of the attending veterinary surgeon. An expectation that diabetic control implies blood glucose concentrations within the range of 5–10 mmol/l throughout each 24-hour period with once daily insulin injections is unrealistic. If a more appropriate goal of control of clinical signs is chosen, more successful management will be achieved. Narrow control of blood glucose concentrations is important in human diabetic management if long-term diabetic complications are to be avoided. In canine or feline diabetes, such fine control of blood glucose concentration is unnecessary.

Before determining how to investigate and manage an uncontrollable diabetic animal, the nature of the problem needs to be defined. In an uncontrollable diabetic, there are two possible manifestations. Either the animal appears to have dramatic fluctuations in insulin requirement (periods of hypoglycaemia interspersed with periods of polyuria and polydipsia) or persistent, unusually high requirements for insulin exist, commonly defined as >2 IU/kg/injection. Most dogs can be expected to stabilise at insulin doses in the range of 1.0 IU/kg or less for twice-daily regimens and 1.0–1.5 IU/kg for once-daily therapy. Requirements for cats are similar.

There are four categories of potential causes for fluctuating or high insulin requirements in an uncontrollable diabetic:

- Insulin: Past its expiry date, heated, frozen, violently shaken, antigenic in recipient because of species of origin, limited duration of activity or poor absorption
- Administration: Injection technique, improper use of syringes, inappropriate syringe type (should be 40 or 100 IU/ml syringes), and site of injection
- Management: Dose and frequency of insulin, consistency and appropriateness of exercise and dietary regimens, erroneous multi-dosing in households with more than one person responsible for drug administration, appropriateness of monitoring strategy (time of day, blood *versus* urine glucose), effects of stress on glucose results, size of increment/decrement in dose when changes required, and concurrent use of diabetogenic therapies (glucocorticoids, progestogens)
- Endogenous: Stress, metoestrus, hyperadrenocorticism, hypothyroidism, hyperthyroidism, spontaneous remission/'honeymoon' phase, azotaemia, sepsis, obesity, pancreatitis, acromegaly, cirrhosis, glucagonoma, phaeochromocytoma, non-endocrine neoplasia, and hypertriglyceridaemia.

INSULIN

Insulin is a peptide hormone which can be damaged or denatured by extremes of heat or cold or by vigorous or violent shaking. For long-term storage, vials of insulin should be refrigerated but care should be taken to ensure that the vial is not in a place where it will be subject to freezing. Keeping an opened vial at room temperature is permissible if the insulin is used within 4–6 weeks of opening and it is not subjected to extremes of temperature. Insulin kept at room temperature may be better tolerated than cold insulin in animals that object to injections. Insulin pouches, with or without frozen gel packs, can be used to keep insulin cool when travelling. If insulin preparations are diluted to improve accuracy of dosing in cats and small dogs, proprietary insulin diluent, water for injection or normal saline are appropriate but the diluted preparation should be used on the same day. Diluted insulin may deteriorate if stored.

Insulin preparations are of porcine, bovine or recombinant human type, and variations in insulin structure occur between species (Smith, 1966; Hallden *et al.*, 1986). Porcine insulin is identical to canine insulin, but human insulin differs from canine insulin by one amino acid and bovine insulin differs by two amino acids. Compared with feline insulin, bovine insulin differs by one amino acid, porcine insulin by three and human insulin by four amino acids. Therefore, porcine insulin is the least antigenic in dogs and bovine insulin is the least antigenic in cats. Antigenicity, however, is not necessarily a disadvantage. A modest titre of anti-insulin antibodies helps prolong the duration of insulin action, which is a therapeutically useful attribute in many cases. On the rare occasions that high titres of anti-insulin antibodies develop, insulin requirements become persistently high and there may be poor recovery from hypoglycaemic episodes as insulin continues to be released from insulin–antibody complexes (Bolli *et al.*, 1984). If significant anti-insulin antibody production is suspected, a change to the least antigenic insulin available should reduce insulin requirements within a matter of weeks. Because this is a rare cause of insulin resistance, and because of the disruption caused by a change of preparation, such a course should only be undertaken after investigation for the more common problems. It may still be possible to locate a human medical laboratory that can measure antibody levels to different species of insulin. However, this is likely to become less accessible as the use of recombinant human insulin preparations increases for the treatment of human diabetes mellitus.

Insulin preparations of inappropriately short duration may be associated with hyperglycaemia and return of clinical signs in the latter part of the inter-injection period; depending on the dose adjustment strategy, this may promote the development of insulin-induced hyperglycaemia (Somogyi 'overswing') exaggerating the clinical picture (see Chapter 12). Short duration of insulin action may present as a persistent high insulin requirement, but the induction of a prolonged Somogyi response may cause a pattern of dramatic fluctuation in requirement, with days of hypoglycaemic episodes followed by a few days of apparently increased requirement when concentrations of insulin antagonists are still high (Feldman and Nelson, 1996). The generation of a 12–24-hour blood glucose curve will assist in the identification of short duration of insulin action and insulin-induced hyperglycaemia, but to identify a prolonged Somogyi overswing it may be necessary to generate blood glucose curves before, and a number of days after, a 25–30% reduction in insulin dose, or to monitor clinical signs or water consumption over the same period.

In some animals the long-acting insulin preparations, protamine zinc insulin (PZI) and ultralente (crystalline-zinc suspension), may be very poorly absorbed from subcutaneous sites, creating the impression of high insulin requirements (Broussard and Peterson, 1994). Serial post-injection serum insulin concentrations may assist in the documentation of this phenomenon but insulin analyses are expensive and therapeutic concentrations of insulin are not well defined for dogs and cats. A simpler approach would be to change to an intermediate-acting insulin such as lente, twice daily if necessary, and monitor the effect.

INSULIN ADMINISTRATION

Early in any investigation of a difficult diabetic animal assurance is needed that the appropriate dose of insulin is being successfully administered. If client education is adequate at the beginning of therapy and appropriate syringes are supplied, then problems due to insulin administration should be infrequent. Confusion over international units (IU), millilitres (ml) and tenths of a millilitre gradations can be avoided if one syringe type is used consistently. The type of syringe (40 or 100 IU/ml) must match the insulin preparation. If there is doubt about the administration technique, the owner should be asked to demonstrate the injection routine, using sterile saline if necessary, in front of the veterinary surgeon or nurse. If regulatory difficulty is a new aspect of a case which was previously well controlled for a long time, then such a demonstration may be less relevant and the implication of criticism may have a negative effect on client relations.

Injections into large, poorly perfused, subcutaneous fat deposits may be less well absorbed than injections into more lean areas or areas where there is greater movement, e.g. over the thoracic wall.

CASE MANAGEMENT

Both diet and exercise can have considerable effects on blood glucose concentrations in diabetic animals. Persistent overfeeding or the provision of diets high in soluble carbohydrates (semi-moist diets) may cause persistently high insulin requirements. Failure to feed a diet consistent in volume, composition and mealtimes may cause a fluctuating insulin requirement. Similarly, dramatic changes in the level of exercise can also cause fluctuating insulin requirement, e.g. visits from other family members commonly result in increased levels of exercise because of playing or family walks. The effects of exercise are less important in the management of diabetic cats.

Veterinary surgeons familiar with treating small-breed diabetic dogs, may, when faced with their first diabetic Rottweiler, believe that the insulin dose of 50 IU once-daily required to control the condition is excessive although it is still approximately 1.0 IU/kg. Also the timing or method of diabetic monitoring may lead to a diagnosis of poor control when it is adequate. For example, blood glucose concentrations are likely to be elevated above 10 mmol/l 24 hours post-injection in dogs on single daily injections of intermediate-acting insulin, but this does not necessarily mean they were poorly controlled the previous day. Worse still, such misunderstanding can lead to more serious problems such as insulin-induced hypoglycaemia and hyperglycaemia if doses are increased. Large increases in insulin dose (>20%) increase the likelihood of insulin-induced hyperglycaemia, and, particularly in combination with correspondingly large decrements in dose, may cause much confusion when retrospectively reviewing records to determine the cause of fluctuating requirements.

During the diabetic stabilisation period, it may take a few days to obtain a consistent response to a new dose of insulin. Daily dose adjustment strategies have the advantage of shorter stabilisation times (especially important if animals are hospitalised) and earlier recognition of insulin insensitivity. However, the lag time in response means that the stabilisation period has to cover a 3 or 4 day period of daily observation for a consistent glucose response at the 'final' dose before the animal is considered stable. Large daily dose adjustments (>20%) and/or failure to observe a consistent response before terminating the stabilisation strategy may cause dramatic signs of diabetic instability with fluctuating requirements.

ENDOGENOUS CAUSES OF POOR DIABETIC CONTROL

Endogenous causes of poor diabetic control are usually associated with increased insulin requirement (cirrhosis may result in a low requirement). Whether the increased requirement is persistent or fluctuating depends on the dynamic nature of the concurrent illness. For example, the increase in requirement associated with bacterial infections or sepsis may fluctuate as the disease waxes and wanes or resolves, but the increased requirement associated with hyperadrenocorticism is likely to be persistent. Spontaneous remission of diabetes mellitus occurs occasionally, particularly in cats that have been overweight or receiving diabetogenic therapies, and in bitches that became diabetic in association with metoestrus. Early in the course of treatment, insulin requirements may also occasionally reduce or disappear and increase again after a few weeks or months in a manner similar to the common 'honeymoon' phase of human type I diabetes mellitus. Animals that have been diabetic once will be at increased risk of becoming diabetic again, particularly after periods of stress or illness, and owners should be made aware of the signs to look for.

Hyperadrenocorticism

Hyperadrenocorticism is commonly found in association with canine diabetes mellitus. Approximately 20% of diabetic dogs referred to the University of Glasgow during the 5-year period 1989–1994 had concurrent hyperadrenocorticism (Graham, 1995). Hyperadrenocorticism is much less common in diabetic cats than dogs. Diagnostic testing protocols described in Chapters 10, 29 and 34 should be followed, but care should be taken in interpretation of adrenal function tests when poorly controlled diabetes mellitus is present. The diagnosis should be made with regard to clinical signs and historical features in addition to the laboratory results. False-positive results for hyperadrenocorticism are common in poorly regulated or newly diagnosed diabetic dogs. This is attributed to the chronic metabolically stressful nature of diabetes mellitus and consequent pituitary–adrenal hyperactivity.

Cortisol is an insulin antagonist, so diabetic animals with hyperadrenocorticism will tend to have high insulin requirements (Peterson *et al.*, 1981; Blaxter and Gruffydd-Jones, 1990); some animals may still have the ability to produce insulin but once clinical diabetes mellitus appears, insulin therapy is usually required. If further deterioration of endogenous insulin production occurs then an increasing exogenous requirement is seen. When hyperadrenocorticism and diabetes mellitus are present concurrently it is likely that the hyperadrenocorticism causes, or at least contributes to, the development of the diabetic condition.

Removal of the source of insulin antagonism causes a dramatic reduction in insulin requirement, increasing the risk of life-threatening hypoglycaemia if blood or urine glucose is not monitored carefully (Blaxter and Gruffydd-Jones, 1990). If adrenalectomy is considered for the treatment of hyperadrenocorticism, insulin doses following surgery need to be withheld or dramatically reduced depending on blood glucose responses or a pre-surgical endogenous serum insulin concentration. For endogenous serum insulin measurements, exogenous insulin is withheld for 24–30 hours. This should be performed early in the diagnostic work-up and not in the days immediately preceding surgery.

Because of the potential for inducing dramatic reductions in insulin requirement and hypoglycaemia, low-dose mitotane therapy (25 mg/kg instead of 50 mg/kg) plus prednisolone (0.4 mg/kg) has been recommended for induction (Peterson *et al.*, 1981). However, careful diabetic monitoring and insulin dose adjustment can allow the institution of the more usual 50 mg/kg approach. During the maintenance phase of therapy, variable insulin requirements may be noticed between weekly mitotane doses, and so alternate-day or twice-weekly protocols may be more appropriate. Significant suppression of adrenal function must be achieved (post-ACTH stimulation test cortisol <100–130 nmol/l) to ensure a stable insulin requirement. The alternative adrenocorticolytic protocol (Rijnberk and Belshaw, 1988), which aims for adrenal ablation, is particularly appealing for use in dogs with concurrent diabetes mellitus but the author has no direct experience of its use.

In one study, dogs with concurrent diabetes mellitus and hyperadrenocorticism had a median survival time of 0.96 years compared with 2.96 years for dogs with diabetes alone (Graham and Nash, 1995). However, this difference may in part be due to the much older age of dogs with hyperadrenocorticism at the time of diagnosis (10.61 years *versus* 8.14 years for dogs with diabetes alone).

Hypo- or hyperthyroidism

Both canine hypothyroidism and feline hyperthyroidism can be associated with increased insulin requirements in animals with diabetes mellitus (Hoenig and Ferguson, 1992; Ford *et al.*, 1993). Thyroxine (T4) has insulin-antagonistic properties but the mechanisms of insulin resistance in hypothyroid dogs are less clear. The diagnosis of these conditions is made according to the protocols described in Chapters 14, 15 and 34 but care should be taken to account for the potentially suppressive effects of diabetes mellitus on serum T4 concentration. Dynamic tests such as the thyroid stimulating hormone (TSH) stimulation test, triiodothyronine (T3) suppression test or multiple repeat baseline tests (including canine TSH measurement) should be considered before a definitive diagnostic decision is made. Standard therapy for these conditions applies to those animals with concurrent diabetes mellitus, but care should be taken to monitor insulin requirements in the post-treatment period. The decrease in requirement seen in dogs treated with T4 is often less dramatic than is seen following the treatment for other causes of insulin resistance.

Azotaemia or sepsis

Azotaemia and bacterial infections can lead to insulin resistance mediated through an increase in glucagon and perhaps cortisol concentrations (Ihle and Nelson, 1991; McGuinness, 1994). Whether the increase in insulin requirement fluctuates or is persistent depends on the course of the underlying illness.

Endocrine neoplasia

Acromegaly, although rare, is one of the most common forms of endocrine neoplasia associated with persistent insulin resistance in diabetic cats along with hyperthyroidism (Peterson *et al.*, 1990). Acromegaly is also recorded in dogs but usually associated with growth hormone (GH) induction by endogenous or exogenous progestogens (Eigenmann and Venker-van Haagen, 1981). Diagnosis is based on the measurement of insulin-like growth factor 1 (IGF-1) in animals displaying appropriate clinical signs (see Chapter 28). GH analyses can also be used for diagnosis where they are available. The Faculty of Veterinary Medicine at the University of Utrecht in The Netherlands has valid canine and feline GH assays. Elevated concentrations may also be found in bitches in metoestrus and in animals which have been subject to chronic hypoglycaemia due to insulin overdose, since GH secretion forms part of the long-term response to hypoglycaemia (Bolli *et al.*, 1984).

Phaeochromocytoma has been recorded in both dogs (Gilson *et al.*, 1994) and cats, and glucagonoma has been recorded in dogs (Gross *et al.*, 1990). In both cases, diabetes mellitus with a persistently high insulin requirement is likely. In humans, glucagonoma is associated with the development of the hepatocutaneous syndrome. This syndrome is seen in diabetic dogs as a severe crusting dermatopathy affecting the distal limbs, face and perineum, often in association with cirrhosis.

Pancreatitis

The presence of pancreatitis may be associated with both persistently elevated and fluctuating insulin requirements. Recently diagnosed diabetic dogs occasionally have concurrent pancreatitis, and insulin requirements may fall as the condition resolves. This is presumably due to a degree of pancreatic recovery and/or a decrease in the levels of stress hormones. In the case of chronic low-grade or recurring pancreatitis, there may be a history of poor control, variable appetite, fluctuating requirements and/or high requirements. Unfortunately, these cases are often difficult to diagnose because of the poor diagnostic efficiency of serum amylase and lipase measurements; they often respond poorly to therapy.

Obesity

Obesity affects insulin receptor number and affinity, and contributes significantly to the pathogenesis of human type II diabetes mellitus. Some obese diabetic cats recover from the disease following dietary restriction and weight loss. Dietary restriction in obese cats must be gradual to avoid hepatic lipidosis. All obese diabetic animals benefit to some degree from weight loss even if their insulin requirements do not appear excessively high.

Cirrhosis

The presence of cirrhosis in diabetic dogs tends to cause either persistently high insulin requirements or fluctuating low requirements. This depends on a differential failure to metabolise and clear insulin and glucagon from the circulation. The measurement of serum hepatic enzymes is of limited value in diagnosing hepatic disease in diabetic dogs. Controlled diabetic dogs may have elevated enzyme concentrations and animals with advanced cirrhosis may have normal or low enzyme concentrations. Pre- and postprandial bile acid concentrations are useful indicators because these will be normal or only modestly increased in well controlled diabetic animals. Plasma ammonia concentrations are helpful in animals displaying neurological signs that are not associated with hypoglycaemia.

INVESTIGATION

Stage 1

Gather information. This should include:

- Signalment and history — in particular the use of diabetogenic agents, history of ovariohysterectomy, and the nature of the difficulty in regulation. Signalment will assist in assessing the relative likelihood of underlying illnesses. For example, in a 3-year-old insulin-resistant diabetic dog, hypothyroidism is more likely than hyperadrenocorticism
- The owner's impression of the degree of therapeutic success
- Clinical examination
- Diabetic diaries detailing insulin doses, daily water consumption, urine or blood glucose results, and other comments such as level of appetite
- Laboratory indicators of diabetic control such as fructosamine.

Stage 2

Take action indicated by deficiencies identified in Stage 1. For example, replace outdated insulin, re-educate clients concerning consistency of diet and exercise, alter timing of glucose monitoring strategy.

Stage 3

If the problem persists, create a blood glucose curve. Take samples for blood glucose assessment at 2-hourly intervals for 12–24 hours (Figure 4.1).

- Check that single point blood glucose monitoring samples have been being taken at an appropriate time of day (close to nadir concentration is best)
- Identify the duration of insulin effect — a duration of effect <16 hours with once-daily insulin indicates a need for twice-daily therapy when there is poor clinical response; therefore decrease dose slightly and re-stabilise
- Is insulin-induced hyperglycaemia (Somogyi 'overswing') present? If blood glucose falls below 3.5 mmol/l and then rises above 15 mmol/l within one inter-injection period, then insulin-induced hyperglycaemia is likely. Reduce the insulin dose by 25–30% and monitor the clinical effect or repeat the serial glucose analyses
- Little decrease in glucose concentration following injection of a 'normal' or high (>2 IU/kg) dose of insulin indicates the presence of insulin resistance

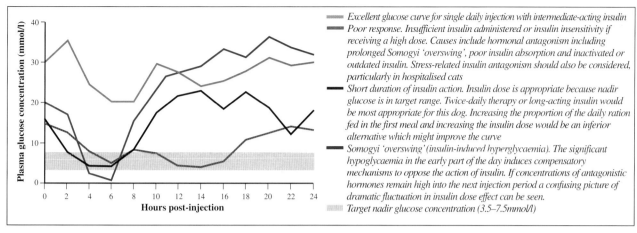

Legend (right of graph):

— Excellent glucose curve for single daily injection with intermediate-acting insulin

— Poor response. Insufficient insulin administered or insulin insensitivity if receiving a high dose. Causes include hormonal antagonism including prolonged Somogyi 'overswing', poor insulin absorption and inactivated or outdated insulin. Stress-related insulin antagonism should also be considered, particularly in hospitalised cats

— Short duration of insulin action. Insulin dose is appropriate because nadir glucose is in target range. Twice-daily therapy or long-acting insulin would be most appropriate for this dog. Increasing the proportion of the daily ration fed in the first meal and increasing the insulin dose would be an inferior alternative which might improve the curve

— Somogyi 'overswing' (insulin-induced hyperglycaemia). The significant hypoglycaemia in the early part of the day induces compensatory mechanisms to oppose the action of insulin. If concentrations of antagonistic hormones remain high into the next injection period a confusing picture of dramatic fluctuation in insulin dose effect can be seen.

▓ Target nadir glucose concentration (3.5–7.5mmol/l)

Figure 4.1: *Example of 24-hour blood glucose curves following single daily administration of intermediate-duration insulin and two evenly divided meals (0 and 6 hours).*

which may be due to concurrent disorders. Defective insulin, prolonged Somogyi 'overswing' (i.e. from previous day), severe hospitalisation/sampling stress or poor insulin absorption will also create little or no response on a blood glucose curve. To investigate poor absorption of PZI or ultralente insulin, change to twice-daily lente insulin and monitor the clinical effect or repeat serial glucose analyses.

Stage 4

If a concurrent disorder is suspected, then an investigation appropriate to the animal's signalment, history and clinical features should be initiated. This should include: Serum chemistry and haematology profiles. These help identify occult sepsis, renal or hepatic dysfunction and perhaps hyperadrenocorticism or hypothyroidism. Urinalysis assists the identification of urinary tract infection or renal dysfunction.

Specific investigations for suspected disorders include:

- ACTH stimulation, low-dose dexamethasone suppression, urinary cortisol/creatinine ratio, ultrasonography, computerised tomography
- Serum ammonia, pre- and post-prandial bile acid concentrations
- Serum total T4, free T4 by dialysis, cTSH, TSH or thyrotropin releasing hormone (TRH) stimulation, T3 suppression
- Serum progesterone, IGF-1 or GH
- Serum amylase, lipase and trypsin-like immunoreactivity concentrations and/or abdominal ultrasonography
- Anti-insulin antibody analyses or test treatment with minimally antigenic insulin — porcine for dogs, bovine for cats
- Urinary catecholamines, serum glucagon measurement (limited information available concerning validity of tests or reference ranges).

On some occasions no cause for resistance or fluctuation can be found and symptomatic therapy is required until more evidence for a particular problem is gathered. Fluctuations in requirement should be followed with frequent changes in dose indicated by close monitoring of blood or urine glucose concentrations. Animals with high insulin requirements need to continue receiving high doses of insulin. There is no maximum or dangerous dose of insulin that applies to all animals. If an animal persistently requires 4 IU/kg of subcutaneous insulin to control its clinical signs and no underlying problem can be identified then that dose is safe for that animal. It may, however, be a lethal dose for a normal dog.

REFERENCES

Blaxter AC and Gruffydd-Jones TJ (1990) Concurrent diabetes mellitus and hyperadrenocorticism in the dog: Diagnosis and management of eight cases. *Journal of Small Animal Practice* **31**, 117–122

Bolli GB, Dimitriadis GD, Pehling GB, Baker BA, Haymond MW, Cryer PE and Gerich JE (1984) Abnormal glucose counterregulation after subcutaneous insulin in insulin-dependent diabetes mellitus. *New England Journal of Medicine* **310**, 1706–1711

Broussard JD and Peterson ME (1994) Comparison of two ultralente insulin preparations with protamine zinc insulin in clinically normal cats. *American Journal of Veterinary Research* **55**, 127–131

Eigenmann JE and Venker-van Haagen AJ (1981) Progestagen-induced and spontaneous canine acromegaly due to reversible growth hormone overproduction: clinical picture and pathogenesis. *Journal of the American Animal Hospital Association* **17**, 813–822

Feldman EC and Nelson RW (1996) Diabetes mellitus. In: *Canine and Feline Endocrinology and Reproduction*, 2nd edn, ed. EC Feldman and RW Nelson, pp. 339–391. WB Saunders, Philadelphia

Ford SL, Nelson RW, Feldman EC and Niwa D (1993) Insulin resistance in three dogs with hypothyroidism and diabetes mellitus. *Journal of the American Veterinary Medical Association* **202**, 1478–1480

Gilson SD, Withrow SJ, Wheeler S and Twedt DC (1994) Pheochromocytoma in 50 dogs. *Journal of Veterinary Internal Medicine* **8**, 228–232

Graham PA (1995) *Clinical and epidemiological studies on canine diabetes mellitus*. PhD Thesis, University of Glasgow, Scotland

Graham PA and Nash AS (1995) How long will my diabetic dog live? *Proceedings of the British Small Animal Veterinary Association Annual Congress*, Birmingham, p. 217

Gross TL, O'Brien TD, Davies AP and Long RE (1990) Glucagon-producing pancreatic endocrine tumors in two dogs with superficial necrolytic dermatitis. *Journal of the American Veterinary Medical Association* **197**, 1619–1622

Hallden G, Gafvelin G, Mutt V and Jornvall H (1986) Characterisation of cat insulin. *Archives of Biochemistry and Biophysiology* **241**, 20–27

Hoenig M and Ferguson DC (1992) Glucose tolerance and insulin secretion in spontaneously hyperthyroid cats. *Research in Veterinary Science* **53**, 338–341

Ihle SL and Nelson RW (1991) Insulin resistance and diabetes mellitus. *Compendium of Continuing Education (Small Animal)* **13**, 197–205

McGuinness OP (1994) The impact of infection on gluconeogenesis in the conscious dog. *Shock* **2**, 336–343

Peterson ME, Greco DS, Randolph JF, Moroff SD and Lothrop CD (1990) Acromegaly in 14 cats. *Journal of Veterinary Internal Medicine* **4**, 192–201

Peterson ME, Nesbitt GH and Schaer M (1981) Diagnosis and management of concurrent diabetes mellitus and hyperadrenocorticism in 30 dogs. *Journal of the American Veterinary Medical Association* **178**, 66–69

Rijnberk A and Belshaw BE (1988) An alternative protocol for the medical management of canine pituitary-dependent hyperadrenocorticism. *Veterinary Record* **122**, 486–488

Smith LF (1966) Species variation in the amino acid sequence of insulin. *American Journal of Medicine* **40**, 662–666

CHAPTER FIVE

The Elderly Cat With Weight Loss

Carmel T. Mooney

INTRODUCTION

Weight loss is a common presenting sign in elderly cats, and in many cases it is the owner's primary concern. Other clinical signs such as polyuria/polydipsia, lethargy, vomiting or diarrhoea may not be as noticeable to cat owners as to dog owners. Cats often have free outdoor access, may live in multicat households, and have a unique ability to adapt their lifestyle and conserve energy to cope with the demands of serious illnesses.

Weight loss is usually evident if greater than 10% of bodyweight has been lost, and progresses to emaciation if greater than 20% has been lost. Emaciation, characterised by prominence of the skeleton, is caused by severe undernutrition resulting in catabolism of body protein and fat (Figure 5.1). Cachexia is the end stage of weight loss and emaciation. Irrespective of underlying cause, cachexia is associated with extreme weakness, depression, and anorexia.

As with many presenting signs, a systematic approach is helpful in achieving a diagnosis. This involves obtaining a detailed history, completing a thorough physical examination, and performing relevant diagnostic tests. In cases where weight loss is the only discernible sign, elimination of the more common causes may be necessary before embarking on specialised diagnostic tests for uncommon disorders.

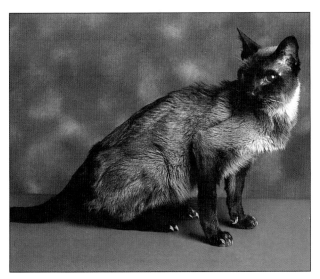

Figure 5.1: *Severe weight loss in a 14 year old Siamese cat. The cat weighed 1.9 kg and had a prolonged history of weight loss and initial polyphagia followed by anorexia. The diagnoses included hyperthyroidism, exocrine pancreatic insufficiency, and hepatic failure.*

HISTORY

A detailed history should contain information on diet type, appetite, and duration of weight loss. Cats may not tolerate abrupt dietary change and the diet type must be appropriate for geriatric animals. There is a significant decline in digestive function as cats age and, provided obesity is not a complicating problem, a highly digestible energy-dense diet is preferred (Harper, 1996). An intact sense of smell is also important in maintaining food intake and its absence may lead to anorexia. Differentiation of weight loss in the face of an increased/normal or decreased appetite is important as specific diseases are associated with each category. In addition, it is important to determine if the cat appears willing to eat but unable to pick up food, masticate, or swallow. Many disorders, for example, hyperthyroidism are associated with gradual and insidious weight loss over months whereas rapid weight loss over a few weeks usually indicates a more severe disease process such as neoplasia. Where weight loss has been rapid it may have to be distinguished from the weight loss associated with dehydration. Skin tenting is unhelpful because of the loss of elasticity associated with ageing, and other variables e.g. appearance of mucous membranes, should be used.

Details of vomiting/diarrhoea, polyuria/polydipsia and any changes in behaviour should be obtained if possible. In addition, details of current medication are important since many drugs, e.g. digoxin, cytotoxic drugs, can result in nausea and anorexia. Cats appear to be less tolerant of environmental change than dogs and it is therefore important to determine if there have been any changes in home or family members or the addition of any new animals.

PHYSICAL EXAMINATION

A thorough physical examination is of vital importance in the investigation of weight loss. Special attention should be given to the mouth, as dental disease, stomatitis, gingivitis, and oral neoplasia are significant causes of illness in older animals. Palpation for goitre becomes a routine part of any physical examination in cats over 6 years of age because of the frequency with which hyperthyroidism occurs in this population of animals. The chest should be auscultated to identify abnormalities in cardiac rate, rhythm and audibility, any murmurs, and abnormal pulmonary sounds. The abdomen should be carefully palpated for unusual masses, organomegaly, thickened intestines, and abnormal kidney size or shape.

DIAGNOSIS

A specific diagnosis may be reached simply on the basis of a detailed history and clinical examination, and subsequently confirmed through the performance of selected diagnostic tests. However, in many cases a definitive diagnosis is not obvious. In addition, because ageing is associated with the progressive and irreversible loss of organ reserve, regenerative powers, and adaptability, one disease may precipitate failure of a number of apparently unrelated organ systems. Thus, screening laboratory tests including urinalysis, haematology, and biochemistry (total protein, albumin, electrolytes, liver enzymes, urea, creatinine, and glucose) are usually indicated. Estimation of circulating total thyroxine (T4) concentration is also warranted because it assists in the diagnosis of hyperthyroidism. In addition, serum total T4 concentrations are inversely correlated with mortality and their measurement provides a useful prognostic indicator in sick cats (Mooney *et al.*, 1996) (Figure 5.2). Examination of viral status is important, particularly for feline immunodeficiency virus (FIV) which is more problematical in the elderly cat. For cases in which clinical and screening laboratory features are unremarkable, thoracic and abdominal radiography and/or ultrasonography may reveal evidence of occult disease.

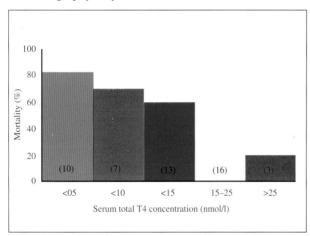

Figure 5.2: Relation of mortality to serum total thyroxine (T4) concentrations in 107 cats with a variety of non-thyroidal illnesses. The number of cats which died or were euthanased are depicted in parentheses.

DISEASES ASSOCIATED WITH POLYPHAGIA

From the history, it is important to determine if the animal has an increased appetite in the face of weight loss as it is associated with fewer differentials than anorexia. Polyphagia associated with weight loss occurs with disorders that result in either negative nutrient balance from excess metabolic demand or a catabolic state from a failure to assimilate or utilise nutrients. Possible diagnoses are detailed in Figure 5.3. Endocrine disorders form the majority of diseases in this category.

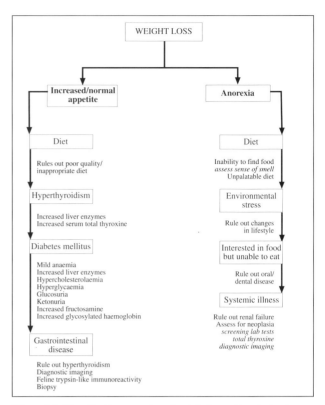

Figure 5.3: Simplified investigation of weight loss with polyphagia or anorexia in the elderly cat.

Hyperthyroidism

Hyperthyroidism (thyrotoxicosis) is the most common endocrine disorder of the cat (see Chapter 15). Excessive concentrations of the thyroid hormones triiodothyronine (T3) and/or T4 are produced, resulting in an overall increase in the metabolic rate. The classical presentation is one of insidious and often marked weight loss despite an increased appetite, polyuria/polydipsia, hyperactivity, and intermittent gastrointestinal signs of vomiting or diarrhoea (Thoday and Mooney, 1992). Signs develop over months or years, and few diseases are capable of inducing such severe weight loss while the animal remains bright and alert. Notable findings on physical examination include enlarged thyroid lobes and an increased heart rate often in association with murmurs. On routine screening laboratory tests, there may be marked elevations of the liver enzymes, and in the elderly cat this is probably the most common reason for such an abnormality. The diagnosis is confirmed by demonstrating an elevation in the circulating concentration of total T4 which occurs in approximately 95% of cases. In a small number of cases, serum total T4 concentrations are not diagnostically elevated because of random fluctuations in hormone concentrations in mildly affected and early cases, or the suppressive effect of concurrent non-thyroidal illness. Although further diagnostic tests (free T4 analyses, T3 suppression test, thyrotropin releasing hormone (TRH) stimulation test) have been recommended for such equivocal cases, serum total T4 concentrations usually increase into the diagnostic thyrotoxic range upon recovery from the non-thyroidal illness or upon retesting 3–6 weeks later.

Diabetes mellitus

Diabetes mellitus is the second most common endocrine disorder in cats (see Chapter 13). Weight loss, despite a normal or increased appetite, is a common presenting sign in uncomplicated cases and occurs because of impaired carbohydrate metabolism and increased fatty acid oxidation (Crenshaw and Peterson, 1996). Polyuria and polydipsia are also significant features because of the osmotic diuretic effect of glucosuria. On physical examination there may be obvious hepatomegaly resulting from hepatic lipidosis. The uncommon finding of a peripheral neuropathy, as evidenced by a plantigrade stance together with a history of polyuria/polydipsia, usually indicates a diagnosis of diabetes mellitus. A stress leucogram, mild non-regenerative anaemia, hypercholesterolaemia, and elevations of the hepatic enzymes are frequent findings on routine screening laboratory tests. Occasionally, hyperbilirubinaemia may also be found. Hyperglycaemia and glucosuria are the biochemical hallmarks of diabetes mellitus. However, because cats are peculiarly sensitive to stress-induced hyperglycaemia, a definitive diagnosis of diabetes mellitus can only be made if there is associated ketonuria, the hyperglycaemia/glucosuria is persistent, or there are elevations in the circulating concentrations of fructosamine or glycosylated haemoglobin (Crenshaw et al., 1996; Elliott et al., 1997).

Hyperadrenocorticism

Hyperadrenocorticism is rare in the cat but is typically associated with polyphagia, weight loss, 'pot belly', muscle weakness, hepatomegaly, and a variety of dermatological changes including alopecia and thin friable skin (see Chapter 29); almost all cats also have diabetes mellitus which could account for most of these signs (Nelson et al., 1988). Hyperadrenocorticism without diabetes mellitus is rare and usually associated with weight gain rather than weight loss (Watson and Herrtage, 1998)

Gastrointestinal disease

A variety of gastrointestinal disorders often associated with a decreased appetite may occasionally result in an increased appetite because of malassimilation (maldigestion/malabsorption) of nutrients (Sherding, 1994). Although traditionally associated with poor condition, helminth infestations are rarely severe enough in the elderly cat to cause significant weight loss and can easily be ruled out by faecal examination. Therefore, the most common differential diagnoses include inflammatory bowel disease (IBD) and exocrine pancreatic insufficiency (EPI), although the latter is considered rare. The history is typical of small intestinal diarrhoea but vomiting may also be a predominant sign. On physical examination, thickened intestines may be palpable in cases of IBD or an oil-stained perineum may be present in cases of EPI. Screening laboratory tests are generally unhelpful and usually more specific tests of gastro-intestinal function are required. These may include diagnostic imaging and assessment of serum trypsin-like immunoreactivity (TLI) which has recently become available for cats (Steiner et al., 1996). For IBD, histopathological examination of the gastrointestinal tract is necessary for a definitive diagnosis and differentiation from neoplasia. Biopsies taken at the time of endoscopy or biopsy are therefore required. Before embarking on these tests, it is important that a diagnosis of hyperthyroidism is ruled out by assessing circulating total T4 concentrations, because the variety of clinical features are indistinguishable among these diseases.

DISEASES ASSOCIATED WITH ANOREXIA

The diseases associated with anorexia and weight loss are numerous, and even those disorders classically associated with polyphagia will eventually develop anorexia if left to progress untreated, for example the hyperthyroid cat developing congestive cardiac failure or the diabetic animal becoming ketoacidotic. It is beyond the scope of this book to detail the possible infectious, inflammatory, neoplastic, toxic, or metabolic disorders capable of inducing anorexia, and a simplified route for investigation is outlined in Figure 5.3. Obviously in the elderly cat, chronic renal disease and neoplasia are significant causes of illness.

Elderly cats with chronic renal failure tend to be presented by owners because of lethargy, anorexia and weight loss rather than noticeable polyuria/polydipsia (DiBartola et al., 1987). There is usually a prolonged history of selective anorexia whereby the cat refuses its normal food but initially remains interested in gourmet-type food or homemade rations. By contrast to the situation in the dog, vomiting appears to be uncommon. Clinical findings tend to be non-specific, relating mainly to weight loss and possibly dehydration. Assessment of kidney size by palpation is generally unrewarding, unless enlarged, although this occurs rarely. Only 25% of affected cats have small, irregular kidneys, but such a finding is also common in older cats without demonstrable renal failure. Pallor of the mucous membranes, mouth ulceration, uraemic halitosis, and retinal detachment may be apparent in severely affected cases. A definitive diagnosis usually relies on the results of routine clinicopathological tests. Abnormalities include non-regenerative anaemia, azotaemia (increased urea and creatinine concentrations), and hyperphosphataemia. Serum total calcium concentration is usually within the reference range, but may be depressed or elevated. Cholesterol concentration is commonly increased without evidence of hypoalbuminaemia, and this appears to be a non-specific finding in renal failure in cats regardless of cause. Mild hyperglycaemia is common, and glucosuria can develop without hyperglycaemia, presumably because of renal tubular dysfunction. Urine samples can be obtained by cystocentesis rapidly and simply with minimal restraint, and provide an inexpensive starting point in the investigation of renal disease (Sparkes and Gruffydd-Jones, 1993). Urine specific gravity is usually within the isosthenuric range (1.007–1.015) and almost 90% of cases have a urine specific gravity <1.025 at presentation (DiBartola et al., 1987). However, in experimental studies of renal failure, cats deprived of water retained the ability to concentrate urine, and therefore such a finding should not preclude a diagnosis of renal failure without adequate biochemical back-up.

Tumours, in general, are more common in dogs than in cats, but the frequency of malignant tumours is considerably higher in the cat (Couto and Hammer, 1994). Most tumours affect cats above 5 years of age, although certain types, e.g. lymphosarcoma have a bimodal age at presentation. Thus, if neoplasia is suspected in the elderly cat, malignancy should be presumed unless proved otherwise. The more common types of tumour, in approximate descending order of frequency, affect the skin and subcutis, digestive system, mammary glands, and respiratory tract. Weight loss and anorexia are relatively common non-specific presenting features, while other signs may relate to the primary tumour, e.g. vomiting and diarrhoea with gastrointestinal neoplasia, or metastatic spread, e.g. liver failure because of hepatic infiltration. In some cases, the diagnosis may be readily apparent on physical examination while in others more detailed investigations including screening laboratory tests and diagnostic imaging procedures are required. These investigations are also of importance in defining metastatic spread. Assessment of viral status (FeLV and FIV) may also be warranted as this may ultimately affect the prognosis or the owner's desire to attempt any treatment if such a course is possible.

REFERENCES

Couto CG and Hammer AS (1994) Oncology. In: *The Cat. Diseases and Clinical Management, 2nd edn*, Vol 2, ed. RG Sherding, pp. 755–818. Churchill Livingstone, New York

Crenshaw KL and Peterson ME (1996) Pretreatment clinical and laboratory evaluation of cats with diabetes mellitus: 104 cases (1992–1994). *Journal of the American Veterinary Medical Association* 209, 943–949

Crenshaw LW, Peterson ME, Heeb LA, Moroff SD and Nichols R (1996) Serum fructosamine concentration as an index of glycaemia in cats with diabetes mellitus and stress hyperglycaemia. *Journal of Veterinary Internal Medicine* 10, 360–364

DiBartola SP, Rutgers HC, Zack PM and Tarr MJ (1987) Clinicopathologic findings associated with chronic renal disease in cats: 74 cases (1973–1984). *Journal of the American Veterinary Medical Association* 190, 1196–1202

Elliott DA, Nelson RW, Feldman EC and Neal LA (1997) Glycosylated haemoglobin concentration for assessment of glycemic control in diabetic cats. *Journal of Veterinary Internal Medicine* 11, 161–165

Harper J (1996) The energy requirements of senior cats. *Waltham Focus* 6, 32

Mooney CT, Little CJL and Macrae AW (1996) Effect of illness not associated with the thyroid gland on serum total and free thyroxine concentrations in cats. *Journal of the American Veterinary Medical Association* 208, 2004–2008

Nelson RW, Feldman EC and Smith MC (1988) Hyperadrenocorticism in cats: 7 cases (1978–1986). *Journal of the American Veterinary Medical Association* 193, 245–250

Sherding RG (1994) Diseases of the intestine. In: *The Cat. Diseases and Clinical Management. 2nd edn*, Vol 2. ed. RG Sherding, pp. 1211–1286. Churchill Livingstone, New York

Sparkes A and Gruffydd-Jones TJ (1993) Laboratory diagnostic aids. In: *Handbook of Feline Medicine*, ed. J Wills and A Wolf, pp. 91–112. Pergamon Press, Oxford

Steiner JM, Medinger TL and Williams DA (1996) Development and validation of a radioimmunoassay for feline trypsin-like immunoreactivity. *American Journal of Veterinary Research* 57, 1417–1420

Thoday KL and Mooney CT (1992) Historical, clinical and laboratory features of 126 hyperthyroid cats. *Veterinary Record* 131, 257–264

Watson PJ and Herrtage ME (1998) Hyperadrenocorticism in six cats. *Journal of Small Animal Practice* (In press)

CHAPTER SIX

Pseudopregnancy in the Bitch

Gary C.W. England

INTRODUCTION

Many non-pregnant bitches exhibit signs that are similar to those normally seen during the prepartum and postpartum periods. These clinical events occur most commonly between 6 and 12 weeks after the end of oestrus, and may develop occasionally, or following every oestrus in an individual bitch.

The condition has been termed pseudopregnancy, phantom pregnancy, false pregnancy, and pseudocyesis. None of these terms is truly accurate since lactation and mothering behaviour are common clinical signs, and these are characteristics of the postpartum period.

The clinical signs of pseudopregnancy are not associated with any endocrine abnormality. They are related to a normal elevated plasma concentration of prolactin, the large polypeptide hormone secreted by the anterior pituitary gland.

There are several options for the management of bitches with pseudopregnancy, and in some cases drug therapy is warranted. The choice of the most suitable agent depends upon the intensity of the clinical signs, and whether previous treatment has been successful.

REPRODUCTIVE PHYSIOLOGY

The bitch is a monoestrous, non-seasonal breeder in which follicular development occurs at the end of a variable period of anoestrus. After ovulation, progesterone profiles are similar in both pregnant and non-pregnant bitches (Figure 6.1). Values may be slightly higher for pregnant bitches,

and elevated progesterone concentration declines earlier, but is of a slightly longer duration in non-pregnant bitches. Both luteinising hormone (LH) and prolactin are luteotrophic factors and therefore promote progesterone secretion by the corpora lutea, especially during the second half of the luteal phase. The uterus does not appear to be involved in the regulation of the corpus luteum.

The long luteal phase of the non-pregnant cycle has been called pseudopregnancy, because of its similarity to pseudopregnancy in other species following a sterile mating. However, the long luteal phase in bitches occurs spontaneously and is not dependent upon a mating-induced ovulation, nor upon initial maternal recognition of pregnancy. The term physiological pseudopregnancy may therefore be used, since in every non-pregnant bitch the luteal phase is long, and there is some degree of mammary gland enlargement. Clinical pseudopregnancy (sometimes referred to as overt pseudopregnancy) is considered to be the development of extensive mammary gland enlargement, combined with lactation and behavioural changes typical of pregnancy and lactation. The incidence of clinical pseudopregnancy in the bitch is not known.

The clinical signs that occur during pregnancy are associated with a rise in plasma prolactin concentration, which commences at 30–35 days after the LH surge. Prolactin concentration continues to increase during late pregnancy to reach a plateau at approximately day 60. Prolactin concentration surges during the prepartum decline in progesterone, and reaches a peak at, or shortly after, parturition.

In the non-pregnant bitch there is a rise in plasma concentration of prolactin when progesterone concentration

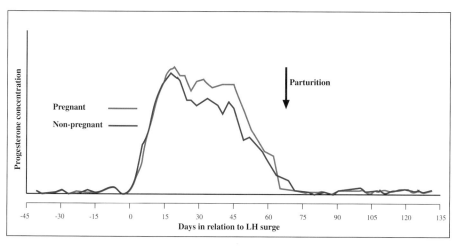

Figure 6.1: Schematic representation of progesterone concentrations in pregnant and non-pregnant bitches.

starts to decline during the late luteal phase. This rise is not as marked as that observed during late pregnancy and lactation, but values are increased by 2–3 times baseline. Prolactin is a known luteotrophic factor in the bitch, and it appears that the mechanisms regulating its release are similar to those of other species. Prolactin release is increased by thyrotropin releasing hormone (TRH) and is reduced by dopamine agonists.

It is common for non-pregnant, non-domestic bitches to exhibit clinical pseudopregnancy with lactation. These bitches will nurse pups born to another bitch, and thus ensure the survival of more of the pack's offspring.

CLINICAL SIGNS

The clinical signs of pseudopregnancy are variable and may include anorexia, nervousness, aggression, nest making, nursing of inanimate objects, lactation and occasionally false parturition. In the majority of non-pregnant bitches mammary gland development is associated with the production of milk. In some cases lactation may result in mastitis.

Pseudopregnancy is generally noted between 6 and 12 weeks after the end of oestrus, during the decline in plasma progesterone concentration. It may also occur should plasma progesterone concentration decline for other reasons. Removal of the ovaries (ovariectomy or more commonly ovariohysterectomy) during the luteal phase will result in a rapid reduction in plasma concentration of progesterone, and a subsequent rise in plasma concentration of prolactin. Similarly, lysis of the corpora lutea may result in a rise in plasma prolactin concentration; this may be seen, for example, following spontaneous abortion in late pregnancy, or following the pharmacological termination of pregnancy. In each of these cases, the induced rise of plasma prolactin may potentiate the development of clinical pseudopregnancy.

In many cases pseudopregnancy undergoes spontaneous remission, especially if there is no stimulus for continued lactation (no sucking). However, in some cases either the physical or the psychological signs, or the effect of these signs upon the owner, may warrant treatment of the condition.

In some cases pseudopregnancy may persist for many months, or even several years. This appears to be most common in cases induced iatrogenically by ovariectomy (commonly ovariohysterectomy) during the luteal phase. The reason for this is unknown, but presumably relates to a lack of hormonal interaction between the pituitary/ hypothalamus and the ovary. In other cases, when pseudopregnancy is inadequately treated, it may appear to persist. Bitches may show no clinical signs during treatment but relapse when treatment is terminated. In these cases treatment has usually been terminated too rapidly allowing a further rise in prolactin concentration.

It is often mistakenly stated that clinical pseudopregnancy predisposes to pyometra, infertility and ovarian abnormalities; this is untrue.

TREATMENT

In the majority of cases, clinical pseudopregnancy requires no treatment. Once the owner has been reassured that the condition is normal, spontaneous resolution can be allowed to occur.

It is always important to ensure that a correct diagnosis of pseudopregnancy has been reached, since the administration of certain drugs to pregnant bitches can produce severe sequelae, including delayed parturition and fetal abnormalities.

Conservative treatment

The administration of sedative agents may be useful in some bitches with marked behavioural changes associated with clinical pseudopregnancy. The agents should be chosen carefully, and phenothiazines for example may be inappropriate, since they are dopamine antagonists and may therefore produce a rise in prolactin concentration.

Some workers have suggested bathing the mammary glands and removing the milk by massage, but stimulation of the mammary glands is likely to potentiate a further rise in prolactin concentration, and may not be therapeutic. Indeed, many bitches stimulate themselves by licking, and the application of an Elizabethan collar around the neck may be useful.

The administration of diuretic agents, or the withholding of fluids has also been suggested; while these may produce minor improvement, they should be performed with care, especially if the bitch is anorexic.

Administration of steroid preparations

Progestogens

The administration of progesterone (or progestogens) to bitches rapidly reduces the signs of clinical pseudopregnancy (Table 6.1). The mechanism of action is likely to be the suppression of pituitary release of prolactin.

Drug	Classification	Dose and route
Agents available in the UK		
Megoestrol acetate	Progestogen	2 mg/kg orally for 5 days
Proligestone	Progestogen	33 mg/kg subcutaneously
Delmadinone acetate	Progestogen	1.5 mg/kg subcutaneously
Methyl testosterone	Androgen	0.66 mg/kg orally for 5–10 days
+ ethinyloestradiol	+ oestrogen	+ 0.0008 mg/kg
Bromocriptine	Prolactin antagonist	Increasing to 0.01–0.1 mg/kg for up to 10 days
Agents available elsewhere		
Mibolerone	Androgen	0.016 mg/kg orally for 5 days
Cabergoline	Prolactin antagonist	5.0 µg/kg daily orally for 5–10 days

Table 6.1: Medical treatment of pseudopregnancy. Some of these agents do not have a product licence for this purpose.

Progestogens may be administered either orally daily as megoestrol acetate, or by depot injection of proligestone or delmadinone acetate, although the latter is not licensed for this purpose. First-generation progestogens such as medroxyprogesterone acetate are not recommended, since they have marked effects upon the uterus and might potentiate the development of pyometra.

In general, depot progestogen therapy works well, since the progestogen concentration gradually reduces in the circulation. Oral therapy is often associated with relapse of the clinical signs if therapy is terminated too quickly; this can usually be prevented by gradually reducing the dose over a period of approximately 7–10 days.

The adverse effects of progestogens include increased appetite, weight gain, lethargy, mammary gland enlargement, and coat and temperament changes. The greatest clinical concern is the risk of inducing cystic endometrial hyperplasia and pyometra. This effect depends upon the particular progestogen, and both the amount of agent used and the duration of treatment. Administration of progestogens may also result in the clinical signs of acromegaly and diabetes mellitus. Progestogen therapy may induce the formation of benign mammary nodules and produce adrenocortical suppression. During pregnancy, progestogen therapy may delay or prevent parturition and may produce masculinised female and cryptorchid male pups.

It is likely that the return to oestrus will be delayed following the administration of progestogens.

Oestrogens and androgens

Oestrogens and androgens, and combinations of these steroids are also effective at reducing the signs of clinical pseudopregnancy (see Table 6.1). Their mechanism of action is likely to be the same as that of progesterone.

In clinical practice administration of these agents alone is uncommon, although a synthetic androgen, mibolerone, unavailable in the UK but available in the USA, is effective and potentially has less adverse uterine effects than the progestogens.

Orally administered combinations of ethinyl oestradiol and methyltestosterone are commercially available to treat clinical pseudopregnancy in the bitch. The treatment regimen is empirical, but the response is usually good and the risk of adverse effects is low. Relapse following cessation of treatment may occur in a similar manner to that after oral progestogens.

Oestrogens may produce bone marrow suppression, and androgens may produce clitoral enlargement and aggression, although when used in combination the individual drug doses are reduced and the risk of adverse effects is low.

Administration of prolactin antagonists

Several synthetic ergot alkaloids which are dopamine agonists have been shown to be inhibitors of prolactin secretion in the dog (see Table 6.1)

Bromocriptine has been used for some time to reduce the circulating concentration of prolactin and therefore to control the signs of clinical pseudopregnancy. Bromocriptine is not specific in its action and oral administration causes vomiting in a large percentage of bitches. These effects can be reduced by starting with a very low dose and increasing this gradually over several days until a clinical effect occurs. The incidence of vomiting may be reduced by mixing the drug with food, or by the prior administration of metoclopramide, although the latter does not make pharmacological sense since bromocriptine and metoclopramide have opposing dopaminergic actions.

The ergot alkaloid cabergoline also reduces the plasma concentration of prolactin, and whilst it is not presently available in the UK it is widely available in Europe. Cabergoline has a higher activity, longer duration of action, and better tolerance, and produces less vomiting than bromocriptine.

The adverse effects of these agents include a reduction in plasma progesterone concentration (prolactin is a major luteotrophic agent in the bitch), and thus if they are administered to pregnant animals resorption or abortion will result. Both agents have been demonstrated to reduce the interval to the next fertile oestrus; owners should be warned of this effect.

Ovariohysterectomy

Ovariectomy (or more commonly ovariohysterectomy) has no value for the treatment of clinical pseudopregnancy. Removal of the ovaries will cause a further reduction in plasma progesterone concentration and potentiate the rise of plasma prolactin.

Whilst it is clear that ovariohysterectomy will prevent the occurrence of pseudopregnancy, caution should be exercised in performing surgery too soon after hormonal treatment, as the suppression of prolactin may only be temporary. Should surgery be performed during clinical pseudopregnancy, the signs may persist, unless treated, for a considerable period of time, often several years. The safest time to perform ovariohysterectomy is during deep anoestrus (at least 3 months after the end of oestrus), although obviously surgery cannot be delayed in the case of pyometra or acute parturient crisis. In bitches that have repeated clinical pseudopregnancy the best time to perform surgery is during the subsequent oestrus.

CONCLUSION

Pseudopregnancy can be regarded as a normal physiological event, and clinical pseudopregnancy should be expected in a proportion of normal bitches. Pseudopregnancy does not predispose to diseases of the reproductive tract, and in the majority of cases treatment is not warranted. Prevention can be achieved by ovariohysterectomy performed in deep anoestrus or during the subsequent oestrus. In those cases in which treatment is necessary, it is prudent to use agents that have minimal effects upon the uterus, such as androgen/oestrogen combinations or the new-generation progestogens. The use of prolactin antagonists has not found wide acceptance in the UK because the only available agent, bromocriptine, has unsatisfactory adverse effects. Nevertheless bromocriptine is the drug of choice for cases of recurrent clinical pseudopregnancy. In other European countries cabergoline is widely used, and has become the drug of first choice.

FURTHER READING

Allen WE (1986) Pseudopregnancy in the bitch: the current view on aetiology and treatment. *Journal of Small Animal Practice* **27**, 419–424

Jochle W, Arbeiter K, Post K, Ballabio R and D'Ver AS (1989) Effects on pseudopregnancy, pregnancy and interoestrous intervals of pharmacological suppression of prolactin secretion in female dogs and cats. *Journal of Reproduction and Fertility* Supplement 39, 199–207

Simpson G, England GCW and Harvey M (1998) *Manual of Small Animal Reproduction and Neonatology*. BSAVA Cheltenham

CHAPTER SEVEN

Prevention of Breeding in the Bitch and Queen

Gary C.W. England

INTRODUCTION

Unwanted and uncontrolled pets are major sources of ecological and social problems which include zoonotic disease, pollution, and damage to public areas, livestock and man.

There are also valid welfare reasons for controlling reproduction since several million unwanted dogs and cats are destroyed each year in the UK alone.

There are several ways by which reproduction may be prevented and these can be divided into surgical, hormonal and immunological methods.

REPRODUCTIVE PHYSIOLOGY

The reproductive cycle in the bitch is unusual in that the luteal phase has a similar duration in both pregnant and non-pregnant animals. The luteal phase is invariably followed by a period of sexual inactivity, termed anoestrus, which lasts an average of 4 months; the interoestrous interval is therefore approximately 7 months. In the queen, a luteal phase rarely follows oestrus, unless mating has occurred, since this species is a coitally induced ovulator. Most queens enter anoestrus at the beginning of winter and remain sexually inactive for 3–4 months each year; anoestrus does not necessarily follow a luteal phase.

In both species, pro-oestrous and oestrous behaviour are not displayed during the luteal phase, since gonadotropin secretion is basal and follicular development is absent. This effect is related to the high concentration of progesterone producing a negative feedback effect upon the hypothalamus and pituitary gland. Similarly, during anoestrus, gonadotropin secretion and follicular development are absent, until just prior to the subsequent pro-oestrus. Clearly the bitch and queen are unlike many other domestic species in that gonadotropin secretion, follicular growth and pro-oestrous behaviour are not initiated by the decline in plasma progesterone that occurs at the end of the luteal phase. These differences are relevant because pro-oestrous and oestrous behaviour can be abolished by suppression of gonadotropin secretion using either gonadotropin releasing hormone (GnRH) antagonists (and agonists), progestogens, androgens, or immunisation against gonadotropins and GnRH. In addition, cyclical activity may be abolished in the bitch by inducing a state of anoestrus following an artificial luteal phase (prolonged administration of progestogens).

SURGICAL OPTIONS

A variety of surgical procedures have been described to prevent reproduction in the bitch and queen. The procedure most frequently performed in the UK is ovariohysterectomy. Removal of the ovaries prevents cyclical activity, and in many other countries a simple ovariectomy is performed. Removal of the uterus prevents the problem of pyometra that might be induced following the administration of progestogens.

Ovariohysterectomy should be considered in any bitch or queen that is not required for breeding as it has several advantages. These include a reduction in the incidence of mammary gland tumours, elimination of the problems of pyometra, and in the bitch pseudopregnancy, in addition to the obvious advantages of absence of oestrous behaviour and inability to produce offspring. There are, however, several claimed adverse effects, including an increased incidence of incontinence, changes in coat texture and a tendency to gain weight. While little can be done regarding the former two conditions, the latter may be controlled by correct dietary management.

Transplantation of a section of the removed ovary has been advocated in bitches as a method for reducing some of the potential adverse effects of ovariohysterectomy, but severe abnormalities at the site of transplantation, including neoplasia, have been observed, and this technique cannot be recommended.

There is considerable discussion concerning the correct time to perform an ovariohysterectomy. There is no doubt that surgery is technically easier and recovery is more rapid in young animals. Some workers advocate surgery at 4 months of age, but it has been suggested that when this procedure is performed before puberty (the first oestrus) in the bitch there is an increased tendency for underdevelopment of the secondary sexual characteristics, and there may also be effects on the closure time of the growth plates, increasing the risk of physeal fractures. Delaying the procedure until after the first oestrus risks pregnancy and pseudopregnancy.

Other surgical options include occlusion or resection of the uterine tubes. These techniques suffer the disadvantage of failing to abolish normal cyclical activity, and are not suitable for clinical practice.

HORMONAL OPTIONS

A variety of compounds may be used to inhibit normal cyclical activity. Their actions are to influence gonadotropin secretion directly and, in some cases in the bitch, to induce a state of anoestrus.

Progestogens

Administration of progestogens to bitches and queens in anoestrus prevents gonadotrophin secretion increasing above basal values, and therefore prevents a return to cyclical activity. If progestogens are given when there is follicular activity (pro-oestrus or early oestrus), ovulation is inhibited and the female returns to a phase of sexual inactivity. This action of progestogens is probably mediated by inhibition of increasing concentration of gonadotrophins, although in other species there is evidence that progestogens may have a direct action upon the ovary. Progestogens also mimic a normal luteal phase, and in the bitch this is followed by a state of anoestrus, comparable in duration to that of the normal cycle. Therefore cyclical activity is inhibited for longer than the duration of progestogen treatment.

There are a large number of progestogenic compounds for use in controlling reproduction, which include progesterone, the original progestogens such as medroxyprogesterone acetate, norethisterone acetate, megoestrol acetate, and the newer generation progestogens such as proligestone and delmadinone acetate (Table 7.1).

All progestogens have adverse effects, although these are reduced in the newer generation progestogens such as proligestone. Unwanted effects include increased appetite, weight gain, lethargy, mammary gland enlargement, and coat and temperament changes. The greatest clinical concern is the risk of inducing cystic endometrial hyperplasia and pyometra. This depends upon the particular progestogen, the amount of agent used and the duration of treatment. All progestogens may potentially induce the production of growth hormone. Chronic oversecretion of growth hormone may result in the clinical signs of acromegaly and peripheral insulin antagonism which may result in diabetes mellitus. Progestogen therapy may also induce the formation of benign mammary nodules and produce adrenocortical suppression. Progestogen therapy during pregnancy may delay or prevent parturition and may produce masculinised female and cryptorchid male fetuses.

Progestogens are available in four formulations including short-duration progesterone in oil for injection, progestogen implants for subcutaneous administration, depot progestogens for injection, and orally active progestogens. Only the last two are routinely used. These are generally administered in one of four regimens to control reproduction.

Subcutaneous administration of depot preparations during anoestrus

Depot progestogens (medroxyprogesterone acetate,

Drug	Classification	Dose and route
Agents available in the UK for bitches		
Megoestrol acetate	Progestogen	0.5 mg/kg/day orally during anoestrus for up to 40 days (may be repeated) 2 mg/kg/day orally during pro-oestrus for 8 days or 2 mg/kg for 4 days and then 0.5 mg/kg for 16 days
Medroxyprogesterone acetate	Progestogen	10–20 mg/day orally during pro-oestrus for 4 days then 5–10 mg/day for 12 days
Proligestone	Progestogen	10–33 mg/kg subcutaneously during anoestrus 10–33 mg/kg subcutaneously during pro-oestrus
Delmadinone acetate	Progestogen	2 mg/kg subcutaneously during anoestrus
Testoterone esters + methyl testosterone	Androgens + androgens	5 mg/kg esters subcutaneously during anoestrus combined with 10 mg/day methyl testosterone orally
Methyl testosterone	Androgen	0.5–1.0 mg/kg/day
Agents available elsewhere Mibolerone	Androgen	0.016 mg/kg/day orally during anoestrus
Agents available in the UK for queens Megoestrol acetate	Progestogen	2.5 mg/kg/week orally during anoestrus for up to 30 weeks. 5 mg/kg/day orally during pro-oestrus for 3 days
Medroxyprogesterone acetate	Progestogen	5 mg/week orally during anoestrus
Proligestone	Progestogen	10–33 mg/kg subcutaneously during anoestrus 10–33 mg/kg subcutaneously during pro-oestrus

Table 7.1: *Medical control of breeding in bitches and queens.*

delmadinone acetate, and proligestone) administered subcutaneously during anoestrus will prevent a subsequent oestrus and regular repeated dosing can be used to prevent oestrus on a long-term basis. Medroxyprogesterone acetate and proligestone are licensed for this purpose in the bitch, whilst proligestone is the sole depot progestogen licensed for use in the queen.

It may be unadvisable to prevent oestrus for more than 2 years but, provided that a breakthrough cycle does not occur, prolonged prevention may have few adverse effects, especially when the more recently developed progestogens are used. Indeed it has been reported that incidence of pyometra and mammary gland tumours is reduced compared with untreated females. When therapy ceases most females cycle normally, although progestogens may induce cystic endometrial hyperplasia and therefore reduce fertility.

Oral administration of progestogens during anoestrus

Low doses of orally active progestogens (megoestrol acetate, medroxyprogesterone acetate, norethisterone acetate) can be used to prevent oestrus for as long as administration is continued.

Megoestrol acetate and medroxyprogesterone acetate are licensed for this purpose in the bitch, whilst megoestrol acetate is the only orally active progestogen licensed for use in the queen.

The drugs are best given during late anoestrus before the anticipated oestrus. However, should the animal enter pro-oestrus during the first few days of treatment, the dosage can be increased.

In bitches, a period of anoestrus usually follows therapy, so oestrus does not return immediately after cessation of treatment.

Oral administration of progestogens during pro-oestrus

High doses of orally active progestogens (megoestrol acetate, medroxyprogesterone acetate, norethisterone acetate) may be given during pro-oestrus to suppress the signs of oestrus. Megoestrol acetate and medroxyprogesterone acetate are licensed for this purpose in the bitch, and megoestrol acetate is licensed for use in the queen.

Usually the signs of pro-oestrus/oestrus disappear in approximately 5 days. Treatment during late pro-oestrus may not prevent ovulation in the bitch, although conception is unlikely to occur.

However, treatment too early may lead to a return to oestrus soon after dosing. A reducing dose regimen administered from the first signs of pro-oestrus and continued for up to 16 days is usually efficacious. This regimen is usually followed by a variable period of anoestrus, and oestrus will return between 4 and 6 months after the end of medication.

Subcutaneous administration of depot preparations during pro-oestrus

Administration of the new-generation depot progestogens (proligestone) to bitches and queens in early pro-oestrus may be used to suppress the signs of that oestrus. Older generation progestogens (medroxyprogesterone acetate) that have potent effects upon the uterus are not recommended, since they increase the risk of uterine disease, especially pyometra. The signs of pro-oestrus/oestrus disappear within approximately 5 days. Following the depot progestogen, there is a variable anoestrus, and oestrus returns approximately 6 months later (range 3–9 months).

Androgens

Administration of androgens to bitches and queens in anoestrus may be used to prevent a return to cyclical activity. The endocrine mechanism of this action has not been determined, although it is likely to be similar to that of progestogens in preventing the increase in gonadotrophin secretion above basal values. Androgens are not useful for inhibiting oestrus in females with follicular activity (pro-oestrus or early oestrus), and therefore administration must be planned to commence in late anoestrus, at least 30 days before the onset of pro-oestrus.

When androgens are used in this manner they do not mimic the normal luteal phase, and therefore there is no subsequent anoestrus. Therefore cyclical activity returns rapidly after the termination of treatment.

Androgens have certain adverse effects and these include clitoral hypertrophy, vaginitis and aggression. If inadvertently administered to pregnant animals, masculinisation of female fetuses may occur. The advantage of androgens is that they have no adverse effects upon the uterus and do not stimulate the development of cystic endometrial hyperplasia or pyometra.

Oral administration of synthetic androgens during anoestrus

A synthetic androgen, mibolerone, which is not available in the UK has been shown to be effective for the long-term prevention of oestrus in bitches and queens (see Table 7.1). Mibolerone is formulated as a liquid for daily oral administration. The compound has adverse effects typical of other androgens, including clitoral hypertrophy, vaginitis and behavioural changes. In addition, anal gland abnormalities, obnoxious body odour and obesity have also been recorded.

Administration of depot androgens during anoestrus

The administration of testosterone either as a prolonged release implant or depot injection of mixed testosterone esters may be used to prevent oestrus in bitches (see Table 7.1). In clinical practice it is not uncommon for depot therapy to be supplemented by daily oral therapy. For example, mixed testosterone esters may be given intramuscularly every 4–6 weeks, with supplemental therapy of daily oral testosterone administration.

GnRH antagonists

GnRH antagonists may be used to prevent cyclical activity in the bitch, but their use has not been described in the queen. The commonly investigated agent detirelix is not available in the UK.

These agents have an immediate onset of action and have most commonly been administered during pro-oestrus, when they produce a reduction in circulating gonadotropins within a few hours. Bitches therefore rapidly return to anoestrus, and are no longer attractive to male dogs.

Problems with the use of these agents are that following continuous dosing there may be potent mast cell degranulating actions. However, single doses may be given during pro-oestrus to produce a rapid return to anoestrus lasting approximately 18 days, before return to a fertile oestrus.

GnRH agonists

The administration of GnRH produces stimulation and then downregulation of GnRH receptors. Agonist analogues of GnRH, such as nafarelin, may therefore be used to prevent reproductive cyclicity. In early studies oestrus was prevented using GnRH implants placed subcutaneously each month, or GnRH was administered daily by osmotic pump. Oestrus was often initially induced although this occurred in fewer bitches when therapy commenced in early metoestrus (dioestrus) or when bitches were treated from less than 4 months of age. Following these studies successful prevention of oestrus was achieved using subcutaneously implanted sialastic devices providing a sustained release of GnRH for up to one year. Upon withdrawal bitches returned to cyclical activity within approximately 2 months.

GnRH agonists have not been evaluated in cats, and generally suitable preparations of these agents are not commercially available.

IMMUNISATION

Immunisation of bitches against zona pellucida proteins, gonadotropins and GnRH may provide an effective means of contraception. A reliable GnRH protein conjugate antigen has recently been developed; however, such methods require further investigation before they become clinically useful.

CONCLUSION

Control of reproduction in the bitch and queen is of paramount importance to reduce the problem of pet overpopulation. The commonly available methods are ovariohysterectomy, or the administration of depot or orally active progestogens, in a variety of regimens. When the use of progestogens is contemplated, their potential adverse effects should be carefully considered. Androgens may be suitable alternatives in certain cases, especially since they do not produce the same adverse effects as progestogens.

It seems likely that in the future gonadotropin agonists and antagonists, or possibly immunological contraception, will be the preferred option.

FURTHER READING

Evans JM and Sutton DJ (1989) The use of hormones, especially progestagens, to control oestrus in bitches.*Journal of Reproduction and Fertility* Supplement 39, 163-173.

Simpson G, England GCW and Harvey M (1998) *Manual of Small Animal Reproduction and Neonatology*. BSAVA, Cheltenham

CHAPTER EIGHT

Timing of Mating in the Bitch

Gary C.W. England

INTRODUCTION

In the bitch, the time of ovulation is variable in relation to the onset of pro-oestrus. Many breeders, however, impose standard mating regimens, usually a defined number of days after the onset of vulval bleeding, upon their animals. Therefore bitches are often mated at an inappropriate time, and this constitutes the commonest cause of apparent infertility.

There are several investigative methods for identifying the optimal mating time, including measurement of plasma hormone concentrations, examination of exfoliated vaginal cells, and vaginal endoscopy. Failure to detect the time of ovulation and achieve pregnancy is a significant problem in this species because the bitch is a monoestrous animal and the mean interoestrus interval is 31 weeks.

REPRODUCTIVE PHYSIOLOGY

The oocyte of the bitch is ovulated in an immature state and, unlike other species, cannot be fertilised immediately. Fertilisation can only occur following maturation of the primary oocytes, extrusion of the polar body, and completion of the first meiotic division. These events are not completed until at least 48 hours after ovulation. Ovulation occurs 2 days after the surge of plasma luteinising hormone (LH). Oocytes remain viable within the reproductive tract for a further 4–5 days before degenerating. The 'fertilisation period' of the bitch therefore extends from 4 to 7 days after the preovulatory surge of LH (i.e. 2–5 days after

ovulation). A further time interval, the 'fertile period', can also be identified. This is the time during which a mating could result in a conception. This period includes the fertilisation period but precedes it by several days, due to sperm survival within the female reproductive tract before ovulation and oocyte maturation. The fertile period extends from 3 days before, until 7 days after, the preovulatory LH surge and may be even longer for dogs with exceptional semen quality (Figure 8.1).

ASSESSING THE OPTIMAL TIME FOR MATING

The optimal time for mating is likely to be during, or immediately preceding the fertilisation period. The period of peak fertility for natural matings ranges from one day before until 6 days after the LH surge. Determination of the optimal time to mate can be assessed by measuring the LH surge, or by methods that reliably indicate the fertile or preferably the fertilisation period. When the use of preserved semen is contemplated, insemination should be performed only during the fertilisation period, to ensure success.

Clinical assessments

Many dog breeders rely upon counting the number of days from the onset of pro-oestrus, and many believe that bitches always ovulate a defined number of days from the onset of this event. This is not the case, and while the 'average

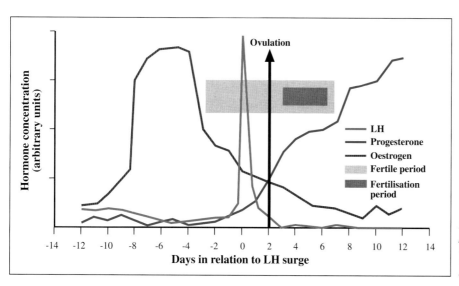

Figure 8.1: Schematic representation of plasma changes in oestrogen, luteinising hormone (LH) and progesterone in relationship to ovulation, and the fertile and fertilisation periods of the bitch.

bitch' may ovulate 12 days after the onset of pro-oestrus (and should therefore be mated on days 14 and 16), some bitches ovulate as early as day 5, or as late as day 30 after the onset of proestrus. It can be seen, therefore, that mating on the 12th and 14th days, which is common breeding practice, fails to result in conception.

Initial studies on laboratory-kept bitches suggested that the onset of standing oestrus occurred at the same time as the LH surge. Using these data, mating 4 days after the onset of standing oestrus would be a suitable time. However, in many bitches the behavioural events have been shown to correlate poorly with the underlying hormonal events, and this method therefore has little value.

One clinical assessment that may be useful in the bitch is the timing of vulval softening. During pro-oestrus the vulva and perineal tissues become enlarged, oedematous and somewhat turgid. Distinct vulval softening often occurs at the time of the LH surge, when there is a change from high oestrogen concentration to low oestrogen concentration with rising progesterone concentration.

When clinical assessments alone are available for the prediction of the optimal mating time, the combination of the onset of standing oestrus and the timing of vulval

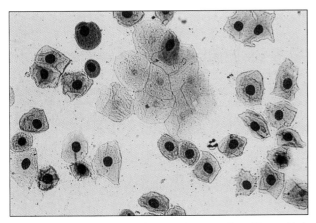

Figure 8.2: Photomicrograph of a vaginal smear collected from a bitch in early oestrus and stained with a modified Wright–Giemsa stain. A range of epithelial cell types are present, ranging from small epithelial cells with a small cytoplasm, to cells which have a large cytoplasm with either pyknotic or absent nuclei.

softening may be useful, since each event occurs on average 2 days before ovulation.

Measurement of plasma hormones

Measurement of the peripheral plasma concentration of LH is a reliable and accurate method for determining the optimum time to mate. There is no readily available commercial assay for canine LH, and at present measurement requires radioimmunoassay (RIA). This method is time-consuming and expensive, and there is frequently a delay in obtaining the results, because samples are assayed in batches. Should LH concentration be measured, mating or insemination can be planned between 4 and 6 days after the LH surge.

In the bitch, the unusual phenomenon of preovulatory luteinisation may be useful for predicting the time of ovulation. The plasma progesterone concentration begins to increase from the baseline level approximately 2 days before ovulation. Serial monitoring of plasma progesterone concentration therefore allows anticipation of ovulation, confirmation of ovulation and detection of the fertilisation period. Since the initial rise in progesterone is gradual, it is only necessary to collect blood samples every second or third day, unlike the daily regimen required to detect the LH surge. Mating or insemination should be planned between 4 and 6 days after the plasma progesterone concentration exceeds 6.5 nmol/l (the value at the time of the LH surge), or should preferably commence one day after values exceed 25.0–32.0 nmol/l (the beginning of the fertilisation period). Progesterone may be measured by RIA, though several enzyme-linked immunosorbent assay (ELISA) test kits have recently become commercially available. These kits allow progesterone concentrations to be assessed either qualitatively or quantitatively within 45–60 minutes of sample collection. They have found wide clinical acceptance and have produced a significant increase in pregnancy rate.

Vaginal cytology

Collection, staining and microscopic examination of

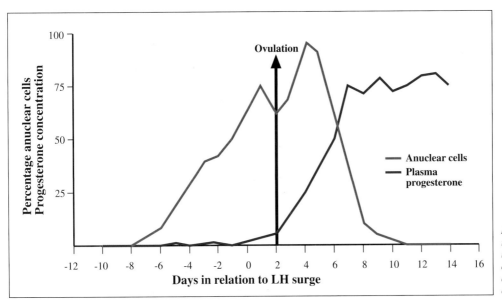

Figure 8.3: Schematic representation of the changes in the percentage of anuclear cells in relationship to ovulation and plasma concentrations of progesterone.

exfoliated vaginal cells is a simple method for monitoring the stage of the oestrous cycle. Vaginal cells may be collected using either a moistened cotton swab rolled within the vagina, or by aspiration of the vaginal cavity using a plastic catheter. When using the former method it is important not to allow contact of the swab with the vestibule, since collection of these cells will give erroneous results; it is prudent to use a small speculum or guard. Once collected, cells are placed on to a glass microscope slide by rolling the cotton swab, or by application of the aspirated fluid which is then spread into a thin film. The smear can be stained using either a simple stain (e.g. Diff-Quik® or a modified Wright–Giemsa stain), or a modified trichrome stain. The former is readily available and has the advantage that sample preparation may take only seconds; the latter has the advantage of identification of keratinised cells, although the staining technique is laborious.

During pro-oestrus, peripheral plasma concentrations of oestrogen are increased, causing thickening of the vaginal mucosa, and an increase in the number of cell layers. The mucosa changes from a cuboidal epithelium into a keratinised squamous epithelium. As the mucosa thickens, the surface cells change in their shape, size and staining character, becoming larger, irregularly shaped and ultimately anuclear (Figure 8.2). The relative proportions of different types of epithelial cell can be used as markers of the endocrine environment. Several indices of cornification and keratinisation have been used; in general, the fertile period can be predicted by calculating the percentage of epithelial cells that appear anuclear when using Diff–Quik® or a modified Wright–Giemsa stain. Mating should be attempted throughout the period when more than 80% of epithelial cells are anuclear (the fertile period) (Figure 8.3).

At the end of the fertilisation period, the plasma progesterone concentration remains at a high value and there is sloughing of much of the vaginal epithelium. The number of cell layers decreases, deeper cells are uncovered and the percentage of large irregularly shaped anuclear cells decreases.

Polymorphonuclear leucocytes are generally absent from the vaginal smear during the fertile period, however they reappear in large numbers at the end of the fertilisation period when plasma progesterone concentrations are high. At this time the vaginal smear is dominated by small epithelial cells, cellular debris, bacteria and polymorphonuclear leucocytes.

While vaginal cytology is a useful technique, polymorphonuclear leucocytes may be found throughout the fertile period in some bitches and in others peak values of only 60% anuclear cells are reached.

Vaginal endoscopy

Vaginal endoscopy (vaginoscopy) is the examination of the vaginal mucosa using a rigid endoscope. The procedure is well tolerated in the non-sedated, standing bitch. The examination can take as little as 2 minutes, and valuable information may be collected quickly and with minimal expense.

Vaginoscopic assessment is based upon observation of the mucosal fold contours and profiles, the colour of the mucosa and of any fluid present. During anoestrus the vaginal mucosa is relatively flat, dry and red in appearance. At the onset of pro-oestrus and during early oestrus the mucosal folds are enlarged, oedematous, and pink or pink/white in colour. These changes are due to thickening of the mucosal epithelium and oedema within the submucosa, both of which are effects of oestrogen. At approximately the time of the LH surge there is progressive shrinking of the folds, accompanied by pallor. These effects are probably the result of an abrupt withdrawal of the water-retaining effect of oestrogen, during its preovulatory decline. Subsequently, mucosal shrinkage is accompanied by wrinkling of the mucosal folds which become distinctly angulated and a dense cream to white colour.

The onset of the fertile period can be detected by observing mucosal shrinkage without angulation, whilst shrinkage with angulation is characteristic of the fertilisation period. Mating or insemination should be planned during the fertilisation period, or 4–6 days after first detecting mucosal shrinkage. The termination of the fertilisation period can be detected by observing a decline or cessation of mucosal shrinkage, combined with sloughing of the vaginal epithelium.

Vaginoscopic changes are useful in clinical practice because they are progressive, therefore it is not necessary to examine the bitch each day.

Ultrasound examination

It has been clearly demonstrated that the ovaries of a bitch can be identified using real-time diagnostic B-mode ultrasound. With careful and repeated examination it is possible to monitor follicular growth and to detect the time of ovulation. In general, however, ovulation is difficult to identify because follicles do not collapse and corpora lutea have a central fluid-filled cavity. Ovulation might be suggested by the detection of a decrease in the number of follicles, and a subjective decrease in follicle size, although the technique appears to have little clinical application at present.

Examination of cervicovaginal secretion

In a small number of bitches it has been shown that the electrical resistance of the vaginal secretions decreases during late oestrus. These changes might therefore be useful for indicating the fertile period. The technique has been poorly investigated in the domestic bitch, although it is used widely to detect the optimal time of insemination in vixen.

Some workers have examined changes in the concentration of glucose within the vaginal discharge of the bitch, and this method is used by several dog breeders for the prediction of mating time. However, the technique has failed to stand up to scientific investigation, and appears to be almost useless.

Crystallisation of mucus collected from the anterior vagina has been described in the bitch and occurs after the peak in plasma oestrogen concentration. Assessment of the mucus, which originates from cervical glandular tissue, may be useful in combination with vaginal cytology for determining the optimal mating time.

CONCLUSION

The majority of bitches presented for fertility investigation are normal, healthy, fertile animals whose apparent infertility is related to a misunderstanding of the physiology of reproduction. Many bitches are mated at inappropriate times, and accurate monitoring of each bitch during each oestrous cycle enables the optimal time for mating or insemination to be detected.

Mating should be planned during the fertile or fertilisation period; these periods can be readily detected using measurement of plasma progesterone, assessment of vaginal cytology, or vaginal endoscopy. In most bitches it is sufficient to start monitoring from approximately 7 days after the onset of pro-oestrus. Following this strategy will result in a significant increase in pregnancy rate and litter size (England, 1992).

When it is necessary to use semen of a suboptimal quality, for example where there is male factor infertility, or when semen has been cryopreserved, it is essential that mating or insemination occurs during the fertilisation period.

REFERENCES AND FURTHER READING

England GCW (1991) ELISA determination of whole blood and plasma progestogen concentration in bitches. *Veterinary Record* **129**, 221–222

England GCW (1992) Vaginal cytology and cervicovaginal mucus arborisation in the breeding management of bitches. *Journal of Small Animal Practice* **33**, 577–582

Jeffcoate I A and Lindsay FEF (1989) Ovulation detection and timing of insemination based on hormone concentrations, vaginal cytology and the endoscopic appearance of the vagina of domestic bitches. *Journal of Reproduction and Fertility* Supplement **39**, 277–287

CHAPTER NINE

Unwanted Mating in the Bitch

Gary C.W. England

INTRODUCTION

Unwanted mating is a common clinical problem in veterinary practice. Its great frequency is probably due to the prolonged period of oestrus, during which time the bitch will accept mating and may actively seek a male dog. In many cases the owner may be uncertain whether mating has occurred, and careful inspection of the bitch, including collection of material for cytological examination, may be necessary to confirm their suspicions.

There are several options available to prevent the birth of pups, and these may be divided into those which prevent or interfere with implantation, those which alter the normal endocrine environment and induce resorption or abortion, and those which are directly embryotoxic.

The choice of the most suitable agent will depend upon the risk factor for pregnancy becoming established, the time interval between presumed mating and veterinary examination, and the likely adverse effects of the agents chosen.

REPRODUCTIVE PHYSIOLOGY

Pro-oestrus is characterised by increased plasma concentration of oestrogen which causes swelling of the vulva and the development of a serosanguinous vulval discharge. Oestrogens also induce the release of specific pheromones which are responsible for attracting male dogs. During pro-oestrus the bitch will not allow mating but may show increased receptivity to the male. This period lasts for approximately 7 days, although this may vary considerably. During pro-oestrus, oestrogen has a negative feedback effect upon the release of the pituitary gonadotropins; concentrations of follicle stimulating hormone (FSH) and luteinising hormone (LH) are reduced compared with late anoestrus. During oestrus the bitch demonstrates characteristic behaviour towards the male dog, including deviation of the tail and presentation of the vulva and perineum. The bitch will stand to be mated. This period lasts for approximately 7 days. The onset of oestrus is associated with a decline in the concentration of plasma oestrogen and at the same time the production of progesterone. The bitch is unusual in that progesterone is produced in low concentrations by luteinisation of the follicle prior to ovulation. It is this decline in the concentration of oestrogen and the increase in the concentration of progesterone which is responsible for stimulating a surge of both FSH and LH. Ovulation of primary oocytes occurs 2 days

after the LH surge, and oocytes are fertilisable from 2 to 5 days after ovulation. In laboratory dogs, the onset of oestrus often occurs simultaneously with the preovulatory surge in LH. Thus, peak fertility might be expected to be within the time period 11–14 days after the onset of pro-oestrus. However this is not always the case, and bitches may have fertile eggs present within their reproductive tracts as early as 4 days, or as late as 30 days, after the onset of pro-oestrus. This large variation is important because the possibility of pregnancy cannot be ruled out simply by estimating the time of mating in relation to the clinical and behavioural characteristics exhibited by the bitch. In addition, many owners do not know accurately when pro-oestrus began.

An important consideration when collecting a history is the time interval between the presumed mating and veterinary examination of the bitch, since this may influence the choice of any treatment administered.

EXAMINATION OF THE BITCH FOLLOWING PRESUMED UNWANTED MATING

While it is clear that the 'blind' treatment of all bitches presumed to have had an unwanted mating may, in certain circumstances, be appropriate, the potential adverse effect of any treatment should be considered. A more satisfactory approach is the careful examination of bitches and the application of treatment in appropriate cases.

Clinical evaluation of the bitch should involve: the collection of a vaginal smear to evaluate the stage of the oestrous cycle and to try to detect spermatozoa; the use of a modified vaginal smear technique to detect spermatozoa; and the measurement of plasma concentration of progesterone to establish accurately the stage of the oestrous cycle.

Vaginal cytology

Collection of exfoliative vaginal cells, and study of the epithelial cell morphology combined with an assessment of the numbers of white and red blood cells, may determine the stage of the oestrous cycle. These results should be used in combination with measurement of plasma concentration of progesterone (see below). Vaginal cells are most conveniently collected either via aspiration of the cranial vagina with a short bovine insemination pipette attached to a 5 ml syringe, or by rolling a moistened cotton swab against the vaginal wall. Once collected, cells are placed on to a glass microscope slide and stained using Diff–Quik® or a modified Wright–Giemsa stain.

In recently mated bitches, spermatozoa may be identified within the vaginal smear. However, there is a rapid reduction in the number of spermatozoa and they may not be identified if the interval from mating exceeds 24 hours.

Bitches that are found to be in cytological pro-oestrus (in these cases plasma progesterone concentrations are low) may not have been mated, since mating is usually refused at this time, and therefore do not warrant treatment. This is not always the case, and some early matings may result in a pregnancy if the spermatozoa are able to remain viable within the female reproductive tract until after ovulation. Assessment of the presence or absence of spermatozoa is essential in these cases.

Bitches that are found to be in cytological oestrus (in these cases plasma progesterone concentration is usually intermediate or high) may have been mated, and in most cases should receive treatment, although reference to the presence or absence of spermatozoa may influence whether treatment is instituted.

Bitches that are found to be in cytological metoestrus (dioestrus) (in these cases plasma progesterone concentration is high) may have been mated. These should be examined for the presence of spermatozoa; however, the most important factor is the time interval from mating to examination, since it is rare for matings occurring after the onset of cytological metoestrus (dioestrus) to be fertile.

Plasma progesterone measurement

Plasma concentrations of progesterone can be measured by radioimmunoassay, but this technique is time-consuming, expensive and frequently there is a delay in obtaining the results. Recently, several enzyme-linked immunosorbent assay (ELISA) techniques have become commercially available. These ELISA kits allow assessment of progesterone concentration either qualitatively or quantitatively within 45-60 minutes of sample collection.

In the bitch, plasma concentrations of progesterone are low during anoestrus and pro-oestrus. Concentrations increase when preovulatory follicular luteinisation occurs, and thereafter there is a rapid rise in progesterone concen-

tration following ovulation. Progesterone concentrations should be interpreted in the light of the clinical history and assessment of vaginal cytology.

Detection of spermatozoa within the vagina

The technique for studying vaginal cytology is unreliable for detecting spermatozoa if the interval between mating and veterinary examination exceeds 24 hours. After this time spermatozoa are only present in small numbers, and many of the spermatozoa will be degenerating and detectable only by the presence of the spermatozoal head.

Accurate detection of spermatozoa requires a modified technique. A saline-moistened swab should be placed into the vagina for 1 minute. The swab tip should be placed in a small test tube with 0.5 ml physiological saline, and allowed to stand for 10 minutes. The swab is then squeezed dry, and the test tube containing the saline is centrifuged at 2000 rpm for 10 minutes. Collection of the sediment and microscopic examination after staining with a modified Wright–Giemsa stain allows detection of spermatozoal heads. Using this technique spermatozoa are found in 100% of samples in which mating occurred within the previous 24 hours, and in 75% of samples in which mating occurred within the previous 48 hours.

TREATMENT OPTIONS

There are several treatment options, even when mating has occurred at a time likely to result in conception. If the bitch is not required for breeding the simplest option is ovariohysterectomy after the end of oestrus. The second option is to treat the bitch in an attempt to prevent implantation, while the third option is to wait until a positive diagnosis of pregnancy can be made before instituting therapy. The latter requires examination of the bitch (usually with diagnostic B-mode ultrasound) at approximately 28 days after mating. If a pregnancy is identified it may be terminated by inducing resorption or abortion after this time.

Treatment options can be considered with respect to the risk of conception (Table 9.1).

Spermatozoa present in vagina	Plasma progesterone concentration	Vaginal cytology examination	Risk of conception*
No	Low	Pro-oestrus	Low
No	Low	Oestrus	Low
No	Intermediate/high	Oestrus	Intermediate
No	High	Metoestrus	Low
Yes	Low	Pro-oestrus	Low
Yes	Low	Oestrus	Intermediate
Yes	Intermediate/high	Oestrus	High
Yes	High	Metoestrus	Low

Table 9.1: Risk of conception in bitches presumed to have been mated.
* The risk should be considered in relation to the time interval between presumed mating and veterinary examination. In low-risk cases, the animal may be examined 28 days after 'mating' for pregnancy diagnosis and, if positive, the pregnancy may be abolished at this time.

Prevention of implantation

Oestrogens

Oestrogens have been used for several years to prevent unwanted pregnancies in several species. It is thought that they act to alter the transport time of zygotes, and to impair implantation. It is interesting that early luteolysis has been noted in some pregnant bitches treated with oestrogen during oestrus, an effect which might be mediated either directly upon luteal progesterone production or by inhibition of LH which is luteotrophic.

In clinical practice in the UK, diethylstilboestrol was commonly used to prevent conception, although this regimen has been replaced by the use of oestradiol benzoate. In other countries, oestradiol cypionate and mestranol have been widely used. Silastic capsules containing oestradiol administered subcutaneously during midpregnancy will produce resorption or abortion, presumably by a luteolytic action.

Only oestradiol benzoate is licensed for the treatment of unwanted mating in the UK. This agent may be administered once at a relatively high dose within 4 days of mating, or at a low dose, using a repeated administration regimen, at 3 and 5 days (and possibly also 7 days) after mating. Both regimens appear to be efficacious; the low-dose regimen was advocated in an attempt to reduce the possibility of adverse effects.

Oestrogens may potentiate the stimulatory effects of progesterone on the uterus, producing cystic endometrial hyperplasia. Oestrogens also cause cervical relaxation, thus allowing vaginal bacteria to enter the uterus. These two events may result in the development of pyometra. Oestrogens also produce dose-related bone marrow suppression, and the toxic dose for an individual may lie within the therapeutic range. Other less severe effects include alopecia, skin hyperpigmentation and mammary gland and vulval enlargement.

There is some concern that the low-dose oestrogen regimen for the treatment of unwanted mating may result in oestrogen administration when plasma progesterone concentrations are elevated, therefore increasing the risk of cystic endometrial hyperplasia and pyometra. To date, no increase in the incidence of uterine disease has been demonstrated.

Tamoxifen

Tamoxifen is an anti-oestrogen which can be used to prevent or terminate pregnancy in the bitch, although the exact mechanism of action is unknown. It may interfere with zygote transport and/or implantation. Relatively high doses of the drug given twice daily orally during pro-oestrus, oestrus, or early dioestrus are efficacious. A high incidence of pathological changes of the bitch's reproductive tract are induced by tamoxifen, including ovarian cysts and endometritis.

Termination of pregnancy

Once pregnancy has become established it may be terminated either by altering the endocrine environment or by direct effects upon the embryo.

The bitch is dependent upon ovarian production of progesterone throughout gestation. Methods that produce premature luteolysis may therefore be used to terminate pregnancy. Since both LH and prolactin have luteotrophic actions, therapy may also be directed against these hormones to cause lysis of the corpora lutea and the termination of pregnancy.

Prostaglandins

When administered to the bitch, prostaglandins lyse the corpora lutea and reduce the plasma concentration of progesterone. The corpora lutea of the bitch are more resistant to prostaglandins than those of other species, and repeated therapy is necessary to achieve this effect. Prostaglandins also produce contraction of smooth muscle, having an ecbolic effect that may be part of the mechanism of inducing abortion. The actions on smooth muscle also account for the adverse effects of prostaglandins, including salivation, vomiting, pyrexia, hyperpnoea, ataxia and diarrhoea; high doses may be lethal.

Pharmacological doses of prostaglandin ($PGF-2\alpha$) can be used to produce luteal regression since the duration of treatment is more important than the dose. Repeated low doses of prostaglandin will significantly reduce plasma progesterone concentration and induce abortion, especially when given later than 25 days after the LH surge. Mature corpora lutea are more sensitive to the effects of prostaglandin than developing corpora lutea. Recent studies have, however, shown that daily treatment commencing 5 days after the onset of metoestrus (dioestrus) using high doses of prostaglandin may be efficacious, although adverse effects are common.

Cloprostenol can be used to produce abortion 25 days after the LH surge when given intravaginally as a 24-hour release plastic device. The slow-release formulation provides a long luteolytic effect and appears to reduce the incidence of adverse reactions.

A prostaglandin analogue (TPT) has also been shown to produce luteolysis and pregnancy termination. This compound is useful because only a single administration is required, but it has similar adverse effects to the natural prostaglandins and it is not commercially available.

Prolactin antagonists

Prolactin antagonists such as bromocriptine and cabergoline reduce plasma concentration of progesterone, especially when administered during the late luteal phase.

These agents are dopamine agonists which inhibit the release of prolactin from the anterior pituitary gland. Bromocriptine is the least specific agent and tends to produce the most adverse effects, especially vomiting. Bromocriptine is, however, the only product available in the UK, although it is not licensed for use in the dog. Cabergoline appears to be more specific than bromocriptine and produces fewer side effects. When administered during midpregnancy both agents produce a significant reduction in plasma progesterone concentration, resulting in resorption or abortion; earlier treatment is less efficacious.

Combination of prostaglandin and prolactin antagonists

The combination of the dopamine agonist cabergoline and the synthetic analogue of prostaglandin PGF-2α, cloprostenol, induces pregnancy termination from day 25 after the LH surge. Cabergoline can be administered orally daily, and cloprostenol subcutaneously every other day. This regimen reduces the adverse effects of prostaglandin therapy alone, and increases the efficacy of prolactin antagonists, which alone work best from 40 days after the LH surge. When bitches are treated for approximately 9 days, 100% will resorb, and there are generally no adverse effects. This regimen would appear to be promising, especially if cabergoline becomes available in the UK.

Progesterone antagonists

Mifepristone (RU486) is a progesterone and glucocorticoid receptor antagonist. Administration of this agent produces an antiprogestogenic effect. Following its administration progesterone concentrations are initially unaltered. When administered to pregnant bitches later than 30 days from the LH surge, fetal death occurs within 5 days of treatment. Earlier administration requires a longer treatment period. Pregnancy loss is characterised by resorption during early pregnancy or abortion during late pregnancy. Adverse effects have not been noted with this treatment. A similar progesterone antagonist (RU534) has recently been marketed for use in bitches in France.

Progesterone synthesis inhibitors

Epostane is a hydroxysteroid dehydrogenase isomerase enzyme inhibitor which prevents the conversion of pregnenolone to progesterone. Plasma progesterone concentrations therefore decrease, whilst concentrations of pregnenolone, which is biologically inactive, increase. Epostane does not have intrinsic oestrogenic, androgenic or progestogenic activity, and after use subsequent fertility is usually normal.

In the bitch a single subcutaneous injection of epostane at the onset of metoestrus (dioestrus) will prevent or terminate pregnancy, although injection site abscessation is common. High doses given orally for 7 days will successfully terminate pregnancy without apparent adverse effects. Epostane is not available in the UK.

GnRH agonists and antagonists

Continuous administration of gonadotropin releasing hormone (GnRH), or GnRH agonists causes a downregulation effect which may be used to withdraw gonadotropin support of the corpus luteum. This results in a decline in progesterone concentration and abortion or resorption.

Similarly, the daily administration of GnRH antagonists successfully suppresses luteal function. The GnRH antagonist, detirelix, has been administered daily to produce abortion or resorption depending upon the stage of pregnancy. Administration very early in the pregnancy is not efficacious even when the dose is increased. This reflects the relative independence of gonadotropin support during early pregnancy, and attempts to overcome this have been made by combining the GnRH antagonists with prostaglandin. These agents are thought to be synergistic, and may be useful for the termination of pregnancy as early as day 4 of metoestrus (dioestrus), although reported success rates are only 80%.

Corticosteroids

In many species glucocorticoid administration during pregnancy induces abortion. The mechanism requires the fetoplacental unit to produce oestrogen and prostaglandin when glucocorticoids are administered. Single doses of glucocorticoids are not efficacious in the bitch; however, dexamethasone administered twice daily for 10 days, commencing after 30 days from the LH surge, produces low progesterone concentrations and abortion. The mechanism of action is uncertain, however the repeated administration and high doses required make the method impractical and the risk of adverse effects must be carefully assessed before this regimen is contemplated.

Non-hormonal embryotoxic agents

Several novel embryotoxic agents have been evaluated in the bitch. These phenyltriazole isoindole and isoquinoline compounds can be administered orally or by injection. They are most effective when given around the time of implantation and often only a single administration is required. One agent, lotrifen, has a slow release from depot injection and may be efficacious when administered any time during the first 15 days after mating. Many of these agents are not available because of their toxicity which includes vomiting, diarrhoea and weight loss. Success rates have been shown to be up to 90%. However unsuccessful cases may end in the birth of stillborn pups or weak pups which rapidly die. In addition, a variety of adverse effects have been reported in bitches including pyrexia, lethargy, purulent meningitis and immunosuppression. These agents are therefore unacceptable in clinical practice.

CONCLUSION

It is important to remember that the majority of bitches presented because of presumed unwanted mating will probably not have been mated. Blanket treatment of all bitches at the time of veterinary examination may therefore be inappropriate. Careful examination of the history, combined with assessment of vaginal cytological findings and the measurement of plasma progesterone concentration, may detect those bitches in which immediate treatment is appropriate.

In certain instances it will be necessary to wait until a diagnosis of pregnancy can be made before instituting therapy, while in others ovariohysterectomy may be the treatment of choice. In those cases where it is necessary to terminate pregnancy, attention should be paid to the adverse effects of various drug regimens, as well as their efficacy. Abortion induction may be unacceptable for the owners of some bitches, and in these cases the induction of resorption may be necessary. At present the regimen that shows most promise is the combination of prolactin antagonists and prostaglandin, and although cabergoline is not yet available in the UK, it is likely that this situation will change in the near future.

FURTHER READING

Bowen RA, Olson PN, Behrendt MD, Wheeler SL, Husted PW and Nett TM (1985) Efficacy and toxicity of estrogens commonly used to terminate canine pregnancy. *Journal of the American Veterinary Medical Association* **186**, 783–788

Concannon PW, England GCW, Verstegen JP and Russell HA (1993) Fertility and infertility in dogs, cats and other carnivores. *Journal of Reproduction and Fertility* Supplement 47, R9–R11

Concannon PW, Morton DB and Weir BJ (1989) Dog and cat reproduction, contraception and artificial insemination. *Journal of Reproduction and Fertility* Supplement 39, R5–R6

Onclin K, Silva LDM and Verstegen JP (1995) Termination of unwanted pregnancy in dogs with the dopamine agonist, cabergoline, in combination with a synthetic analog of PGF2alpha, either cloprostenol or alphaprostol. *Theriogenology* **43**, 813–822

PART TWO

Common Endocrine Disorders

CHAPTER TEN

Canine Hyperadrenocorticism

Michael E. Herrtage

INTRODUCTION

Each adrenal gland is composed of a cortex and a medulla, which are embryologically and functionally separate endocrine glands. Only the cortex is essential for life. The most common disorders of the adrenal gland affect the adrenal cortex and cause either hyperadrenocorticism (Cushing's disease) or hypoadrenocorticism (Addison's disease). Conditions affecting the adrenal medulla are rare, the most common being a tumour (phaeochromocytoma). Hyperadrenocorticism is associated with excessive production or administration of glucocorticoids, and is one of the most commonly diagnosed endocrinopathies in the dog. Hyperadrenocorticism is rare in the cat and is described in Chapter 29.

PHYSIOLOGY OF THE ADRENAL CORTEX

The adrenal cortex (Figure 10.1) produces about 30 different hormones, many of which have little or no clinical significance. The hormones can be divided into three groups based on their predominant actions: mineralocorticoids, which are important in electrolyte and water homeostasis (see Chapter 11); glucocorticoids, which promote gluconeogenesis; and small quantities of sex hormones, particularly male hormones that have weak androgenic activity and are rarely significant clinically. The principal glucocorticoid, cortisol, is produced in the zona fasciculata and zona reticularis. Sex hormones are also produced in these two zones.

Regulation of glucocorticoid release

Glucocorticoid release is controlled almost entirely by adrenocorticotropic hormone (ACTH) secreted by the anterior pituitary, which in turn is regulated by corticotropin releasing hormone (CRH) from the hypothalamus (Figure 10.2). CRH is secreted by the neurons in the anterior portion of the paraventricular nuclei within the hypothalamus and is transported to the anterior pituitary by the portal circulation, where it stimulates ACTH release. There is probably an internal or 'short loop' negative feedback control by ACTH on CRH. ACTH secreted into the systemic circulation causes cortisol release, with concentrations rising almost immediately. Cortisol has direct negative feedback effects on the hypothalamus to decrease formation of CRH, and on the anterior pituitary

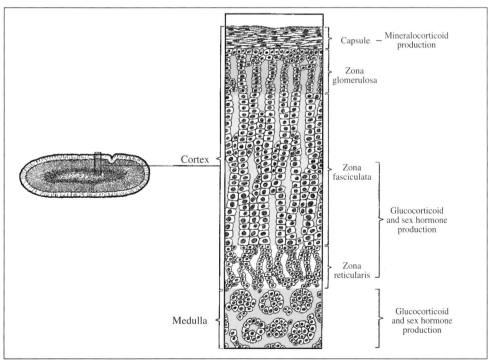

Figure 10.1: Anatomy of the normal adrenal gland.

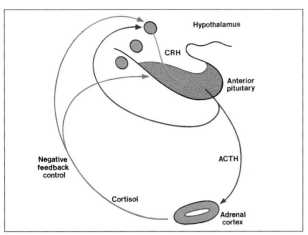

Figure 10.2: Regulation of glucocorticoid release. ACTH, adrenocorticotropic hormone; CRH, corticotropin releasing hormone.

gland to decrease the formation of ACTH. These feedback mechanisms help regulate the plasma concentration of cortisol.

Secretion of CRH and ACTH is normally episodic and pulsatile, which results in fluctuating cortisol levels during the day. Diurnal variation is superimposed on this type of release. It is usually stated that, in the dog, CRH, ACTH and thus cortisol levels, are highest in the early hours of the morning and that, in the cat, they are greatest in the evening. However, a true circadian rhythm of cortisol concentrations has been difficult to confirm in either dogs or cats (Kemppainen and Sartin, 1984; Kemppainen and Peterson, 1996). The episodic release of CRH and ACTH is perpetuated by the reciprocal effect of cortisol acting through negative feedback control. This reciprocal arrangement does not persist during periods of stress when both ACTH and cortisol are maintained at high levels, because the effects of stress tend to override the normal negative feedback control. Challenges to the immune system also activate the hypothalamic–pituitary–adrenal axis since cytokines, principally interleukin-1, stimulate the release of CRH from the hypothalamus.

Functions of glucocorticoids

Cortisol has diverse effects on the body. Its main effect is on the metabolism of carbohydrate, protein and fat, to promote gluconeogenesis.

Effect on carbohydrate metabolism

Cortisol stimulates gluconeogenesis in the liver by inducing the formation of hepatic gluconeogenic enzymes. One of the effects of increased gluconeogenesis is a marked increase in glycogen stores within the hepatocytes. Cortisol also causes a moderate decrease in the rate of glucose utilisation by cells everywhere in the body. Both the increased rate of gluconeogenesis and the moderate reduction in the rate of glucose utilisation by cells cause the blood glucose concentration to rise. The increase in blood glucose causes secondary hyper-insulinism that counters glucocorticoid activity. The net result in the normal animal is a balance between these opposing factors.

Effect on protein metabolism

Cortisol reduces protein stores in essentially all cells except those of the liver. This reduction is caused by decreased protein synthesis and increased catabolism. The catabolic actions of glucocorticoids on muscle result in muscle wasting and weakness. Cortisol depresses amino acid transport into muscle cells and probably into other extrahepatic cells. This effect, combined with increased catabolism, leads to a rise in blood amino acid concentrations. The increased plasma concentration of amino acids, plus the fact that cortisol enhances transport of amino acids into the hepatic cells could also account for enhanced utilisation of amino acids by the liver to cause such effects as:

* Increased conversion of amino acids to glucose (gluconeogenesis)
* Increased protein synthesis in the liver
* Increased formation of plasma proteins by the liver
* Increased deamination of amino acids by the liver.

Effects on fat metabolism

Cortisol increases lipolysis which results in the release of free fatty acids and glycerol from adipose tissue. Insulin counters this effect by inhibiting lipolysis and stimulating lipogenesis. Ketogenesis occurs if the effects of insulin are exceeded. Adipose tissue tends to be redistributed to the abdomen and back of the neck in dogs with excess levels of glucocorticoids.

Anti-inflammatory effects

Glucocorticoids modify the inflammatory process and the immune response by:

* Stabilising lysosomal membranes to reduce the release of proteolytic enzymes by damaged cells
* Decreasing capillary permeability, which prevents loss of plasma into the tissues and also reduces the migration of white cells into the inflamed area
* Depressing the ability of white blood cells to digest phagocytosed tissues, thus blocking further release of inflammatory materials
* Suppressing the immune system, especially the T cells. Glucocorticoids decrease the number of circulating lymphocytes and eosinophils. Cortisol in excess can decrease antibody production, but anamnestic antibody production, for example, after booster vaccination, is relatively resistant compared with initial responses
* Reducing fever
* Suppressing wound healing and scar formation.

The effects of glucocorticoids on different body systems and organ functions are summarised in Table 10.1.

AETIOLOGY

Hyperadrenocorticism can be spontaneous or iatrogenic. Spontaneously occurring hyperadrenocorticism may be associated with inappropriate secretion of ACTH by the

Liver
Increased gluconeogenesis
Increased glycogen stores
Induction of certain enzymes

Liver
Increased gluconeogenesis
Increased glycogen stores
Induction of certain enzymes

Muscle
Increased protein catabolism — muscle wasting and weakness

Bone
Osteoporosis associated with increased protein catabolism and negative calcium balance

Skin
Increased protein catabolism — thin skin, poor wound healing, and poor scar formation

Blood
Erythrocytosis
Decrease in circulating lymphocytes
Decrease in circulating eosinophils
Increase in circulating neutrophils

Kidney
Increased glomerular filtration rate or interference with antidiuretic hormone release or action (polyuria)
Increased calcium excretion

Immune system
Diminished inflammatory response
Reduced immune response

Adipose tissue
Increased lipolysis
Redistribution of fat deposits

Pituitary and hypothalamus
Suppression of adrenocorticotropic hormone and corticotropin releasing hormone secretion

Table 10.1: Effects of glucocorticoids on different body systems.

pituitary (pituitary-dependent hyperadrenocorticism) or with a primary adrenal disorder (adrenal-dependent hyperadrenocorticism) (Figure 10.3).

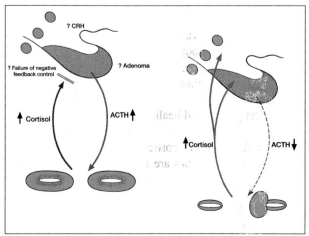

Figure 10.3: Pituitary–adrenal axis in (left) pituitary-dependent and (right) adrenal-dependent hyperadrenocorticism. ACTH, adrenocorticotropic hormone; CRH, corticotropin releasing hormone.

Pituitary-dependent hyperadrenocorticism

Pituitary-dependent hyperadrenocorticism accounts for over 80% of dogs with naturally occurring hyperadrenocorticism. Excessive ACTH secretion results in bilateral adrenocortical hyperplasia and excess cortisol secretion. There is a failure of the negative feedback mechanism of cortisol on ACTH. However, episodic secretion of ACTH results in fluctuating cortisol levels that may at times be within the normal range. The presence of excess cortisol secretion can be confirmed by urine cortisol excretion over a 24-hour period.

It is generally considered that more than 90% of dogs with pituitary-dependent hyperadrenocorticism have a pituitary tumour. Adenomas of the corticotrophs of the pars distalis and pars intermedia are the most common canine pituitary tumour. The pathological changes in pituitary-dependent hyperadrenocorticism include microadenomas, macroadenomas, and primary failure of the feedback response.

Microadenomas

Microadenomas are <10 mm in diameter. Although the reported incidence of corticotroph adenomas associated with pituitary-dependent hyperadrenocorticism varies, this is probably more to do with the fact that detection of small tumours requires careful microdissection, experience, and special stains. In one study using immunocytochemical staining, more than 80% of dogs with pituitary-dependent hyperadrenocorticism were positive for pituitary adenomas (Peterson *et al.*, 1982a).

Macroadenomas

Macroadenomas are >10 mm in diameter. Only about 10–15% of dogs have large corticotroph adenomas (Duesberg *et al.*, 1995). These may compress the remaining pituitary gland and extend dorsally into the hypothalamus (Figure 10.4). However, they are generally slow growing and may not produce neurological signs. Although reported, corticotroph adenocarcinomas are rare.

Primary failure of the feedback response

The defect responsible for pituitary-dependent

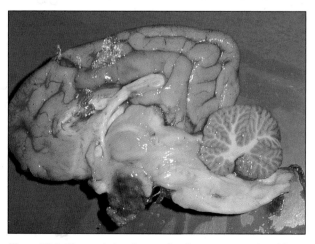

Figure 10.4: Chromophobe adenoma found at post-mortem in a 13 year old Golden Retriever which had been successfully treated for hyperadrenocorticism for 5 years. There were no neurological signs associated with this tumour.

hyperadrenocorticism not associated with pituitary neoplasia is unknown, but may be associated with excessive stimulation of pituitary corticotrophs because of a hypothalamic disorder. A primary failure of the negative feedback response by cortisol has been proposed. Others suspect an overproduction of CRH from the hypothalamus, which may cause diffuse hyperplasia of the corticotroph cells in the anterior pituitary.

From a clinical point of view, the precise pituitary pathology is not of great importance unless neurological signs are present at the time of diagnosis or become apparent during the initial treatment.

Adrenal-dependent hyperadrenocorticism
The remaining 15–20% of spontaneous cases of hyperadrenocorticism are caused by unilateral or, occasionally, bilateral adrenal tumours. Adrenocortical tumours may be benign or malignant, although it can be difficult histologically to distinguish between an adrenocortical adenoma and a carcinoma.

Adrenocortical adenomas
Adrenocortical adenomas are small, well circumscribed tumours that do not metastasise and are not locally invasive. Approximately 50% are partially calcified (Reusch and Feldman, 1991).

Adrenocortical carcinomas
Adrenocortical carcinomas are usually large, locally invasive, haemorrhagic and necrotic. Tumour calcification also occurs in 50% of dogs (Reusch and Feldman, 1991). Carcinomas, especially of the right adrenal, frequently invade the phrenicoabdominal vein and caudal vena cava and metastasise to the liver, lung and kidney (Figure 10.5).

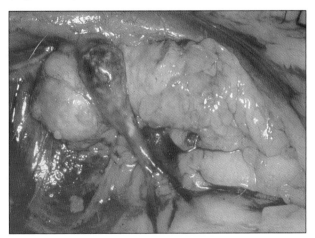

Figure 10.5: An adrenocortical carcinoma of the right adrenal gland invading the phrenicoabdominal vein. The caudal vena cava can be seen at the top of the photograph.

In dogs, adrenocortical adenomas and carcinomas occur with approximately equal frequency. The cortex contiguous to the tumour, and that of the contralateral gland, atrophy in the presence of functional adenomas and carcinomas (Figure 10.6). This is important if the tumour is to be removed surgically, as postoperatively the animal may not be able to secrete sufficient glucocorticoids and

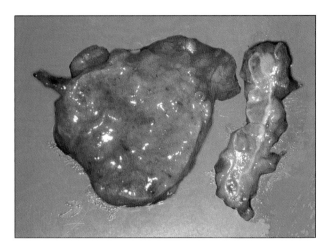

Figure 10.6: Cut surface of both adrenal glands from the case in Figure 10.5. Note the severe cortical atrophy (pale rim) in the contralateral adrenal.

may require temporary supplementation. Function of the zona glomerulosa should not be affected.

Other potential causes
Ectopic ACTH production has not been recognised in the dog, but in humans a number of tumours, for example oat cell carcinomas of the lung, are capable of synthesising and secreting excessive quantities of ACTH.

SIGNALMENT

Breed
Any breed can develop hyperadrenocorticism but Poodles, Dachshunds and small terriers, for example the Yorkshire Terrier, Jack Russell Terrier and Staffordshire Bull Terrier, seem at increased risk of developing pituitary-dependent hyperadrenocorticism. Adrenocortical tumours occur more frequently in larger breeds, with about 50% of affected dogs weighing more than 20 kg (Reusch and Feldman, 1991).

Age
Pituitary-dependent hyperadrenocorticism is usually a disease of the middle-aged to older dog, with an age range of 2 to 16 years and a median age of 7 to 9 years. Dogs with adrenal-dependent hyperadrenocorticism tend to be older, ranging between 6 and 16 years with a median age of 11 to 12 years (Meijer, 1980; Reusch and Feldman, 1991).

Sex
There is no significant difference in sex distribution in pituitary-dependent hyperadrenocorticism; however, female dogs are more likely to develop adrenal tumours than males. In one survey, between 60% and 65% of dogs with functional adrenocortical tumours were female (Reusch and Feldman, 1991).

CLINICAL FEATURES

Affected dogs usually develop a classic combination of

clinical signs associated with increased glucocorticoid levels, and these are listed in Table 10.2 in approximate decreasing order of frequency. Larger breeds of dogs and those with recent onset of disease, however, may not show all of these signs.

Polydipsia and polyuria
Polyphagia
Abdominal distension
Liver enlargement
Muscle wasting/weakness
Lethargy, poor exercise tolerance
Skin changes
Alopecia
Persistent anoestrus or testicular atrophy
Calcinosis cutis
Myotonia
Neurological signs

Table 10.2: Clinical signs of canine hyperadrenocorticism in approximate decreasing order of frequency.

Hyperadrenocorticism has an insidious onset and is slowly progressive over months or even years. Many owners consider the early signs as part of the normal ageing process of their dog. In a few cases, clinical signs may be intermittent, with periods of remission and relapse (Peterson *et al.*, 1982b) and in others there may be apparent rapid onset and progression of clinical signs.

Polydipsia and polyuria

Polydipsia, defined as water intake in excess of 100 ml/kg body weight per day, and polyuria, defined as urine production in excess of 50 ml/kg body weight per day, are seen in virtually all cases of hyperadrenocorticism. Excessive thirst, nocturia, incontinence and/or urination in the house are usually noted by owners.

Polydipsia occurs secondary to the polyuria, which is only partially responsive to water deprivation. The precise cause of the polyuria remains obscure, but may be due to increased glomerular filtration rate, inhibition of the release of antidiuretic hormone (ADH), inhibition of the action of ADH on the renal tubules, or possibly accelerated inactivation of ADH.

Polyphagia

Increased appetite is common but most owners often assess this as a sign of good health. A voracious appetite, scavenging, or stealing food, however, may give rise to concern, especially if the dog previously had a poor appetite.

Polyphagia is assumed to be a direct effect of glucocorticoids.

Abdominal distension

A 'pot-bellied' appearance is very common in hyperadrenocorticism but may be so insidious that owners fail to recognise its significance (Figure 10.7).

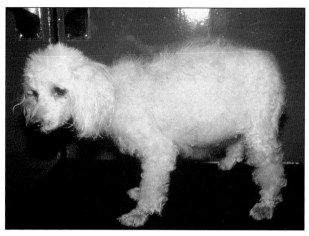

Figure 10.7: A 6 year old female Poodle with pituitary-dependent hyperadrenocorticism. Note the abdominal distension, muscle wasting, alopecia and thin skin.

The abdominal distension is associated with redistribution of fat to the abdomen, liver enlargement, and wasting and weakness of the abdominal muscles. The weakness of the abdominal muscles makes palpation of the pendulous abdomen easier and more rewarding.

Muscle wasting/weakness

The gradual onset of lethargy and poor exercise tolerance are usually considered by owners to be compatible with ageing. Only when muscle weakness is severe, as reflected by an inability to climb stairs or jump into the car, does the owner become concerned. Lethargy, excessive panting and poor exercise tolerance are probably an expression of muscle wasting and weakness. Apart from the development of a pendulous abdomen, decreased muscle mass may be noted around the limbs, over the spine or over the temporal region. Muscle weakness is the result of muscle wasting caused by protein catabolism.

Occasionally, dogs with hyperadrenocorticism develop myotonia, characterised by persistent active muscle contractions that continue after voluntary or involuntary stimuli. All limbs may be affected, but the signs are usually more severe in the hindlegs. Animals with myotonia walk with a stiff, stilted gait. The affected limbs are rigid and rapidly return to extension after being passively flexed. In some cases, passive flexion may be difficult or impossible to achieve because of the persistent muscle tone. Spinal reflexes are difficult to elicit because of the rigidity, but pain sensation is normal. The muscles are usually slightly hypertrophied rather than being atrophied and a myotonic dimple can be elicited by percussion of the affected muscle. Bizarre high frequency discharges are noted on electromyography (Duncan *et al.*, 1977). These bizarre myotonic and pseudomyotonic discharges may be found in some dogs with hyperadrenocorticism that do not show obvious clinical manifestations of myotonia.

Dermatological features

The skin, particularly over the ventral abdomen, becomes thin and inelastic. Elasticity can be assessed clinically by tenting the skin between the thumb and forefinger

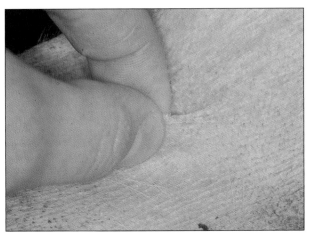

Figure 10.8: *Tenting of the skin of the ventral abdomen to assess elasticity.*

Figure 10.9: *In hyperadrenocorticism, the skin is thin and inelastic and remains tented. Note the abdominal veins are visible through the thin skin.*

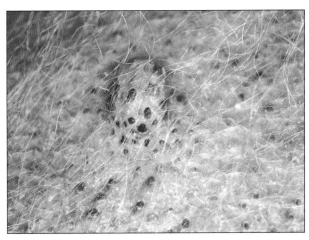

Figure 10.10: *Comedones are seen around a nipple. The skin is thin and abdominal veins are visible.*

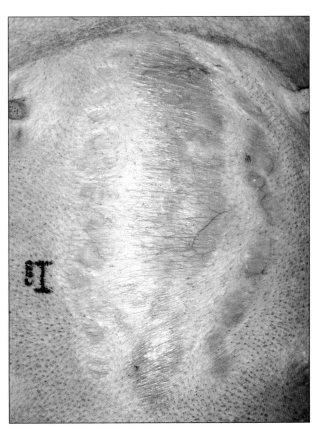

Figure 10.11: *Partial breakdown of an abdominal incision in a Boxer with hyperadrenocorticism. Note the striae to the right of the cranial end of the incision. The mark to the left represents 1 cm.*

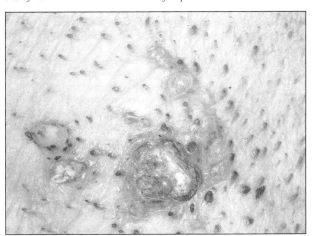

Figure 10.12: *Skin in the inguinal area of a Poodle with hyperadrenocorticism. Focal areas of calcinosis cutis can be seen eroding through the epidermis. Comedones are also present.*

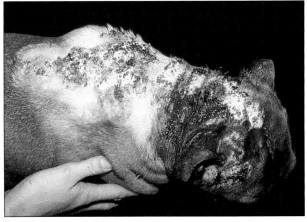

Figure 10.13: *Diffuse calcinosis cutis involving the dorsal aspect of the neck of a Staffordshire Bull Terrier. The skin is ulcerated and secondarily infected.*

(Figure 10.8). In the normal dog, the skin will flow back to a smooth contour but in hyperadrenocorticism it remains tented. Striae can form as a result of this inelasticity. The abdominal veins are prominent and easily visible through the thin skin (Figure 10.9). There is often excessive surface scale, and comedomes caused by follicular plugging are seen, especially around the nipples (Figure 10.10). Hyperpigmentation of the skin is rare in canine hyperadrenocorticism.

Protein catabolism causing atrophic collagen also

leads to excessive bruising following venepuncture or other minor trauma. Wound healing is extraordinarily slow, presumably because of inhibition of fibroblast proliferation and collagen synthesis. Healing wounds often undergo dehiscence and even old scars may start to break down (Figure 10.11).

Calcinosis cutis is a frequent finding in biopsy material from the skin, however clinical evidence of calcinosis cutis is less common. The gross appearance can vary but the sites of predilection are the neck, axilla, ventral abdomen, and inguinal areas (Figures 10.12 and 10.13). Calcinosis cutis usually appears as a firm, slightly elevated, white or cream plaque surrounded by a ring of ery-thema. Large plaques tend to crack, become secondarily infected, and develop a crust containing white powdery material. The exact pathogenesis is unknown but plasma calcium and phosphate levels are usually normal.

Thinning of the haircoat leading to bilaterally symmetrical alopecia is frequently seen with hyperadrenocorticism, and occurs because of the inhibitory effect of cortisol on the anagen or growth phase of the hair cycle. The remaining hair is dull and dry because it is in the telogen or resting phase of the hair cycle. The alopecia is non-pruritic and affects mainly the flanks, ventral abdomen and thorax, perineum and neck. The head, feet, and tail are usually the last areas to be affected (see Figure 10.7). The coat colour is often lighter than normal. Occasionally, affected dogs may not lose their haircoat, but retain it and become hypertrichotic.

When hair has been clipped in dogs with hyperadrenocorticism it will frequently fail to regrow or the regrowth will be poor or sparse.

Anoestrus/testicular atrophy

Entire bitches with hyperadrenocorticism usually cease to cycle. The length of anoestrus, often years, indicates the duration of the disease process. In the intact male both testes become soft and spongy.

Anoestrus and testicular atrophy occur due to the negative feedback effect of high levels of cortisol on the pituitary which also suppresses secretion of gonadotrophic hormones.

Neurological features

Although uncommon at the time of presentation, a few cases will develop neurological signs associated with a large functional pituitary tumour. The most common clinical signs are dullness, depression, loss of learned behaviour, anorexia, aimless wandering, head pressing, circling, ataxia, blindness, anisocoria and seizures. More often, however, neurological signs develop during initial treatment of pituitary-dependent hyperadrenocorticism with mitotane. This is thought to involve removal of the negative feedback of cortisol, which then allows some pituitary tumours to enlarge rapidly.

LABORATORY FINDINGS

The main haematological, biochemical, and urinalysis findings are listed in Table 10.3.

Haematology
Lymphopenia (<1.5 × 10^9/l)
Eosinopenia (<0.2 × 10^9/l)
Neutrophilia
Monocytosis
Erythrocytosis
Biochemistry
Increased alkaline phosphatase (ALP) (often markedly elevated)
Increased alanine aminotransferase (ALT)
High normal fasting blood glucose (rarely diabetic)
Decreased blood urea
Increased cholesterol (>8 mmol/l)
Lipaemia
Increased bile acids
Increased bromosulphothalein retention
Low thyroid hormone concentrations
Reduced response to thyroid stimulating hormone stimulation
Urinalysis
Urine specific gravity <1.015
Glycosuria (<10% of cases)
Urinary tract infection

Table 10.3: Laboratory findings in canine hyperadrenocorticism.

Haematology

The most consistent haematological finding is a stress leucogram with a relative and absolute lymphopenia (<1.5 × 10^9/l) and eosinopenia (<0.2 × 10^9/l). Lymphopenia is most likely the result of steroid lymphocytolysis and eosinopenia results from bone marrow sequestration of eosinophils (Feldman and Nelson, 1996). A mild to moderate neutrophilia and monocytosis may be found and is thought to result from decreased capillary margination and diapedesis associated with excess glucocorticoids.

The red cell count is usually normal, although mild polycythaemia may occasionally be noted. Platelet counts may also be elevated. These findings are thought to result from stimulatory effects of glucocorticoids on the bone marrow.

Biochemistry

Alkaline phosphatase
Serum alkaline phosphatase (ALP) concentrations are increased in over 90% of cases of canine hyperadrenocorticism. The increase in serum ALP concentration is commonly 5 to 40 times the upper end of the reference range, and is perhaps the most sensitive biochemical screening test for hyperadrenocorticism. The increased concentration occurs because glucocorticoids, both endogenous or exogenous, induce a specific hepatic isoenzyme of ALP, which is unique to the dog. However, a normal serum ALP concentration does not exclude a diagnosis of hyperadrenocorticism, and increases in serum

ALP do occur in a variety of other conditions.

It was believed that discrimination between the gluco-corticoid-induced and liver isoenzymes of alkaline phosphatase would provide a useful screening test for canine hyperadrenocorticism. The glucocorticoid-induced ALP is more heat stable than other serum isoenzymes of alkaline phosphatase in the dog. Initial studies were encouraging and suggested that it provided a more accurate assessment of elevated serum ALP activity (Oluju *et al.*, 1984). However, subsequent studies have concluded that while measurement of the glucocorticoid-induced iso-enzyme of ALP is quite sensitive, it is not specific for spontaneous canine hyper-adrenocorticism since the glucocorticoid-induced isoen-zyme can be increased in primary hepatopathies, diabetes mellitus, anticonvulsant therapy, and with exogenous gluco-corticoid therapy (Teske *et al.*, 1989).

Alanine aminotransferase

Alanine aminotransferase (ALT) is commonly elevated in hyperadrenocorticism, but the increase is usually only mild and is believed to result from liver damage caused by swollen hepatocytes due to glycogen accumulation.

Glucose

Blood glucose concentration is usually in the high–normal range. About 10% of cases develop overt diabetes mellitus which is caused by antagonism to the action of insulin by the gluconeogenic effects of excess glucocorticoids. Initially, serum insulin concentrations increase to maintain normoglycaemia, but the pancreatic islet cells may become exhausted and the β cells are destroyed giving rise to overt diabetes mellitus.

Urea and creatinine

Circulating urea concentration is usually normal to decreased due to the continual urinary loss associated with glucocorticoid-induced diuresis. Serum creatinine concen-tration also tends to be in the low–normal range.

Cholesterol and triglyceride

Serum cholesterol and triglyceride concentrations are usu-ally increased due to glucocorticoid stimulation of lipo-lysis. Cholesterol is usually >8 mmol/l but this is not a specific finding as cholesterol is also raised in hypo-thyroidism, diabetes mellitus, cholestatic liver disease, and protein-losing nephropathy, all of which may be differential diagnoses. Lipaemia is less common but is particularly important as it can interfere with the accurate assessment of a number of laboratory parameters.

Electrolytes

Serum sodium, potassium, calcium and phosphate con-centrations are usually in the normal range.

Bile acids

Serum bile acid concentration may be mildly to moder-ately elevated in some cases. Although the bromosulpho-thalein (BSP) retention test has been generally replaced by bile salt measurements as a test of liver function, BSP retention is also mildly or moderately elevated. Thus,

when abnormal results are obtained, these tests cannot be used to differentiate primary liver disorders.

Thyroid hormones

Basal total thyroxine (T4) and/or triiodothyronine (T3) concentrations are decreased in approximately 70% of dogs with hyperadrenocorticism (Peterson *et al.*, 1984). Serum free T4 concentrations are also depressed in many cases (Ferguson and Peterson, 1992). The effects of cortisol on thyroid function are complex but may involve pituitary suppression, altered hormone binding to plasma proteins and enhanced metabolism of thyroid hormones. The recent development of the endogenous canine thyrotropin (thyroid stimulating hormone, TSH) assay will allow further evaluation of the proposed mechanisms. The T4 response to exogenous TSH stimu-lation usually parallels a normal response, but both pre- and post-TSH concentrations are subnormal (Peterson *et al.*, 1984).

Urinalysis

Urine specific gravity

The specific gravity of urine of dogs with hyperadreno-corticism is usually <1.015 and is often hyposthenuric (<1.008) provided water has not been withheld. Dogs with hyperadrenocorticism can concentrate their urine if water is withheld, but their concentrating ability is usually reduced.

Urine glucose

Glucosuria is present in the 10% of cases with overt diabetes mellitus.

Urinary tract infection

Urine collected by cystocentesis should be analysed for infection, because urinary tract infections occur in about 50% of cases of hyperadrenocorticism. Urinary tract infection occurs because urine is retained in the over-distended bladder, as voiding is never complete due to muscle weakness. There is often little evidence of inflam-matory cells in the sediment of the urine due to the immunosuppressive action of excess glucocorticoids.

DIAGNOSTIC IMAGING

Advances in diagnostic imaging over the past decade have enabled clinicians to identify the cause of spontaneous hyperadrenocorticism and the extent of the underlying pathology, so that treatment can be directed more specifi-cally to the individual patient.

Radiography

Radiographic examination of the thorax and abdomen is advisable in all cases of suspected or proven hyperadreno-corticism. Although positive diagnostic information is only obtained in the small number of cases in which adrenal enlargement or mineralisation can be detected, the number and frequency of radiological changes consistent with hyperadrenocorticism provide a useful aid to diagnosis. In addition, survey radiographs may reveal significant intercurrent disease, which might alter the prognosis. The radiological signs of hyperadrenocorticism have been reviewed (Huntley *et al.*, 1982) and the common changes are listed in Table 10.4.

Liver enlargement

Hepatomegaly is the most consistent radiographic finding in hyperadrenocorticism. There is good radiographic contrast to permit easy identification of the abdominal structures because of the large deposits of intra-abdominal fat. Hepatomegaly may be mild to severe and the ventral lobe borders vary between distinctly rounded and sharply wedge-shaped. The 'pot-bellied' appearance is usually very obvious on the recumbent lateral projection (Figure 10.14).

Abdominal radiographs
Liver enlargement
Good radiographic contrast
'Pot-bellied' appearance
Calcinosis cutis/soft tissue mineralisation
Distended bladder
Cystic calculi
Adrenal enlargement/mineralisation
Osteoporosis

Thoracic radiographs
Tracheal and bronchial wall mineralisation
Pulmonary metastasis from adrenocortical carcinoma
Osteoporosis
Congestive heart failure (rare)
Pulmonary thromboembolism (rare)

Table 10.4: Radiological signs compatible with hyperadrenocorticism.

Adrenal enlargement/mineralisation

Normal adrenal glands are not visible on abdominal radiographs. Although adrenomegaly is the least common finding on abdominal radiographs, gross enlargement is suggestive, though not diagnostic, of an adrenocortical carcinoma. Unilateral mineralisation in the region of an adrenal gland also suggests the possibility of an adrenal tumour, although the presence of mineralisation cannot be used to distinguish benign from malignant tumours since both adrenocortical adenomas and adrenocortical carcinomas can become calcified.

Calcinosis cutis and soft tissue mineralisation

Calcinosis cutis tends to have a nodular mineralisation pattern, whereas calcification in the fascial planes, for example, just dorsal to the thoracolumbar spine, tends to be linear (see Figure 10.14). Mineralisation may also be seen in the renal pelvis, liver, gastric mucosa and abdominal aorta.

Urinary bladder

A grossly distended urinary bladder may be seen radiographically, even when the animal has been allowed to urinate before the radiographic examination. Cystic calculi may also be present and are usually associated with urinary tract infection.

Osteoporosis

Objective evaluation of skeletal demineralisation is notoriously difficult. However, occasionally the impression of osteoporosis is gained from a distinct reduction in radiographic density of the lumbar vertebral bodies relative to the vertebral end plates (see Figure 10.14).

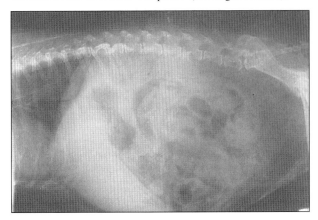

Figure 10.14: Abdominal radiograph of a Cairn Terrier with pituitary-dependent hyperadrenocorticism. The radiographic signs include hepatomegaly, 'pot-bellied' appearance, calcinosis cutis, dystrophic calcification in the soft tissues along the spine, enlarged bladder, and osteoporosis.

Tracheal and bronchial wall mineralisation

This is frequently seen radiographically in cases of hyperadrenocorticism. Calcification of these structures, however, can be seen in normally ageing animals and is not considered highly significant (Owens and Drucker, 1977; Huntley *et al.*, 1982).

The thoracic radiographs should also be examined for evidence of lung metastasis from an adrenocortical carcinoma, congestive heart failure, osteoporosis of the thoracic spine and pulmonary thromboembolism. The last is a rare complication of hyperadrenocorticism and may be suspected when the radiographic signs include pleural effusion, increased diameter and blunting of the pulmonary arteries, decreased vascularity of the affected lobes, and overperfusion of the unobstructed pulmonary vasculature (Fluckiger and Gomez, 1984; LaRue and Murtaugh, 1990). However in some cases of pulmonary thrombo-embolism, the radiographs may reveal no abnormalities.

Skull

Plain radiographs of the skull are usually unrewarding. Cavernous sinus venography, however, can be used to identify large pituitary tumours (Lee and Griffiths, 1972).

Abdominal ultrasonography

With improved ultrasound equipment, it is now possible for an experienced ultrasonographer to image the normal adrenal glands of most dogs. Large, obese and

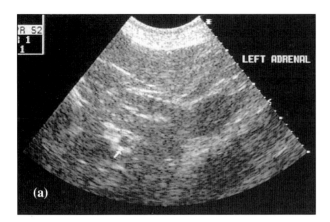

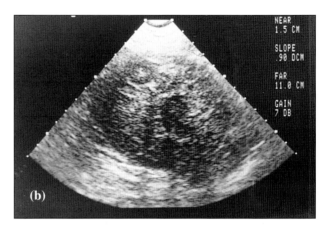

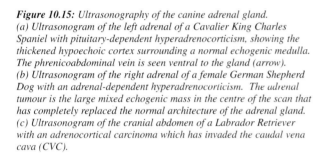

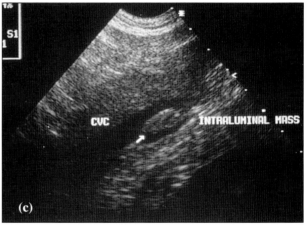

Figure 10.15: *Ultrasonography of the canine adrenal gland. (a) Ultrasonogram of the left adrenal of a Cavalier King Charles Spaniel with pituitary-dependent hyperadrenocorticism, showing the thickened hypoechoic cortex surrounding a normal echogenic medulla. The phrenicoabdominal vein is seen ventral to the gland (arrow). (b) Ultrasonogram of the right adrenal of a female German Shepherd Dog with an adrenal-dependent hyperadrenocorticism. The adrenal tumour is the large mixed echogenic mass in the centre of the scan that has completely replaced the normal architecture of the adrenal gland. (c) Ultrasonogram of the cranial abdomen of a Labrador Retriever with an adrenocortical carcinoma which has invaded the caudal vena cava (CVC).*

deep-chested dogs still provide the most challenge. The best images of the adrenals are obtained by scanning from the right and left lateral intercostal and abdominal approaches. The right adrenal gland is more difficult to image than the left. It is located craniomedial to the right kidney, lying between the cranial pole of the kidney and caudal vena cava. The left adrenal gland is more variable in location. It may be found anywhere from craniomedial to the left kidney to a more midline position near the aorta adjacent to the first or second lumbar vertebra. The left adrenal gland is ventrolateral to the aorta between the origin of the cranial mesenteric artery and the left renal artery.

The normal adrenal gland is somewhat flattened, bilobed, and hypoechoic compared with the surrounding tissues. The cranial lobe is larger, with a spatulate shape, and the caudal lobe tapers distally. The mid-region of the adrenal is narrowed and frequently has a groove in which the phrenicoabdominal vein lies. The medulla of the normal adrenal is slightly hyperechoic compared with the cortex. The maximum dimensions (length × thickness) of normal canine adrenal glands are usually in the range 12–33 mm × 3–7 mm. There is poor correlation between these dimensions and body weight (Douglass *et al.*, 1997).

The challenge for the ultrasonographer is to consistently distinguish between normal, hyperplastic and neoplastic glands. Although the adrenal glands of dogs with pituitary-dependent hyperadrenocorticism have been characterised as being symmetrically enlarged and of normal conformation, the diagnosis of adrenal hyperplasia is a somewhat subjective evaluation. The measurement of the

thickness (ventrodorsal dimension) of the adrenal gland is considered more sensitive than the either the length or width of the gland. The hyperplastic adrenal is larger and much easier to image than a normal one, but has a normal, homogeneous hypoechoic pattern (Figure 10.15a). A thickness of >7.5 mm for the left adrenal gland is considered to provide the best sensitivity and specificity as a diagnostic test for pituitary-dependent hyperadrenocorticism (Bartez *et al.*, 1995).

Abdominal ultrasonography can also detect large adrenocortical tumours (Kantrowitz *et al.*, 1986). Adrenal masses are diagnosed by the location of the mass and clinical signs exhibited by the animal (Figure 10.15b). There is a propensity for adrenal tumours to invade nearby vessels and surrounding tissues, therefore a thorough ultrasonographic examination of adjacent vessels and tissues should be performed (Figure 10.15c). Mineralisation is frequently associated with benign and malignant adrenocortical tumours in the dog, and acoustic shadowing may aid in localising the adrenal tumour. If an adrenal mass is identified, the liver should also be examined ultrasonographically for evidence of hepatic metastases.

Other imaging techniques

Computerised tomography (CT) and magnetic resonance imaging (MRI) have proved useful in the diagnosis of adrenal tumours, adrenal hyperplasia, and large pituitary tumours but both techniques are expensive and not widely available (Voorhout *et al.*, 1988; Bertoy *et al.*, 1995; Duesberg *et al.*, 1995). In a study comparing abdominal survey radiography with CT for the detection of adreno-cortical tumours, CT accurately localised all tumours whereas abdominal radiography only accurately localised 55% of the cases (Voorhout *et al.*, 1990). This was due to the fact that tumours <20 mm in diameter could not be seen on abdominal radiographs. CT can also identify invasion of the caudal vena cava by the tumour, and adhesions between the adrenal gland and the caudal vena cava.

Although no comparative studies have been carried out in dogs, MRI has been found to be superior to CT in detecting ACTH-secreting tumours of the pituitary gland in humans. MRI is extremely sensitive and can detect pituitary tumours as small as 3 mm at their greatest height (Bertoy *et al.*, 1995). Large pituitary tumours (up to 12 mm in diameter) have been shown to be present without causing neurological signs, whereas in another study pituitary masses ranging in size from 8–24 mm were associated with neurological signs (Duesberg *et al.*, 1995). In those cases with neurological signs, MRI or CT examination of the brain is essential for accurately planning therapy if pituitary irradiation is to be considered.

Gamma camera imaging of the adrenal glands has also been reported (Mulnix *et al.*, 1976).

CONFIRMATORY DIAGNOSTIC TESTS

A presumptive diagnosis of hyperadrenocorticism can be made from clinical signs, physical examination, routine laboratory tests, and diagnostic imaging findings, but the diagnosis must be confirmed by hormonal assay. A single resting or basal plasma or serum cortisol determination is of very limited diagnostic value because of the overlap in cortisol concentrations between healthy and disease states. Plasma or serum cortisol values are only useful after dynamic manipulation with ACTH or dexamethasone. The most commonly used screening tests are the ACTH stimulation test or the low-dose dexamethasone suppression test, however, the urinary corticoid:creatinine ratio has also proved a useful screening test. None of these tests is perfect and all are capable of giving false negative and false positive test results. If a dog with clinical signs compatible with hyperadrenocorticism produces a negative result with one screening test, an alternative screening test should be used. False positive results can be obtained in dogs suffering from non-adrenal disease (Kaplan *et al.*, 1995). Thus, a definitive diagnosis of hyperadrenocorticism should never be made purely on the basis of results of one or more of these screening tests, especially in dogs without classic signs of hyperadrenocorticism or in dogs with known non-adrenal disease.

The protocols for these tests are given in Table 10.5. The relative merits of each test and interpretation are discussed below. The author's preference is to use the ACTH stimulation test as the first screening test and the low-dose dexamethasone suppression test if the ACTH stimulation test gives a normal result in a dog with clinical signs suspicious of hyperadrenocorticism.

ACTH stimulation test

Advantages
The ACTH stimulation test is the best screening test for distinguishing spontaneous from iatrogenic hyperadrenocorticism. In spontaneous hyperadrenocorticism, the ACTH stimulation test reliably identifies more than 50% of dogs with adrenal-dependent hyperadrenocorticism,

---

The ACTH stimulation test
1. Collect 3 ml plasma or serum sample for basal cortisol concentration.*
2. Inject 0.25 mg of synthetic ACTH intravenously or intramuscularly to dogs >5 kg. Use only 0.125 mg in dogs <5 kg.
3. Collect a second sample for cortisol concentration 30–60 minutes after intravenous administration of ACTH. Some authors recommend that samples are collected 60–90 minutes after intramuscular administration.

The recent administration of glucocorticoids such as hydrocortisone, prednisolone, or prednisone may result in elevated cortisol concentrations due to cross-reactivity in many cortisol assays. For this reason glucocorticoids should be withheld for at least 24 hours before testing. There is no cross-reactivity with dexamethasone, but dexamethasone will suppress cortisol concentrations in patients with an intact hypothalamic–pituitary–adrenal axis.

The low-dose dexamethasone screening test
1. Collect 3 ml plasma or serum sample for cortisol determination
2. Inject 0.01 mg/kg (some authors prefer 0.015 mg/kg) of dexamethasone intravenously
3. Collect a second sample for cortisol concentration 3–4 hours later and a third sample 8 hours after dexamethasone administration.

The urine corticoid:creatinine ratio
Urine (5 ml) is collected in the morning for cortisol and creatinine measurements. It is preferable for the dog to be at home for this test so that it is minimally stressed. The urine corticoid:creatinine ratio is determined by dividing the urine cortisol concentration (in μmol/l) by the urine creatinine concentration (in μmol/l).

Table 10.5: Protocols for screening tests for hyperadrenocorticism.

and about 85% of dogs with pituitary-dependent hyperadrenocorticism.

It is a simple and quick test to perform and documents excessive production of glucocorticoids by the adrenal cortex in cases of hyperadrenocorticism. The information gained is also useful in providing baseline information for monitoring mitotane therapy, although different criteria are used to interpret cortisol results during treatment.

Disadvantages

The ACTH stimulation test does not reliably differentiate adrenal-dependent from pituitary-dependent hyperadrenocorticism. A diagnosis of hyperadrenocorticism should not be excluded on the basis of a normal ACTH response if the clinical signs are compatible with the disease. Occasionally, an animal under chronic stress may develop some degree of adrenal hyperplasia, which produces an abnormal ACTH response. This may be seen, for example, with diabetes mellitus or pyometra, and a normal cortisol response to ACTH stimulation will be obtained after treatment of the underlying disease in these cases.

Interpretation

It is essential to use absolute values for pre- and post-ACTH plasma cortisol concentrations rather than a ratio or percentage increase in post-ACTH cortisol concentration over the basal concentration. In normal dogs, pre-ACTH cortisol concentrations are usually between 20 and 250 nmol/l with post ACTH cortisol concentrations between 200 and 450 nmol/l. Regardless of the pre-ACTH cortisol value, a diagnosis of hyperadrenocorticism can be confirmed by demonstrating a post-ACTH cortisol concentration >600 nmol/l in dogs with compatible clinical signs (Figure 10.16).

Low-dose dexamethasone suppression test

Advantages

The low-dose dexamethasone suppression test is more reliable than the ACTH stimulation test in confirming hyperadrenocorticism, as the results are diagnostic in all adrenal-dependent cases and in 90–95% of dogs with pituitary-dependent hyperadrenocorticism.

Disadvantages

The low-dose dexamethasone suppression test is not suitable for the detection of iatrogenic hyperadrenocorticism. The test is also affected by more variables than the ACTH stimulation test, takes 8 hours to complete, and does not provide pre-treatment information that may used in monitoring the effects of mitotane therapy. The low-dose dexamethasone suppression test does not reliably differentiate pituitary-dependent from adrenal-dependent hyperadrenocorticism.

Interpretation

Interpretation of the results of a low-dose dexamethasone suppression test must be based on the laboratory's normal range for the dose and preparation of dexamethasone administered. If the dose of dexamethasone fails to suppress circulating cortisol concentrations adequately in

a dog with compatible clinical signs, a diagnosis of hyperadrenocorticism is confirmed. While basal and 8-hour post-dexamethasone samples are most important for interpretation of the test (Figure 10.17), one or more samples taken at intermediate times, for example, 2, 4 or 6 hours, during the test period may also prove helpful. If a plasma cortisol concentration determined 2–6 hours after dexamethasone injection is suppressed normally or near-normally (to <40 nmol/l), while the 8-hour sample shows escape from cortisol suppression, then a diagnosis of pituitary-dependent hyperadrenocorticism is indicated (Peterson, 1984).

Urinary corticoid:creatinine ratio

Evaluation of urinary corticoid:creatinine ratio rather than the more laborious 24-hour urinary corticoid excretion has

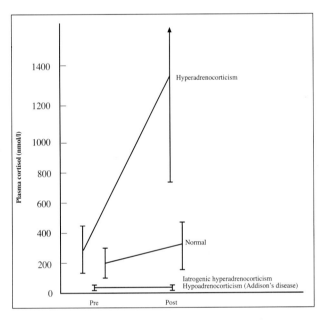

Figure 10.16: Adrenocorticotropic hormone (ACTH) stimulation test. Interpretation of plasma cortisol concentrations determined before and after administration of synthetic ACTH.

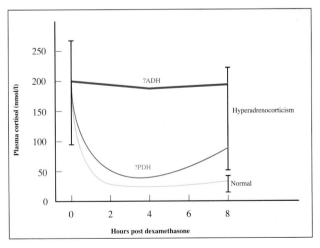

Figure 10.17: Low-dose dexamethasone suppression test. Interpretation of plasma cortisol concentrations determined during low-dose dexamethasone screening. ?ADH represents the type of response seen in cases of adrenal-dependent hyperadrenocorticism. ?PDH represents a possible response in pituitary-dependent cases.

been shown to be a simple and valuable screening test (Rijnberk *et al.*, 1988).

Cortisol and its metabolites are excreted in urine. By measuring urine cortisol in the morning sample, the concentration will reflect cortisol release over a period of several hours, thereby adjusting for fluctuations in plasma cortisol concentrations. The concentration of cortisol in urine increases with increased plasma concentrations. Relating the urine cortisol concentration to urine creatinine concentration provides a correction for any differences in urine concentration.

Urine is collected in the morning for cortisol and creatinine estimations. It is preferable for the dog to be at home for this test so that the dog is subjected to as little stress as possible, otherwise abnormal cortisol concentrations will be found in the urine. The urine corticoid:creatinine ratio is determined by dividing the urine cortisol concentration (in μmol/l) by the urine creatinine concentration (in μmol/l).

Interpretation

The reference ratio for healthy dogs is <10 × 10⁻⁶ (Stolp *et al.*, 1983). The urine cortisol:creatinine ratio is increased above the normal (>10 × 10⁻⁶) in dogs with hyperadrenocorticism. However, the ratio is also increased in many dogs with non-adrenal illness (Smiley and Peterson, 1993). Therefore, while this simple test appears highly sensitive in detecting hyperadrenocorticism in dogs, it is not specific. Values within the reference range make a diagnosis of hyperadrenocorticism highly unlikely, but high values may be associated with other non-adrenal illnesses. The urine cortisol:creatinine ratio does not reliably differentiate pituitary-dependent from adrenal-dependent hyperadrenocorticism, although ratios above 100 × 10⁻⁶ are more commonly associated with pituitary-dependent hyperadrenocorticism (Galac *et al.*, 1997). The test is of little value in monitoring the response to mitotane therapy in dogs with hyperadrenocorticism (Angles *et al.*, 1997; Guptill *et al.*, 1997).

DISCRIMINATORY DIAGNOSTIC TESTS

The ability to differentiate between pituitary-dependent and adrenal-dependent hyperadrenocorticism can have important implications in providing the most effective method of management for the disease. An accurate test is therefore required to differentiate pituitary from adrenal causes of hyperadrenocorticism. The high-dose dexamethasone suppression test was the most commonly used test for differentiating the cause of hyperadrenocorticism, but its accuracy has recently been brought into question. Canine ACTH assays are now readily available, and the determination of the plasma ACTH concentration has been shown to provide reliable discrimination between pituitary and adrenal causes of hyperadrenocorticism. Diagnostic imaging techniques, particularly abdominal ultrasonography, have also proved sensitive in distinguishing dogs with pituitary-dependent hyperadrenocorticism from dogs with adrenocortical tumours.

The high-dose dexamethasone suppression test
1. Collect 3 ml serum or plasma sample for cortisol determination.
2. Inject 0.1 mg/kg (although some authors recommend 1.0 mg/kg) of dexamethasone intravenously.
3. Collect two post-dexamethasone samples, one at 3–4 hours and a second at 8 hours after the dexamethasone.

Plasma endogenous adrenocorticotropic hormone (ACTH) concentration
1. Blood (5 ml) is collected into a cooled plastic EDTA tube and centrifuged at 4°C immediately.
2. The plasma should then be harvested and stored frozen (at less than -20°C) in a plastic tube.
3. Samples must be transported to the laboratory frozen and must be kept frozen until assayed.

- Stringent and meticulous sample handling is crucial since hormone activity in the plasma will reduce rapidly resulting in falsely low values and incorrect interpretation.
- The endogenous ACTH assay must be validated for use in dogs, otherwise the test may provide spurious results that could be misleading.

Table 10.6: *Protocols for endocrine tests to differentiate the cause of hyperadrenocorticism.*

Recognition of metastatic lesions with radiography and/or ultrasonography, however, is the only method that can distinguish dogs with adenomas from dogs with carcinomas (Reusch and Feldman, 1991).

The protocols for the endocrine tests that can be used to differentiate pituitary-dependent from adrenal-dependent hyperadrenocorticism are given in Table 10.6.

High-dose dexamethasone suppression test

This test is indicated in those cases where the diagnosis of hyperadrenocorticism has been established by a screening test, but the differentiation of adrenal-dependent and pituitary-dependent hyperadrenocorticism has not been determined. The high dose of dexamethasone inhibits pituitary ACTH secretion through negative feedback in pituitary-dependent hyperadrenocorticism, thus suppressing cortisol concentrations. Adrenocortical tumours are autonomous and thus cortisol is not suppressed. However, it has been shown that approximately 20–30% of pituitary-dependent cases will not show suppression with this test. The high-dose dexamethasone suppression test does not differentiate adrenocortical adenomas from adrenocortical carcinomas.

Plasma endogenous ACTH concentration

Stringent and meticulous sample handling is crucial since ACTH activity in the plasma will reduce rapidly resulting in falsely low values and incorrect interpretation. The endogenous ACTH assay used must be validated for use in dogs.

Measurement of basal endogenous ACTH concentrations is of no value in the diagnosis of hyperadrenocorticism because of the episodic secretion of ACTH in the normal dog and the overlapping values with those dogs with hyperadrenocorticism.

Interpretation

Endogenous ACTH concentrations in normal dogs range from 20 to 80 pg/ml. Dogs with adrenal tumours have very low endogenous ACTH concentrations (<10 pg/ml) whereas cases with pituitary-dependent hyperadrenocorticism tend to have high–normal to high concentrations (>45 pg/ml).

Diagnostic imaging

Abdominal radiography, abdominal ultrasonography, and abdominal and cranial CT/MRI can be used to differentiate between pituitary-dependent hyperadrenocorticism and adrenal-dependent hyperadrenocorticism. Diagnostic imaging can also be used to distinguish between benign and malignant tumours of the adrenal cortex.

TREATMENT OF PITUITARY-DEPENDENT HYPERADRENOCORTICISM

Mitotane therapy

Mitotane (op'-DDD) is the treatment of choice for pituitary-dependent hyperadrenocorticism. During its evaluation as an insecticide, mitotane was discovered to have adrenocorticolytic effects. It selectively destroys the zona fasciculata and zona reticularis while tending to preserve the zona glomerulosa.

Pre-treatment assessment

Mitotane therapy should only be considered once the diagnosis of hyperadrenocorticism has been confirmed. Because of its powerful effects, it should never be used empirically. Before treatment is instigated, the dog's daily water consumption should be measured over at least two consecutive 24-hour periods. If the water intake and appetite are not increased then baseline lymphocyte counts and cortisol concentrations, both before and after ACTH stimulation, are required in order that the effects of treatment can be monitored.

Initial treatment

The author prefers to have his patients hospitalised for the initial course of treatment, although many clinicians have dogs treated by their owners at home, with the owners doing the necessary monitoring.

Mitotane is given orally at a dosage of 50 mg/kg/day. It should be administered with food, since it is a fat-soluble drug and its absorption is poor when administered orally to fasted animals (Watson *et al.*, 1987). Daily mitotane therapy should be continued until any of the following changes are noted:

- Water intake of a polydipsic dog drops to below 60 ml/kg/day

- The dog takes longer to consume its meal than before treatment or stops eating completely
- The dog develops vomiting or has diarrhoea
- The dog becomes listless and depressed.

The initial mitotane course is then stopped and the dog put on maintenance therapy. The importance of close monitoring of the patient during this period cannot be overemphasised.

Mitotane therapy is comparatively safe and adverse effects which occur most frequently, for example, anorexia, vomiting or diarrhoea, are rarely serious provided they are noticed early so that mitotane therapy can be withheld. Some of the problems that can be encountered during treatment are summarised in Table 10.7, together with their suggested management.

Some authors advocate the administration of glucocorticoids during the induction treatment to prevent signs of hypocortisolaemia. However, there is no evidence that this reduces the incidence of adverse effects and it makes interpretation of subsequent ACTH stimulation tests difficult due to the cross-reactivity of prednisolone in most cortisol assays (Dunn *et al.*, 1995). Therefore concomitant glucocorticoid treatment is not advised routinely, although if the dog is being treated at home, the owner should be given a small supply of prednisolone tablets to be used in an emergency.

Rarely, dogs will develop neurological signs during the induction course of treatment with mitotane. These signs are thought to be associated with a rapid expansion in the size of a pituitary macroadenoma when the circulating cortisol concentrations fall, with subsequent removal of negative feedback inhibition. Clinical signs can include ataxia, incoordination, head tilt, circling, blindness and seizures. Most of these cases will respond favourably to treatment with glucocorticoids. If the glucocorticoid therapy is slowly withdrawn over several weeks, the brain can often adapt to the enlargement of the pituitary tumour.

The majority of dogs with pituitary-dependent hyperadrenocorticism require between 6 and 14 days treatment with an average of 10 days before water consumption reduces to below 60 ml/kg/day. If the dog is not polydipsic or polyphagic then treatment should continue until the lymphocyte count is above 1.0×10^9 cells/l or until the serum cortisol concentrations both before and after ACTH stimulation are below 120 nmol/l. A few dogs respond in 2 to 3 days, but, rarely, others require more than 60 consecutive days of treatment. It is important to emphasise that each dog must be treated as an individual if the therapy is to be successful, and that an ACTH stimulation test should be performed to check that the induction course of therapy has adequately suppressed adrenal function before maintenance therapy is introduced. If serum cortisol concentrations are undetectable and do not respond to ACTH stimulation, then the introduction of maintenance therapy should be delayed until the cortisol concentrations are between 20 and 120 nmol/l after ACTH stimulation.

Maintenance therapy

Having produced sufficient adrenocortical damage with

Problem	Management
Vomiting or anorexia within the first few days of treatment (gastric irritation)	Discontinue mitotane and reassess patient. Divide dose and give two to four times per day.
Profound weakness, depression and anorexia usually around the fourth or fifth day of treatment	Discontinue mitotane and reassess patient. Check circulating sodium and potassium concentrations and institute prednisolone (0.2 mg/kg/day) Reassess ACTH stimulation test. Start maintenance therapy with mitotane
Acute onset of neurological signs	Reassess patient Continue mitotane unless the dog is anorexic, vomiting or depressed. Give prednisolone 2.0 mg/kg/day or dexamethasone 0.1 mg.kg/day, and decrease dose slowly once neurological signs have resolved
Failure to resume normal water intake	Recheck urinalysis and blood urea. Reassess ACTH stimulation test. Increase mitotane by 50% if post-ACTH cortisol level is >200 nmol/l
Failure to regrow hair	Reassess ACTH stimulation test. Increase mitotane by 50% if post-ACTH cortisol level is >200 nmol/l. (If <120 nmol/l investigate for hypothyroidism)
Excessive depression or weakness or ataxia related to weekly maintenance therapy	Reassess patient. Check circulating sodium and potassium concentrations. Repeat ACTH stimulation test. If cortisol level post ACTH is <15 nmol/l reduce maintenance dose or give every other week. Consider splitting weekly dose

Table 10.7: Possible problems that may be encountered during mitotane therapy and their management.

daily mitotane treatment, it is important to continue therapy, albeit at a lower dose, otherwise the adrenal cortex will regenerate a hyperplastic zona fasciculata and zona reticularis and the clinical signs will recur.

Mitotane is given at a dose of 50 mg/kg/week with food. Cases that are well controlled may sleep for a few hours after the weekly dose, and for that reason it is often recommended that the treatment is given in the evening. More profound depression or weakness requires re-evaluation using the ACTH stimulation test and possibly a reduction of the maintenance dose. Failure to control the polydipsia may require an increased dose (see Table 10.7).

Re-examination
Treated dogs should be re-examined 6 to 8 weeks after completion of the initial therapy, unless there are any problems. Marked improvement should be noted at this time. The most obvious and rapid response is a reduction in water intake, urine output and appetite, and this is usually obvious at the end of the initial course of therapy. Muscle strength and exercise tolerance improve over the first 3 to 4 weeks. Skin and hair coat changes take longer and the progress is variable. The skin and alopecia may deteriorate markedly before improving; alternatively, there may be gradual and noticeable resolution of the clinical signs. Although improvement should be noted at 8 weeks, the skin and haircoat may not return to normal for 3 to 6 months (Figure 10.18). A few dogs have dramatic

changes in coat colour following successful therapy (Figure 10.19).

Re-evaluation every 3 to 6 months is recommended for the remainder of the animal's life. The dosage of mitotane should be adjusted according to the results of ACTH stimulation testing. The goal of therapy is to achieve an ACTH test result with serum cortisol concentrations between 20 and 120 nmol/l. Relapses and episodes of overdosage do occur. Relapses (serum cortisol >200 nmol/l) may require a short course of daily mitotane therapy or an increase in the maintenance dosage. Overdosage (serum cortisol <15 nmol/l) requires a reduction in the frequency or dose of maintenance therapy.

Primary hypoadrenocorticism with both glucocorticoid and mineralocorticoid insufficiency occurs in 5–17% of treated dogs during maintenance therapy. Although Addison's disease can develop at any time during treatment, most cases of primary hypoadrenocorticism occur during the first year of treatment. There is, unfortunately, no way to predict which dogs will develop complete adrenocortical insufficiency, but if it does develop, maintenance mitotane therapy should be stopped and the dog treated with mineralocorticoid and glucocorticoid supplementation as for primary hypoadrenocorticism.

The mean survival time of treated dogs was 30 months in one study, with a range of a few days to over 7 years (Dunn *et al.*, 1995). The highest mortality was seen in the first 16 weeks of treatment, and dogs which survived this

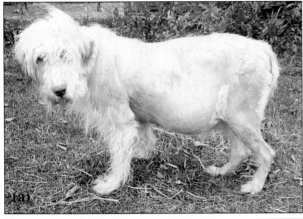

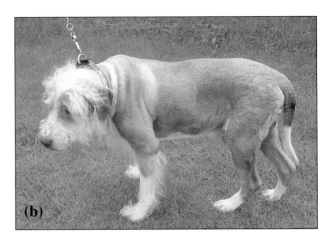

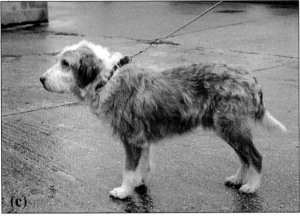

Figure 10.18: (a) A 10 year old crossbred dog with pituitary-dependent hyperadrenocorticism before treatment with mitotane. (b) The same dog after commencing treatment with mitotane. (c) The same dog 6 months later.

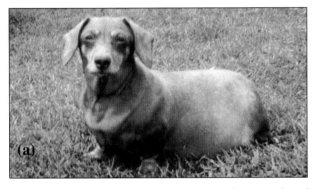

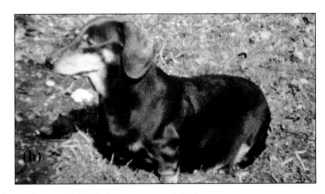

Figure 10.19: (a) A 7 year old female Dachshund with pituitary-dependent hyperadrenocorticism before treatment with mitotane. (b) The same dog 4 months later after commencing mitotane therapy. Note the marked change in coat colour following successful treatment.

period had a longer mean survival time. Other studies have shown similar survival times (Kintzer and Peterson, 1991).

Alternative therapies

L-Deprenyl

L-Deprenyl (selegiline hydrochloride) is a monoamine oxidase inhibitor (MAOI) that inhibits ACTH secretion by increasing dopaminergic tone to the hypothalamic–pituitary axis. The depletion of dopamine and consequent increase in ACTH secretion is considered to be a possible aetiology for pituitary-dependent hyperadrenocorticism in the dog. A veterinary formulation is available in North America. In the United Kingdom, L-deprenyl is likely to be licensed for use in the dog in the near future but only for behaviour modification.

The current recommended dose of L-deprenyl is 1 mg/kg daily. If there is an inadequate response after 2 months, the dosage is increased to 2 mg/kg/day. If this dosage also proves ineffective, alternative treatment should be employed. L-deprenyl is not recommended for dogs with pituitary-dependent hyperadrenocorticism and concurrent diabetes mellitus, pancreatitis, heart failure, renal disease, or other severe illnesses. The drug should not be administered with other MAOIs, opioids or tricyclic antidepressants.

Preliminary trials with L-deprenyl have shown that the efficacy is variable, with about 50% of dogs failing to respond adequately to treatment (Bruyette *et al.*, 1997). However, the advantage of L-deprenyl is that there are no severe adverse effects with this treatment. Accurately monitoring therapy is difficult because there are only minor reductions in serum cortisol concentrations during a low-dose dexamethasone suppression test or an ACTH stimulation test when on this treatment.

Ketoconazole

Ketoconazole is an imidazole antifungal drug that suppresses steroidogenesis. It has a reversible inhibitory effect on glucocorticoid synthesis while having a negligible effect on mineralocorticoid production. Ketoconazole has been used effectively in the management of canine hyperadrenocorticism (Feldman and Nelson, 1996).

The initial dose of ketoconazole is 5 mg/kg twice daily for 7 days to assess drug tolerance. If there are no adverse reactions, the dose is increased to 10 mg/kg twice daily for 14 days. The efficacy of the treatment is determined by an ACTH stimulation test using the same criteria as for monitoring mitotane therapy. If sufficient suppression of cortisol is not achieved, i.e. serum cortisol >120 nmol/l, then the dose should be increased to 15 mg/kg twice daily. Occasionally doses of 20 mg/kg twice daily are required to control the disease.

Adverse effects include anorexia, vomiting, diarrhoea, hepatopathy and jaundice. Higher doses are associated with a higher incidence of adverse effects.

The treatment is expensive and not always effective. About 25% of dogs treated with ketoconazole fail to respond adequately.

Cyproheptadine

Cyproheptadine is a drug with antiserotonin, antihistamine, and anticholinergic properties. Since excess ACTH secretion from the pituitary can be the result of increased serotonin concentrations, cyproheptadine might act to reduce ACTH release in pituitary-dependent hyperadrenocorticism. Although cyproheptadine has been used for the treatment of pituitary-dependent hyperadrenocorticism, the response has been variable, with a low success rate.

Pituitary irradiation

Pituitary irradiation is indicated for dogs with neurological signs associated with pituitary tumours. CT or MR imaging of the brain is required to plan the treatment protocol. Radiotherapy using megavoltage irradiation from a linear accelerator or cobalt 60 source is required to penetrate to the depth of the pituitary gland without seriously injuring overlying soft tissues. Most treatment protocols involve the administration of 40–50 Gy in 3–4 Gy fractions. There is often a dramatic response, although in some cases improvement takes several weeks. The resolution of neurological signs parallels the reduction in size of the tumour which can continue to decrease for a year or more after the completion of the radiotherapy. Reduction in ACTH secretion by the tumour is less predictable and, if it does occur, it may not be evident for 6 to 12 months after therapy. Therefore, medical management of hyper-adrenocorticism with mitotane is indicated initially.

Hypophysectomy

Hypophysectomy has been successfully performed in the dog for the treatment of pituitary-dependent hyperadrenocorticism using the trans-sphenoidal approach, but the operation is technically difficult and associated with high morbidity and mortality. Haemorrhage and incomplete visualisation and removal of larger lesions are common complications. Transient diabetes insipidus may develop which requires treatment, and all dogs will require lifelong thyroid and glucocorticoid replacement therapy.

Bilateral adrenalectomy

Bilateral adrenalectomy has been employed successfully but involves the risk of putting an ill animal with a compromised immune system and poor wound healing, through a difficult surgery procedure. Dogs treated by this approach require lifelong treatment for hypoadrenocorticism.

TREATMENT OF ADRENAL-DEPENDENT HYPERADRENOCORTICISM

Dogs with adrenal-dependent hyperadrenocorticism carry the best prognosis if the tumour can be completely removed surgically, however these dogs are often poor surgical candidates. Mitotane therapy has also been recommended for adrenal-dependent hyperadrenocorticism (Kintzer and Peterson, 1994).

Surgical adrenalectomy

Pre-operative staging of the adrenal tumour should include thoracic radiography and abdominal ultrasonography to assess the presence of vascular invasion and metastatic spread. Administration of mitotane or ketoconazole is recommended by some authors in order to attempt to control the hyperadrenocorticism.

Unilateral adrenalectomy requires considerable experience and expertise because of the complex anatomy. The technique is well described using the paracostal, flank approach (Johnston, 1977, 1983). Glucocorticoid and mineralocorticoid supplementation are required during surgery and postoperatively, since the contralateral adrenal cortex will be atrophic and unable to respond adequately to stress. The surgery should only be performed by experienced surgeons and even so there is a high morbidity and mortality rate. In one study, the perioperative mortality was 30% (van Sluijs et al., 1995). In the same study, the median survival time was just less than 2 years with some dogs surviving for longer than 4 years.

Mitotane therapy

Mitotane is effective and relatively safe in dogs with adrenal-dependent hyperadrenocorticism. Dogs with adrenal tumours, however, tend to be more resistant to mitotane than dogs with pituitary-dependent hyperadrenocorticism (Feldman et al., 1992). Generally, dogs with adrenal-dependent hyperadrenocorticism require higher daily induction doses (50–75 mg/kg/day) and a longer period of induction (>14 days) than dogs with pituitary-dependent hyperadrenocorticism (Kintzer and

Peterson, 1994). However, in this study about 20% of cases responded successfully to the recommended protocol for pituitary-dependent hyperadrenocorticism. Frequent monitoring of treatment, by ACTH stimulation testing, is important to ensure adequate control of the hyperadrenocorticism.

Maintenance doses are also generally higher (75–100 mg/kg/week) and again frequent monitoring of the cortisol response to ACTH stimulation is required to maintain optimal control of the disease. Adverse effects of treatment are similar to those described for pituitary-dependent hyperadrenocorticism. Those dogs requiring higher dose rates tend to be more prone to adverse effects. The adrenal tumour and any metastatic mass will often reduce in size due to the cytotoxic effects of mitotane, but in other cases the tumour will continue to grow despite increasing doses of mitotane. In one study of adrenocortical tumours treated using mitotane therapy, the median survival time was 11 months with a range of a few weeks to more than 5 years (Kintzer and Peterson, 1994).

REFERENCES

Angles JM, Feldman EC, Nelson RW and Feldman MS (1997) Use of cortisol:creatinine ratio versus adrenocorticotropic hormone stimulation testing for monitoring mitotane treatment of pituitary-dependent hyperadrenocorticism in dogs. *Journal of the American Veterinary Medical Association* **211**, 1002–1004

Bartez PY, Nyland T.G. and Feldman E.C. (1995) Ultrasonographic evaluation of the adrenal glands in dogs. *Journal of the American Veterinary Medical Association* **207**, 1180–1183

Bertoy EH, Feldman EC, Nelson RW, Duesberg CA, Kass PH, Reid MH and Dublin AB (1995) Magnetic resonance imaging of the brain in dogs with recently diagnosed but untreated pituitary-dependent hyperadrenocorticism. *Journal of the American Veterinary Medical Association* **206**, 651–656

Bruyette DS, Ruehl WW, Entriken TL, Darling LA and Griffin DW (1997) Treating canine pituitary-dependent hyperadrenocorticism with L-deprenyl. *Veterinary Medicine* August, 711–727

Douglass JP, Berry CR and James S (1997) Ultrasonographic adrenal gland measurements in dogs without evidence of adrenal disease. *Veterinary Radiology and Ultrasound* **38**, 124–130

Duesberg CA, Feldman EC, Nelson RW, Bertoy EH, Dublin AB and Reid MH (1995) Brain magnetic resonance imaging for the diagnosis of pituitary macrotumours. *Journal of the American Veterinary Medical Association* **206**, 675–662

Duncan ID, Griffiths IR and Nash AS (1977) Myotonia in canine Cushing's disease. *Veterinary Record* **100**, 30–31

Dunn KJ, Herrtage ME and Dunn JK (1995) Use of ACTH stimulation tests to monitor the treatment of canine hyperadrenocorticism. *Veterinary Record* **137**, 161–165

Feldman EC, Nelson RW, Feldman MS and Farver TB (1992) Comparison of mitotane treatment for adrenal tumor versus pituitary-dependent hyperadrenocorticism in dogs. *Journal of the American Veterinary Medical Association* **200**, 1642–1647

Feldman EC and Nelson RW (1996) Hyperadrenocorticism In: *Canine and Feline Endocrinology and Reproduction. 2nd edition.* pp. 187–265. WB Saunders, Philadelphia

Ferguson DC and Peterson ME (1992) Serum free and total iodothyronine concentrations in dogs with hyperadrenocorticism. *American Journal of Veterinary Research* **53**, 1636–1640

Fluckiger MA and Gomez JA (1984) Radiographic findings in dogs with spontaneous pulmonary thrombosis or embolism. *Veterinary Radiology* **25**, 124–131

Galac S, Kooistra HS, Teske E. and Rijnberk A (1997) Urinary corticoid/creatinine ratios in the differentiation between pituitary-dependent hyperadrenocorticism and hyperadrenocorticism due to adrenocortical tumour in the dog. *Veterinary Quarterly* **19**, 17–20

Guptill L, Scott-Moncrieff JC, Bottoms G, Glickman L, Johnson M, Glickman N, Nelson R, and Bertoy E (1997) Use of urine cortisol:creatinine ratio to monitor treatment response in dogs with pituitary-dependent hyperadrenocorticism. *Journal of the American*

Veterinary Medical Association **210**, 1158–1161

Huntley K, Frazer J, Gibbs C, and Gaskell CJ (1982) The radiological features of canine Cushing's syndrome: a review of forty-eight cases. *Journal of Small Animal Practice* **23**, 369–380

Johnston DE (1977) Adrenalectomy via retroperitoneal approach in dogs. *Journal of the American Veterinary Medical Association* **170**, 1092

Johnston DE (1983) Adrenalectomy in the dog. In: *Current Techniques in Small Animal Surgery*, ed. MJ Bojrab, pp. 386–388. Lea and Febiger, Philadelphia

Kantrowitz CM, Nyland TG and Feldman EC (1986) Adrenal ultrasonography in the dog: detection of tumours and hyperplasia in hyperadrenocorticism. *Veterinary Radiology* **27**, 91–96

Kaplan AJ, Peterson ME and Kemppainen RJ (1995) Effects of disease on the results of diagnostic tests for use in detecting hyperadrenocorticism in dogs. *Journal of the American Veterinary Medical Association* **207**, 445–451

Kemppainen RJ and Peterson ME (1996) Domestic cats show episodic variation in plasma concentrations of adrenocorticotropin, melanocyte-stimulating hormone (α-MSH), cortisol and thyroxine with circadian variation in α-MSH concentrations. *European Journal of Endocrinology* **134**, 602–609

Kemppainen RJ and Sartin JL (1984) Evidence for episodic but not circadian activity in plasma concentrations of adrenocorticotropin, cortisol and thyroxine in dogs. *Journal of Endocrinology* **103**, 219–226

Kintzer PP and Peterson ME (1991) Mitotane (o,p'-DDD) treatment of 200 dogs with pituitary-dependent hyperadrenocorticism. *Journal of Veterinary Internal Medicine* **5**, 182–190

Kintzer PP and Peterson ME (1994) Mitotane treatment of 32 dogs with cortisol-secreting adrenocortical neoplasms. *Journal of the American Veterinary Medical Association* **205**, 54–60

LaRue MJ and Murtaugh RJ (1990) Pulmonary thromboembolism in dogs: 47 cases (1986–1987). *Journal of the American Veterinary Medical Association* **197**, 1368–1372

Lee R & Griffiths IR (1972) A comparison of cerebral arteriography and cavernous sinus venography in the dog. *Journal of Small Animal Practice* **13**, 225

Meijer JC (1980) Canine hyperadrenocorticism. In: *Current Veterinary Therapy VII*, ed. RW Kirk, pp. 975–979. WB Saunders, Philadelphia

Mulnix JA, Van Den Brom WE and Lubberink AAME, De Bruijne JJ and Rijnberk A (1976) Gamma camera imaging of bilateral adrenocortical tumours in the dog. *American Journal of Veterinary Research* **37**, 1467–1471

Oluju MP, Eckersall PD and Douglas TA (1984) Simple quantitative assay for canine steroid-induced alkaline phosphatase. *Veterinary Record* **115**, 17

Owens JM and Drucker WD (1977) Hyperadrenocorticism in the dog: Canine Cushing's syndrome. *Veterinary Clinics of North America* **7**, 583

Peterson ME (1984) Hyperadrenocorticism. *Veterinary Clinics of North America: Small Animal Practice* **14**, 731–749

Peterson ME, Krieger DT, Drucker WD, and Halmi NS (1982a) Immunocytochemical study of the hypophysis in 25 dogs with pituitary-dependent hyperadrenocorticism. *Acta Endocrinologica* **101**, 15–24

Peterson ME, Gilbertson SR, and Drucker WD (1982b) Plasma cortisol response to exogenous ACTH in 22 dogs with hyperadrenocorticism caused by an adrenocortical neoplasia. *Journal of the American Veterinary Medical Association* **180**, 542–544

Peterson ME, Ferguson DC, Kintzer PP, and Drucker WD (1984) Effects of spontaneous hyperadrenocorticism on serum thyroid hormone concentrations in the dog. *American Journal of Veterinary Research* **45**, 2034–2038

Reusch CE and Feldman EC (1991) Canine hyperadrenocorticism due to adrenocortical neoplasia: pretreatment evaluation in 41 dogs. *Journal of Veterinary Internal Medicine* **5**, 3–10

Rijnberk A, Van Wees A, and Mol JA (1988) Assessment of two tests for the diagnosis of canine hyperadrenocorticism. *Veterinary Record* **122**, 178–180

Smiley LE and Peterson ME (1993) Evaluation of a urine cortisol:creatinine ratio as a screening test for hyperadrenocorticism in dogs. *Journal of Veterinary Internal Medicine* **7** 163–168

Stolp R, Rijnberk A, Meijer JC and Croughs RJM (1983) Urinary corticoids in the diagnosis of canine hyperadrenocorticism. *Research in Veterinary Science* **34**, 141–144

Teske E, Rothuizen J, de Bruijne JJ and Rijnberk A (1989) Corticosteroid-induced alkaline phosphatase isoenzyme in the diagnosis of canine hypercorticism. *Veterinary Record* **125**, 12–14

van Sluijs FJ, Sjollema BE, Voorhout G, van den Ingh TSGAM and Rijnberk A (1995) Results of adrenalectomy in 36 dogs with hyperadrenocorticism caused by adrenocortical tumour. *Veterinary*

Quarterly **17**, 113–116

Voorhout G, Stolp R, Lubberink AAME and Van Waes PFGM (1988). Computed tomography in the diagnosis of canine

hyperadrenocorticism not suppressible by dexamethasone. *Journal of the American Veterinary Medical Association* **192**, 641–646

Voorhout G, Stolp R, Rijnberk A and van Waes PFGM (1990)

CHAPTER ELEVEN

Hypoadrenocorticism

Michael E. Herrtage

INTRODUCTION

Hypoadrenocorticism is a syndrome that results from deficient mineralocorticoid and/or glucocorticoid secretion by the adrenal cortices. Destruction of more than 90% of both adrenal cortices causes a clinical deficiency of all adrenocortical hormones and is termed primary hypoadrenocorticism (Addison's disease). Secondary hypoadrenocorticism is caused by a deficiency in adrenocorticotropic hormone (ACTH) which leads to atrophy of the adrenal cortices and impaired secretion of glucocorticoids. The production of mineralocorticoids, however, usually remains adequate because ACTH has little tropic effect on mineralocorticoid production. Primary and secondary hypoadrenocorticism differ not only in their pathophysiology, but also in their clinical presentation.

PHYSIOLOGY OF THE ADRENAL CORTEX

A knowledge of the normal physiology of the adrenal cortex is crucial to the understanding of hypoadrenocorticism. Regulation of the release of glucocorticoids and their functions are detailed in Chapter 10. Aldosterone is the most important mineralocorticoid, and it is produced by the zona glomerulosa of the adrenal cortex. The regulation of aldosterone release and its function are widely different from glucocorticoids.

Regulation of mineralocorticoid release

Aldosterone release is influenced primarily by the renin–angiotensin system (RAS) and by plasma potassium levels (Fig. 11.1).

Renin is secreted into the blood by the cells of the juxtaglomerular apparatus, which consists of specialised cells in the wall of the afferent arteriole immediately proximal to the glomerulus and the specialised epithelial cells of the distal convoluted tubule adjacent to that arteriole, the macula densa. Renin release may be stimulated by stretch receptors in the juxtaglomerular apparatus in response to hypotension or reduced renal blood flow, or by sodium and chloride receptors in the macula densa. Renin is also released by sympathetic nerve stimulation and is inhibited by angiotensin II, antidiuretic hormone (ADH), hypertension, and increased reabsorption of sodium by the renal tubules.

Renin is a proteolytic enzyme which converts

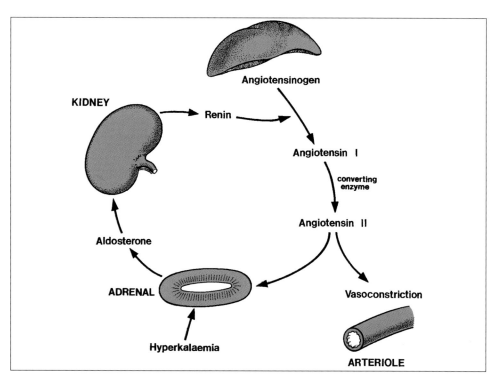

Figure 11.1: Regulation of aldosterone release.

circulating angiotensinogen, an α_2-globulin produced by the liver, into the decapeptide angiotensin I. Angiotensin I is hydro-lysed to the octapeptide, angiotensin II, by angiotensin converting enzyme (ACE) found almost entirely in the pulmonary capillary endothelium.

Angiotensin II is a powerful vasoconstrictor and stimulates aldosterone secretion from the zona glomerulosa. Through its action on the distal convoluted tubule, aldosterone has a negative feedback effect on the juxtaglomerular apparatus.

Potassium has a direct stimulatory effect on the zona glomerulosa cells to release aldosterone.

ACTH and sodium play a less significant role in aldosterone secretion. ACTH is necessary to maintain normal aldosterone output. In the absence of ACTH, the zona glomerulosa partially atrophies, causing mild to moderate aldosterone deficiency compared with almost total atrophy of the other zones.

Functions of mineralocorticoids

The main function of aldosterone is to protect against hypotension and potassium intoxication. Aldosterone promotes sodium, chloride and water reabsorption as well as potassium excretion in many epithelial tissues including the intestinal mucosa, salivary glands, sweat glands and kidneys. Its main site of action is the renal tubule where it promotes sodium and chloride reabsorption in the proximal convoluted tubule and sodium reabsorption by exchange with potassium in the distal convoluted tubule. It is one of the complex systems for the regulation of extracellular fluid electrolyte concentrations, extracellular fluid volume, blood volume, and arterial pressure.

PRIMARY HYPOADRENOCORTICISM (ADDISON'S DISEASE)

Primary hypoadrenocorticism is considered rare in the dog but probably occurs more frequently than is recognised. It is much less common than canine hyperadrenocorticism (Cushing's disease). Hypoadrenocorticism is very rare in the cat; only 10 cases have been reported (Peterson and Greco, 1989). The clinical signs, diagnosis and treatment of hypoadrenocorticism are similar in the dog and cat.

Causes of primary hypoadrenocorticism

Primary hypoadrenocorticism in the dog has been associated with the following conditions.

Idiopathic adrenocortical atrophy

This is the commonest cause in the dog and is thought to be the end result of immune-mediated destruction of the adrenal cortex. Immune-mediated destruction of the adrenal cortices is the most common cause of human hypoadrenocorticism. The presence of antiadrenal antibodies in two dogs and characteristic histopathological findings in another support this hypothesis (Schaer et al., 1986). The increased predisposition of primary hypoadrenocorticism in young to middle-aged female dogs is

also characteristic of an immune-mediated disease.

In humans, hypoadrenocorticism has been found to be associated with other immune-mediated disorders such as Hashimoto's thyroiditis, insulin-dependent diabetes mellitus, hypoparathyroidism, primary gonadal failure and atrophic gastritis. Autoimmune polyglandular disease has also been recognised in the dog and is described in Chapter 29.

Mitotane-induced adrenocortical necrosis

Hypoadrenocorticism is a possible complication of mitotane therapy in canine hyperadrenocorticism (see Chapter 10). Although mitotane usually spares the zona glomerulosa and therefore mineralocorticoid secretion, cases of complete adrenocortical failure can occasionally occur. In these cases, the adrenal cortex does not recover when mitotane therapy is withdrawn, and permanent hormone replacement therapy is required.

Bilateral adrenalectomy

The surgical removal of both adrenals has been used for the treatment of canine pituitary-dependent hyperadrenocorticism. The surgery is technically difficult and there is a high morbidity and mortality rate even with experienced surgeons. These dogs must be treated for hypoadrenocorticism with replacement hormone therapy for the rest of their lives.

Other possible causes

Rarely, canine hypoadrenocorticism can be caused by haemorrhage or infarction of the adrenal glands, granulomatous or neoplastic involvement of the adrenal glands, amyloidosis of adrenal cortices, or by trauma.

The adrenocortical pathology leads to mineralocorticoid and glucocorticoid deficiency. Aldosterone is the major mineralocorticoid; deficiency causes impaired ability to conserve sodium and water; and failure to excrete potassium leading to hyponatraemia and hyperkalaemia. Hyponatraemia induces lethargy, depression, and nausea and leads to the development of hypovolaemia, hypotension, reduced cardiac output, and decreased renal perfusion. Hyperkalaemia causes muscle weakness, hyporeflexia, and impaired cardiac conduction. Glucocorticoid deficiency causes decreased tolerance of stress, loss of appetite, and a normocytic, normochromic anaemia.

Signalment

Breed

Many breeds of dog have been reported with hypoadrenocorticism, but Great Danes, Portuguese Water Dogs, Rottweilers, Standard Poodles, West Highland White Terriers and Soft-coated Wheaten Terriers seem to be at greater risk of developing hypoadrenocorticism compared with dogs of other breeds (Peterson et al., 1996). Evidence of familial occurrence and the possibility of an hereditary factor has been suggested in Standard Poodles (Shaker et al., 1988), Bearded Collies (Ahlgren and Bamberg-Thalen, 1993) and Chinese Crested Dogs.

Anorexia
Lethargy/depression
Weakness, usually episodic
Vomiting
Waxing and waning illness
Weight loss or failure to gain weight
Dehydration
Diarrhoea or occasionally constipation
Polydipsia and/or polyuria
Collapse or syncope
Restlessness/shaking/shivering
Melaena
Weak pulse
Bradycardia
Abdominal pain

Table 11.1: Clinical signs of primary hypoadrenocorticism (Addison's disease).

Age

Hypoadrenocorticism seems to be a disease predominantly of the young and middle-aged dog, with an age range of 3 months to 14 years and a median age of 4 years.

Sex

Approximately 70% of reported cases are female, and sexually intact females have been shown to have a significantly higher risk of developing hypoadrenocorticism than spayed females (Peterson *et al.*, 1996).

Clinical signs

The clinical signs of primary hypoadrenocorticism vary from mild to severe with the progression being either acute or chronic. Chronic hypoadrenocorticism is far more common than the acute disease in the dog.

Acute primary hypoadrenocorticism

The clinical appearance of acute hypoadrenocorticism is that of hypovolaemic shock (an adrenocortical crisis). The animal is usually found in a state of collapse, or collapses when stressed. Other signs include weak pulse, profound bradycardia, abdominal pain, vomiting, diarrhoea, dehydration and hypothermia. The condition is rapidly progressive and life threatening and represents a true medical emergency. Aggressive fluid therapy will help most patients and allow more time to make a diagnosis.

Chronic primary hypoadrenocorticism

The clinical signs in the chronic form are often vague and non-specific and may be exacerbated by stress (Table 11.1). The diagnosis should be considered in any dog with a waxing and waning type of illness or that shows episodic weakness and collapse (Herrtage and McKerrell, 1995). The most consistent clinical signs include anorexia, vomiting, lethargy, depression and/or weakness. The severity of each sign can vary during the course of the disease and may be interspersed with periods of apparent good health often following non-specific veterinary therapy, usually consisting of cage rest, glucocorticoid therapy and/or parenteral fluid administration. Hypoadrenocorticism can easily be mistaken for chronic renal failure, primary neuromuscular disorders and various other causes for signs such as weight loss, weakness, anorexia, vomiting and diarrhoea.

Common findings on physical examination apart from depression and weakness, include dehydration, bradycardia, and weak femoral pulses. The electrocardiographic (ECG) findings are described below. In a few cases, severe gastrointestinal haemorrhage with melaena and occasionally haematemesis can occur resulting in profound anaemia (Medinger *et al.*, 1993).

Routine laboratory abnormalities

The most common haematological, biochemical and urinalysis findings are listed in Table 11.2.

Haematology
Lymphocytosis
Eosinophilia
Relative neutropenia
Anaemia: usually a normocytic, normochromic, non-regenerative anaemia, but can be blood loss anaemia associated with gastrointestinal haemorrhage
Biochemistry
Azotaemia
Hyponatraemia
Hyperkalaemia
Reduced sodium: potassium ratio (<23:1)
Reduced bicarbonate and total carbon dioxide concentrations
Hypochloraemia
Hypercalcaemia
Hypoglycaemia
Urinalysis
Specific gravity variable (usually 1.015–1.030)

Table 11.2: Routine laboratory findings in primary hypoadrenocorticism (Addison's disease).

Haematology

Haematological changes may include lymphocytosis, eosinophilia and mild normocytic, normochromic, non-regenerative anaemia. However, these findings are not consistent. Normal or elevated eosinophil and lymphocyte counts in any sick animal with signs compatible with hypoadrenocorticism are significant, because the expected response to stress would be eosinopenia and lymphopenia. A mild anaemia may not be appreciated until the dog has been rehydrated because of the haemoconcentration effect of dehydration. Profound anaemia (packed cell volume <0.20 l/l) is usually found in association with gastrointestinal haemorrhage.

Biochemistry

The most consistent laboratory findings in

hypoadrenocorticism are prerenal azotaemia, hyponatraemia, hyperkalaemia, and mild to moderate metabolic acidosis. However, approximately 10% of dogs with primary hypoadrenocorticism have normal serum electrolyte concentrations and these cases are referred to as atypical Addison's disease (Sadek and Schaer, 1996).

Urea and creatinine: Circulating urea and creatinine concentrations are increased secondary to reduced renal perfusion and decreased glomerular filtration rate. Reduced renal perfusion results from hypovolaemia, reduced cardiac output and hypotension, which in turn result from chronic fluid loss through the kidneys, acute fluid loss through vomiting and/or diarrhoea, and inadequate fluid intake. Gastrointestinal haemorrhage, which may occur in hypoadrenocorticism, can contribute to the elevation in urea concentration.

Prerenal azotaemia is usually associated with concentrated urine (specific gravity >1.030) whereas the urine in primary renal failure is often isosthenuric or only mildly concentrated (1.008–1.025). The urine specific gravity in hypoadrenocorticism is variable, but is usually between 1.015–1.030 which may cause confusion for the clinician. This reduced urine specific gravity develops in hypoadrenocorticism because of impaired concentrating ability due to chronic sodium loss reducing the renal medullary concentration gradient (Tyler *et al.*, 1987). With adequate fluid therapy, the blood urea and creatinine concentrations will quickly return to normal in cases of hypoadrenocorticism, confirming that the azotaemia is prerenal.

Sodium and potassium: The serum sodium concentration is usually <135 mmol/l and the serum potassium concentration is usually >5.5 mmol/l. However, because of the variability of these two abnormalities, the ratio of sodium to potassium may be more reliable than the absolute values. The normal ratio varies between 27:1 and 40:1, whereas in patients with hypoadrenocorticism, the ratio is usually <23:1 and may be <20:1. Serum chloride concentration is also reduced in association with sodium, and frequently chloride concentrations <100 mmol/l are found in cases of hypoadrenocorticism.

Concurrent hypovolaemia, hyponatraemia, and hyperkalaemia may develop in other conditions apart from hypoadrenocorticism, such as gastrointestinal disease, chronic blood loss, acute and chronic renal failure, chronic hepatic failure, chronic heart failure, repeated drainage of chylous and non-chylous pleural effusions, and lymphangiosarcoma (Lamb and Muir, 1994). Pseudohyperkalaemia, which is defined as a spurious increase in serum or plasma potassium concentration caused by *in vitro* changes, is seen in haemolysed blood samples, especially from Japanese Akitas (Degen, 1987) and in dogs with thrombocytosis or extreme leucocytosis (Reimann *et al.*, 1989).

Approximately 10% of cases of primary hypoadrenocorticism have normal serum electrolyte concentrations at the time of presentation. It is generally believed that these dogs with atypical Addison's disease have early or mild primary hypoadrenocorticism, and that typical electrolyte abnormalities will develop in time. Rarely, isolated primary hypocortisolaemia has been reported in the dog, and these cases never show serum electrolyte abnormalities (Dunn and Herrtage, 1998).

Calcium: Mild to moderate hypercalcaemia is seen in about a third of cases of hypoadrenocorticism, usually in those dogs most severely affected by the disease and in which there is significant hyperkalaemia. The mechanism by which hypercalcaemia occurs in hypoadrenocorticism remains to be elucidated, but haemoconcentration, increased renal tubular reabsorption, and decreased glomerular filtration are thought to play a part. The differential diagnosis of hypercalcaemia includes neoplasia, primary hyperparathyroidism, chronic renal failure and hypervitaminosis D (see Chapter 16). In a study of 40 dogs with hypercalcaemia, hypoadrenocorticism was the second most common cause and accounted for 25% of the cases (Elliot *et al.*, 1991). In the same study, the degree of hypercalcaemia was found to be significantly lower in the cases of hypoadrenocorticism (mean plasma calcium concentration 3.5 ± 0.4 mmol/l) than in lymphoproliferative disease (mean plasma calcium concentration 4.3 ± 0.7 mmol/l).

Glucose: There is a tendency to develop hypoglycaemia because glucocorticoid deficiency reduces glucose production by the liver, and peripheral cell receptors become more sensitive to insulin. Hypoglycaemia is uncommon (Willard *et al.*, 1982) but the potential should remain a concern for the clinician as severe hypoglycaemia may result in clinical signs of ataxia, disorientation, or seizures (Levy, 1994).

Albumin: Moderate to severe hypoalbuminaemia has been noted in some cases of hypoadrenocorticism. The pathogenesis of hypoalbuminaemia in primary hypoadrenocorticism is unknown, but gastrointestinal haemorrhage, impaired intestinal absorption of nutrients, and impaired albumin synthesis may be involved. The major causes of hypoalbuminaemia include increased loss (for example, protein-losing nephropathy or enteropathy, blood loss, severe exudation, or haemorrhage into body cavities) and decreased production (for example, severe malabsorption, maldigestion, malnutrition, or inadequate production in chronic liver disease). In one study, 39% of dogs with hypoadrenocorticism were found to have hypoalbuminaemia (Langlais-Burgess *et al.*, 1995). However other studies have shown the frequency of hypoalbuminaemia to be considerably lower, accounting for between 6% and 12% of cases (Melián and Peterson, 1996; Peterson *et al.*, 1996).

Liver enzymes: Mild to moderate increases in liver enzyme activities, such as alanine aminotransferase (ALT), aspartate aminotransferase (AST), and alkaline phosphatase (ALP), are found in some cases of hypoadrenocorticism. Although the precise cause of the elevation is unknown, reduced cardiac output and poor tissue perfusion probably play a role. Raised liver enzyme

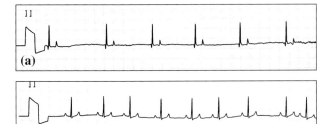

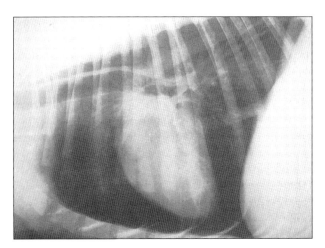

Figure 11.2: *Electrocardiograms (ECGs) from a 4 year old Bearded Collie with primary hypoadrenocorticism taken (a) before and (b) after supplementation with glucocorticoids and mineralocorticoids 1 mV/cm, 25 mm/s). (a) The P waves are absent, the T waves are peaked and there is profound bradycardia. The plasma sodium concentration was 138 mmol/l and the plasma potassium 9.5 mmol/l. (b) ECG after treatment showing sinus arrhythmia. The plasma sodium concentration was 142 mmol/l and the plasma potassium 5.4 mmol/l.*

Figure 11.3: *Thoracic radiograph of a Standard Poodle with primary hypoadrenocorticism, showing the effects of hypovolaemia including microcardia, decreased pulmonary vasculature, and reduced caudal vena cava.*

concentrations, hypoalbuminaemia and hypoglycaemia increase the suspicion of primary hepatic disease in some cases of hypoadrenocorticism, and clinicians should be aware of this potential confusion.

Acid–base balance: Mild to moderate metabolic acidosis is common in dogs with hypoadrenocorticism. Total carbon dioxide concentrations and serum bicarbonate determinations are reduced. The acidosis develops because reduced aldosterone concentrations impair renal tubular secretion of hydrogen ions. Hypotension and poor renal perfusion are likely to contribute to the acidosis.

ECG features

Hyperkalaemia impairs cardiac conduction which can be assessed by ECG (Figure 11.2). Although the ECG changes do not correlate directly with serum potassium concentrations, probably because of the influence of other electrolyte abnormalities, particularly the cardio-protective effects of increased calcium, metabolic acidosis, and impaired tissue perfusion, the following guidelines have proved helpful:

* >5.5 mmol/l: Peaking of the T wave
                 Shortening of the Q–T interval
* >6.5 mmol/l: Increased QRS duration
* >7.0 mmol/l: P wave amplitude decreased
                 P–R interval prolonged
* >8.5 mmol/l: P wave absent (sinoatrial standstill)
                 Severe bradycardia.

In some cases, bizarre QRS complexes are seen, representing ventricular extrasystoles, and these could be the result of hypoxia and/or hyperkalaemia.

ECG can also be used for monitoring the patient during treatment. An improvement in the ECG tracing suggests a reduction in serum potassium concentration.

Radiographic features

Dogs with hypoadrenocorticism may show radiographic signs of hypovolaemia which include: microcardia, decreased size of pulmonary vessels, reduced size of the caudal vena cava, and microhepatica (Figure 11.3). These

changes, however, are not specific and only represent hypovolaemia and dehydration irrespective of the cause.

A few dogs with hypoadrenocorticism develop megaoesophagus as a result of generalised muscle weakness, and this can be seen on thoracic radiographs as an air-filled, dilated oesophagus. Image-intensified fluoroscopy, using barium paste or barium mixed with food, demonstrates a complete absence of oesophageal peristaltic activity. The cause of oesophageal dilatation in hypoadrenocorticism remains unclear, but was considered to be attributable to the effect of abnormal sodium and potassium concentrations on membrane potential and neuro-muscular function (Burrows, 1987). However, in other cases of hypoadrenocorticism with megaoesophagus, abnormal serum electrolytes were never documented, thus suggesting that the oesophageal dilatation was associated with glucocorticoid deficiency (Bartges and Nielson, 1992; Whitley, 1995). The megaoesophagus resolves rapidly with appropriate supplementation.

Ultrasonographic features

In a recent study involving the ultrasonographic examination of the adrenal glands in dogs with hypoadreno-corticism, the adrenal glands were shown to be shorter (median values: left adrenal 12.1 mm, right adrenal 13.1 mm) and thinner (median values: left adrenal 2.4 mm, right adrenal 2.5 mm) than those of healthy dogs (Hörauf and Reusch, 1997). Although ultrasonography could not distinguish between primary and secondary hypoadreno-corticism, the technique was considered to be a useful screening test, especially in emergency cases with acute disease.

Confirmatory diagnostic tests

ACTH stimulation test

The ACTH stimulation test is commonly used to provide definitive confirmation of the presence of hypoadreno-corticism. The intravenous preparation of ACTH should be used, as absorption of depot products such as ACTH gel cannot be relied on, particularly if the patient is collapsed or severe hypotension is suspected. (The protocol is described in Chapter 10.) In dogs with hypoadrenocorticism, the resting cortisol concentration will be low with a subnormal or negligible response to ACTH. The ACTH stimulation test, however, does not distinguish between primary hypoadrenocorticism and secondary hypoadrenocorticism due to pituitary failure or iatrogenic glucocorticoid administration.

Endogenous plasma ACTH concentration

Plasma ACTH concentrations are useful in distinguishing primary from secondary hypoadrenocorticism, but stringent and meticulous sample handling is crucial (see Chapter 10).

Dogs with primary hypoadrenocorticism have very high endogenous ACTH concentrations (>500 pg/ml), whereas those with secondary hypoadrenocorticism have low or even undetectable concentrations of ACTH.

Plasma aldosterone concentrations

Basal aldosterone concentrations are of little or no diagnostic value. Plasma aldosterone concentrations should be measured in response to ACTH stimulation (as in the protocol above). Theoretically, plasma aldosterone concentrations should help differentiate between primary hypoadrenocorticism (with reduced cortisol and aldosterone concentrations) and secondary hypoadrenocorticism (with normal aldosterone and reduced cortisol concentrations). However, aldosterone assays are not widely available and few studies have reported on their use.

After stimulation with ACTH, plasma aldosterone concentrations should double, unless the basal concentration is already in the high–normal range (Golden and Lowthrop 1988). In dogs suffering from primary hypoadrenocorticism with hypoaldosteronism, the basal aldosterone concentration is low with minimal or no increase in the post-ACTH aldosterone concentration. Dogs with atypical Addison's disease may have higher aldosterone concentrations both before and after ACTH stimulation than typical cases of hypoadrenocorticism, but concentrations are still abnormally low.

Treatment

Acute primary hypoadrenocorticism

Treatment is directed at resuscitation of intravascular volume, reversal of hyperkalaemia and hyponatraemia, provision of glucocorticoids, and reversal of any life-threatening cardiac arrhythmias; it is described in Chapter 19. Once the patient is stable, oral maintenance therapy is instigated.

Chronic primary hypoadrenocorticism (maintenance therapy)

This involves the use of mineralocorticoid supplementation, with or without glucocorticoid or salt supplementation, after initial stabilisation for acute hypoadrenocorticism.

Mineralocorticoid therapy: All cases of primary hypo-adrenocorticism with classic electrolyte disturbances, hyponatraemia, hyperkalaemia and hypochloraemia, will require lifelong treatment with mineralocorticoids. The use of mineralocorticoid supplementation in cases of atypical Addison's disease, where the electrolyte concentrations are normal, is more complex. In one study, two dogs with atypical primary hypoadrenocorticism were discharged on glucocorticoid supplementation only and both dogs died within 9 days of a presumed addisonian crisis (Kintzer and Peterson, 1997). However, rarely some dogs with atypical primary hypoadrenocorticism have an isolated glucocorticoid deficiency and normal mineralocorticoid concentrations; these cases respond well to just glucocorticoid replacement therapy as do cases of secondary hypoadrenocorticism (Dunn and Herrtage, 1998). Certainly it is prudent to try and differentiate primary from secondary hypoadrenocorticism or isolated glucocorticoid deficiency with plasma ACTH concentrations and basal and post-ACTH stimulated plasma aldosterone concentrations. While awaiting the results of these tests, it would seem wise to administer both mineralocorticoid and glucocorticoid replacement therapy to reduce the possibility of an acute addisonian crisis developing.

There are two preparations used for mineralocorticoid supplementation, fludrocortisone acetate and desoxycorticosterone pivalate, however only the former is currently available in the United Kingdom.

Fludrocortisone is a potent oral synthetic adrenocortical steroid with mainly mineralocorticoid effects, although it retains some glucocorticoid activity. It is available in 0.1 mg tablets and is the treatment of choice for maintenance therapy in dogs with hypoadrenocorticism in the United Kingdom. An initial dose of 15 µg/kg of fludrocortisone is administered once daily. The response is monitored and serum electrolytes measured after 5 to 7 days. The dose rate should then be adjusted until the sodium and potassium levels are within the normal range. Frequently, the dose of fludrocortisone has to be increased during the first 6 to 18 months of therapy in order to maintain normal electrolyte concentrations and in a few of these cases, fludrocortisone may have to be administered twice daily. In one study, the daily maintenance dose of fludrocortisone increased from an initial median dose of 13 µg/kg to a final median dose of 23 µg/kg (Kintzer and Peterson, 1997). In the same study, the final dose of fludrocortisone administered to more than half the dogs ranged from 15 to 30 µg/kg/day.

Adverse effects develop in some dogs, particularly those requiring high doses of fludrocortisone to maintain serum electrolyte concentrations within the normal range. These include mild signs of iatrogenic hyperadrenocorticism, i.e. polyuria, polydipsia, polyphagia, and weight gain, due to the glucocorticoid effects of fludrocortisone.

Desoxycorticosterone pivalate is a long-acting ester of desoxycorticosterone acetate, a synthetic corticosteroid with only mineralocorticoid activity and no glucocorticoid activity. It is formulated into a microcrystalline suspension for injection. This preparation is not currently available in the United Kingdom, but studies have shown it to be effective in replacing the mineralocorticoid deficiency in dogs with hypoadrenocorticism (Lynn and Feldman, 1991). The recommended dosage is 2.2 mg/kg intramuscularly or subcutaneously every 25 days. In another study, lower doses of between 1.4 and 1.9 mg/kg were found to be effective in controlling electrolyte concentrations and this study also showed that the interval between injections varied among dogs, ranging from 14 days to 35 days (Kintzer and Peterson, 1997).

Signs of iatrogenic hyperadrenocorticism have not been associated with long-term use of desoxycorticosterone pivalate. However, a few cases have developed anorexia and depression in the presence of normal electrolyte concentrations which resolved promptly with glucocorticoid replacement therapy.

Glucocorticoid therapy: The majority of cases do not require daily glucocorticoid supplementation for maintenance therapy after the initial period of treatment and this may be due in part to the inherent glucocorticoid activity of fludrocortisone. Glucocorticoids at replacement dosages are administered for the first one to two weeks of treatment until the animal is stable and then gradually reduced and stopped. However, the owners of dogs with hypoadrenocorticism should always be provided with a supply of prednisolone tablets to be given if the patient appears unwell (depressed, anorexic, or vomiting). Prednisolone at a dose of 0.2 mg/kg daily should be sufficient as glucocorticoid replacement for those cases that do require glucocorticoids. Higher doses (0.5 mg/kg) are more likely to produce signs of iatrogenic hyperadrenocorticism and are usually reserved for periods of severe stress.

Salt supplementation: Sodium chloride tablets or salting of the food should be instigated at a dose of 0.1 mg/kg/day initially to help correct hyponatraemia but can be phased out and are not usually required long term in most cases. Dogs requiring unusually high doses of fludrocortisone, however, may respond to a lower dose of fludrocortisone if concurrently provided with salt supplementation.

The prognosis with hypoadrenocorticism is excellent when oral maintenance therapy has been used, providing owner education is adequate. In one study, the median survival time for dogs with hypoadrenocorticism was 4.7 years with a range of 7 days to 11.8 years (Kintzer and Peterson, 1997). In this study, age, breed and sex were not shown to influence survival time and no significant difference was found in the survival time of dogs treated with fludrocortisone compared to dogs treated with with desoxycorticosterone pivalate.

SECONDARY HYPOADRENOCORTICISM

Secondary hypoadrenocorticism is associated with a deficiency of glucocorticoids caused by a deficiency in ACTH production and/or release. The production of mineralocorticoids, although reduced, generally remains adequate.

Causes of secondary hypoadrenocorticism

Secondary hypoadrenocorticism can be associated with destructive lesions, for example, large non-functional tumours in the hypothalamus or pituitary. More commonly, however, it is an iatrogenic condition associated with prolonged suppression of ACTH by drug therapy with glucocorticoids or progestogens such as megoestrol acetate (van den Broek and O'Farrell, 1994).

Clinical signs

The clinical signs are variable, but may include depression, anorexia, occasional vomiting or diarrhoea, weak pulse, and sudden collapse when stressed. If the secondary hypoadrenocorticism is associated with glucocorticoid therapy, then clinical signs of iatrogenic hyperadrenocorticism (Cushing's disease) are usually present.

Diagnosis

The diagnosis of secondary hypoadrenocorticism is based on a failure of plasma cortisol concentrations to respond to ACTH stimulation together with low or undetectable endogenous plasma ACTH concentrations. If measured, the plasma aldosterone concentrations may be reduced, but basal concentrations will increase with ACTH stimulation.

Treatment

Glucocorticoid replacement, using prednisolone at a dose of 0.2 mg/kg daily, is indicated for immediate correction of the clinical signs. Further treatment and the prognosis depend on the cause of the disease and whether it can be treated. Management of glucocorticoid therapy and the prevention of iatrogenic hyperadrenocorticism are discussed in Chapter 32.

REFERENCES

Ahlgren M and Bamberg-Thalen B (1993) Hypoadrenocorticism in the dog. *European Journal of Companion Animal Practice* **3**, 62–68

Bartges JW and Nielson DL (1992) Reversible megaesophagus associated with atypical primary hypoadrenocorticism in a dog. *Journal of the American Veterinary Medical Association* **201**, 889–891

Burrows CF (1987) Reversible mega-oesophagus in a dog with hypoadrenocorticism. *Journal of Small Animal Practice* **28**, 1073–1078

Degen M (1987) Pseudohyperkalemia in Akitas. *Journal of the American Veterinary Medical Association* **190**, 541–543

Dunn KJ and Herrtage ME (1998) Hypocortisolaemia in a Labrador retriever. *Journal of Small Animal Practice* **39**, 90–93

Elliott J, Dobson JM, Dunn JK, Herrtage ME and Jackson KF (1991) Hypercalcaemia in the dog: a study of 40 cases. *Journal of Small Animal Practice* **32**, 564–571

Golden DL and Lowthrop CD (1988) A retrospective study of aldosterone secretion in normal and adrenopathic dogs. *Journal of Veterinary Internal Medicine* **2**, 121–125

Herrtage ME and McKerrell RE (1995) Episodic weakness. In: *Manual of Dog and Cat Neurology, 2nd edn*, ed. SL Wheeler, pp.189–207. BSAVA, Cheltenham

Hörauf A and Reusch C (1997) Evaluation of ultrasonography in the diagnosis of hypoadrenocorticism in dogs. *Proceedings of the 7th Annual Congress of the European Society of Veterinary Internal Medicine* p. 137

Kintzer PP and Peterson ME (1997) Treatment and long-term follow-up of 205 dogs with hypoadrenocorticism. *Journal of Veterinary Internal Medicine* **11**, 43–49

Lamb WA and Muir P (1993) Lymphangiosarcoma associated with hyponatraemia and hyperkalaemia in a dog. *Journal of Small Animal Practice* **35**, 374–376

Langlais-Burgess L, Lumsden JH and Mackin A (1995) Concurrent hypoadrenocorticism and hypoalbuminemia in dogs: a retrospective study. *Journal of the American Animal Hospital Association* **31**, 307–311

Levy JK (1994) Hypoglycemic seizures attributable to hypoadrenocorticism in a dog. *Journal of the American Veterinary Medical Association* **204**, 526–528

Lynn RC and Feldman EC (1991) Treatment of canine hypoadrenocorticism with microcrystalline desoxycorticosterone pivalate. *British Veterinary Journal* **147**, 478–483

Medinger TL, Williams DA and Bruyette DS (1993) Severe gastrointestinal tract haemorrhage in three dogs with hypoadrenocorticism. *Journal of the American Veterinary Medical Association* **202**, 1869–1872

Melián C and Peterson ME (1996) Diagnosis and treatment of naturally occurring hypoadrenocorticism in 42 dogs. *Journal of Small Animal Practice* **37**, 268–275

Peterson ME and Greco DS (1989) Primary hypoadrenocorticism in ten cats. *Journal of Veterinary Internal Medicine* **3**, 55–58

Peterson ME, Kintzer PP and Kass PH (1996) Pretreatment clinical and laboratory findings in dogs with hyperadrenocorticism: 225 cases (1979–1993). *Journal of the American Veterinary Medical Association* **208**, 85–91

Reimann KA, Knowlen GG and Tvedten HW (1989) Factitious hyperkalemia in dogs with thrombocytosis. *Journal of Veterinary Internal Medicine* **3**, 47–52

Sadek D and Schaer M (1996) Atypical Addison's disease in the dog: a retrospective survey of 14 cases. *Journal of the American Animal Hospital Association* **32**, 159–163

Schaer M, Riley WJ, Buergelt CD, Bowen DJ, Senior DF, Burrows CF and Campbell GA (1986) Autoimmunity and Addison's disease in the dog. *Journal of the American Animal Hospital Association* **22**, 789–794

Shaker E, Hurvitz AJ and Peterson ME (1988) Hypoadrenocorticism in a family of standard Poodles. *Journal of the American Veterinary Medical Association* **192**, 1091–1092

Tyler RD, Qualls CW, Heald RD, Cowell RL and Clinkenbeard KD (1987) Renal concentrating ability in dehydrated hyponatremic dogs. *Journal of the American Veterinary Medical Association* **191**, 1095–1100

van den Broek AHM and O'Farrell V (1994) Suppression of adrenocortical function in dogs receiving therapeutic doses of megestrol acetate. *Journal of Small Animal Practice* **35**, 285–288

Whitley NT (1995) Megaoesophagus and glucocorticoid-deficient hypoadrenocorticism in a dog. *Journal of Small Animal Practice* **36**, 132–135.

Willard MD, Schall WD, Mccaw DE and Nachreiner RF (1982) Canine hypoadrenocorticism: Report of 37 cases and review of 39 previously reported cases. *Journal of the American Veterinary Medical Association* **180**, 59–62

CHAPTER TWELVE

Canine Diabetes Mellitus

Peter A. Graham

INTRODUCTION

Canine diabetes mellitus is not a single disease but a manifestation of diverse pathophysiological processes. The unifying characteristic of these disorders is the presence of hyperglycaemia resulting from an absolute or relative insulin deficiency combined with an absolute or relative excess of glucagon.

Insulin and glucagon are peptides secreted by the β and α islet cells of the pancreas, respectively, and their roles are counter-regulatory, ensuring efficient storage and mobilisation of metabolic fuels.

In the healthy animal, insulin facilitates the uptake of sodium, potassium and glucose by cells. Insulin is secreted in response to increased circulating concentrations of glucose or amino acids. Glucagon secretion is also stimulated by increased concentrations of amino acids. Glucagon prevents hypoglycaemia resulting from protein-stimulated postprandial insulin secretion.

Insulin consists of two peptide chains linked by disulphide bridges; it is formed by the cleavage of a connecting peptide (C peptide) from a precursor molecule (proinsulin) within the secretory granules of the β cell. Insulin and C peptide are therefore secreted in equimolar concentrations following a stimulus for insulin release.

PATHOPHYSIOLOGY

In healthy animals, insulin promotes glucose uptake, glycogen synthesis, and lipid and protein anabolism and storage while inhibiting glycogenolysis, gluconeogenesis, lipolysis, ketogenesis and proteolysis. Glucagon promotes glycogenolysis, gluconeogenesis, lipolysis and ketogenesis while inhibiting glycogen synthesis. The catabolic effects of glucagon are very sensitive to inhibition by insulin which ensures efficient storage of nutrients during the fed state. During starvation, however, glucagon activity predominates, releasing stored fuels and ensuring an adequate level of circulating glucose for optimal central neurological function. This is important because neurological tissue (except for a small section of the hypothalamus) has no insulin-mediated active transport mechanism for glucose, and relies on passive diffusion of its metabolic fuel.

In diabetic animals, insulin deficiency allows glucagon-driven gluconeogenesis by the liver to proceed uncontrolled. This increased glucose production results in hyperglycaemia which is further exacerbated by reduced insulin-dependent uptake of glucose from the circulation. When hyperglycaemia is greater than 10–12 mmol/l, the ability of the renal tubule to resorb glucose is exceeded resulting in glucosuria and consequent osmotic diuresis and compensatory polydipsia.

When the supply of glucose, the body's preferred energy source, is compromised by diabetes mellitus or starvation, alternative energy substrates, ketones, can be generated in the liver from lipids which have been mobilised from peripheral stores. The principal ketones are acetone, acetoacetate and β-hydroxybutyrate. In diabetic animals with severe insulin deficiency or glucagon excess, ketogenesis, regulated by the insulin:glucagon

Failure of insulin production	Failure of insulin transport	Failure of tissue sensitivity
Anti-islet autoimmunity	Insulin antibodies	Obesity
Islet cell hypoplasia	(after exogenous	Hormonal antagonism
Drug/chemical toxicities	insulin therapy)	Glucagon:
Senile islet degeneration		Infection, uraemia, glucagonoma
Pancreatitis		Glucocorticoids:
Pancreatic injury		Stress, hyperadrenocorticism, exogenous
Pancreatectomy		Catecholamines:
Pancreatic neoplasia		Stress, phaeochromocytoma
		Growth hormone:
		Acromegaly, progestogens
		Progestogens:
		Endogenous, exogenous

Table 12.1: Factors that may contribute to the development of, or exacerbate existing, canine diabetes mellitus.

ratio, will be stimulated. If the production of ketones, which are acidic, exceeds the body's buffering capacity then metabolic acidosis ensues and the animal is described as ketoacidotic.

AETIOLOGY AND CLASSIFICATION

Diabetes mellitus can arise from any process which affects insulin production, insulin transport or the sensitivity of target tissues to insulin. Disorders implicated in canine diabetes mellitus are listed in Table 12.1. An animal that has failure of target tissue sensitivity will initially compensate for this by increasing insulin production (Eigenmann, 1981; Selman *et al.*, 1994); depending on the magnitude of this increase relative to the degree of insensitivity, control of blood glucose concentrations may or may not be maintained. After a prolonged period of sustained maximum output, the β cells may become 'exhausted', resulting in both failure of insulin production and target tissue insensitivity (Figure 12.1). An alternative explanation for 'exhaustion' of insulin production is the concept of glucose toxicity whereby the β cells stop responding to elevated concentrations of circulating glucose because of an inhibitory effect of hyperglycaemia on insulin secretion. In such cases, if the source of the insulin insensitivity can be controlled before 'exhaustion' occurs, then the dog need not become permanently diabetic. Bitches with diabetes mellitus associated with high levels of progesterone and growth hormone (GH) during metoestrus may be cured by ovariohysterectomy before β cell exhaustion, or their clinical signs may disappear as progesterone concentrations decrease at the end of metoestrus (Eigenmann, 1981; Reusch *et al.*, 1993; Graham, 1995).

There are no studies which accurately define the relative incidences of the different underlying mechanisms in canine diabetes mellitus. It is likely that hormonal antagonism (Eigenmann, 1981; Eigenmann and Venker-van Haagen, 1981; Peterson *et al.*, 1981; Campbell and Latimer, 1984; Blaxter and Gruffydd-Jones, 1990), pancreatic inflammation (Alejandro *et al.*, 1988), autoimmunity (Sai *et al.*, 1984; Haines and Penhale, 1985; Elie and Hoenig, 1995), obesity (Mattheeuws *et al.*, 1984a,b) and an equivalent of human type II diabetes (Mattheeuws *et al.*, 1984b), all have a role to play in canine diabetes mellitus. Recently, at the University of Glasgow, a mixed (primary stabilisation or secondary investigation) referral population of diabetic dogs had a high frequency (34%) of concurrent hyperadrenocorticism or diabetes associated with metoestrus (Graham, 1995).

In human medicine, diabetes mellitus is broadly classified into idiopathic and secondary forms and several uncommon, specific or prediabetic states such as malnutrition-associated diabetes mellitus, gestational diabetes mellitus and impaired glucose tolerance. Within the idiopathic category are insulin-dependent (IDDM) and non-insulin-dependent (NIDDM) forms of diabetes mellitus. Secondary diabetes mellitus can arise from a number of causes such as generalised pancreatic disease or injury,

effects of antagonistic hormones or drug toxicities. In very general terms, idiopathic IDDM affects young lean people who then have a tendency to develop ketosis and who require insulin to prevent life-threatening ketoacidosis. IDDM is now known in many cases to be caused by idiopathic immune-mediated islet cell destruction in genetically susceptible individuals. NIDDM, however, tends to affect mature, often overweight, individuals who retain sufficient insulin production to prevent ketosis and may be managed by oral hypoglycaemics, diet and weight control alone. The aetiologically descriptive terms type I and type II diabetes mellitus have commonly been used synonymously with IDDM and NIDDM, respectively; however, confusion arises because many restrict the use of the term type I to cases of documented immune-mediated islet cell toxicity and type II to refer to those diabetics who do not have immune-mediated islet cell toxicity or any other known cause of diabetes mellitus, but have a form commonly associated with insulin insensitivity. These classifications may not even be stable within individual patients. Many type I (immune-mediated) diabetics may experience periods when exogenous insulin therapy is not required and, conversely, type II patients may sometimes require insulin injections as adjunctive management. In 1985, the World Health Organization suggested that the terms type I and type II should lose their aetiopathological connotations and be used synonymously with the clinically descriptive terms IDDM and NIDDM. This proposal met with controversy and has not been uniformly followed.

In canine medicine, it is likely that a large percentage of diabetic dogs fit into the 'secondary' category since immune-mediated diabetes mellitus and type II disease are infrequently reported. In addition, nearly all diabetic dogs can be said to be insulin dependent. Unfortunately, in attempts to have a classification system similar to that for human medicine, some veterinary diabetologists have used the term type I in reference to all those forms of diabetes mellitus in which insulin production failure appears to be the primary problem and type II to all those in which insulin insensitivity seems to be the principal component, regardless of the underlying aetiologies. The term type III has even been proposed to describe a condition which most closely resembles the impaired glucose tolerance category in human diabetic medicine (Mattheeuws *et al.*, 1984b).

More appropriate language for the description of canine diabetics may include reference to the status of insulin dependency and the principal underlying aetiology, when it is known or can be surmised. Examples of such descriptions might include: 'spontaneous insulin-dependent diabetes mellitus', 'insulin-dependent diabetes mellitus in association with hyperadrenocorticism', 'suspected islet cell hypoplasia' and 'transient diabetes mellitus associated with metoestrus'.

INCIDENCE AND EPIDEMIOLOGY

The prevalence of canine diabetes mellitus has been estimated to be between 0.0005 and 1.5% (Krook *et al.*, 1960;

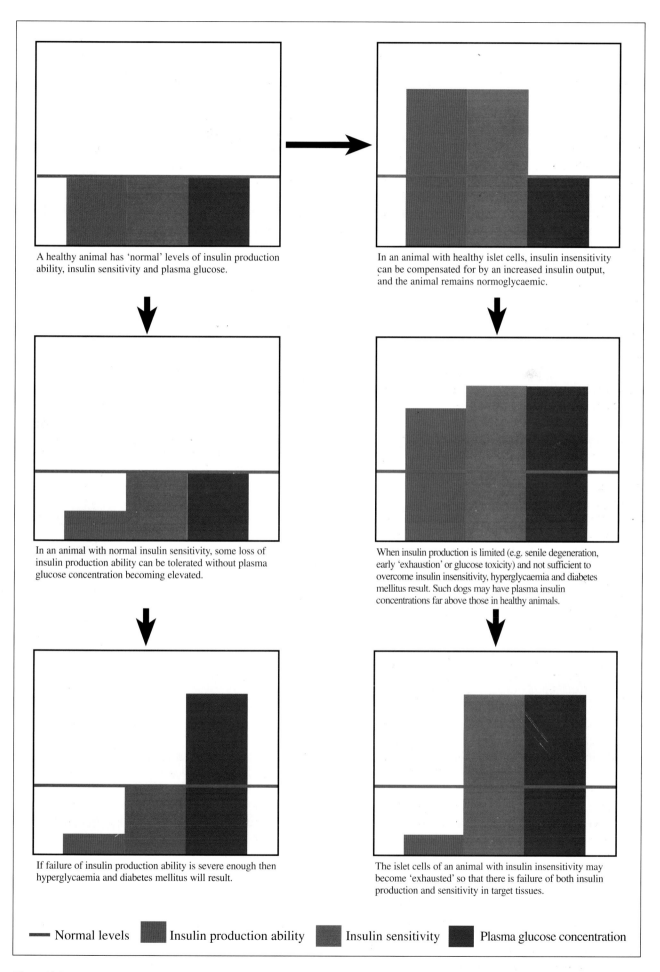

A healthy animal has 'normal' levels of insulin production ability, insulin sensitivity and plasma glucose.

In an animal with healthy islet cells, insulin insensitivity can be compensated for by an increased insulin output, and the animal remains normoglycaemic.

In an animal with normal insulin sensitivity, some loss of insulin production ability can be tolerated without plasma glucose concentration becoming elevated.

When insulin production is limited (e.g. senile degeneration, early 'exhaustion' or glucose toxicity) and not sufficient to overcome insulin insensitivity, hyperglycaemia and diabetes mellitus result. Such dogs may have plasma insulin concentrations far above those in healthy animals.

If failure of insulin production ability is severe enough then hyperglycaemia and diabetes mellitus will result.

The islet cells of an animal with insulin insensitivity may become 'exhausted' so that there is failure of both insulin production and sensitivity in target tissues.

— Normal levels   ▮ Insulin production ability   ▮ Insulin sensitivity   ▮ Plasma glucose concentration

Figure 12.1: *Conceptual pathways to diabetes mellitus.*

Wilkinson, 1960; Mattheeuws *et al.*, 1984b).

Diabetes can occur at any age but the peak prevalence is in animals of 7 years or older. Females may be at greater risk of developing diabetes than males but this relationship is age associated; in dogs <7 years old, males are at an equivalent or greater risk (Marmor *et al.*, 1982; Mattheeuws *et al.*, 1984b; Graham, 1995). The difference in the prevalence of diabetes mellitus between entire and neutered bitches is also age dependent. Entire females in the 8–10 year old age group are over three times more likely to be diabetic than neutered females (Graham, 1995). The explanation for this age/gender effect is probably that the necessary degree of metoestrus-associated islet cell exhaustion (either on its own or in combination with other processes) will take many oestrous cycles to develop and result in a late middle age onset of the disease. Mammary tissue has been identified as the source of progesterone-induced GH secretion (Selman *et al.*, 1994), and neoplastic mammary tissue may also be responsible for greater production of GH (a powerful insulin antagonist) than is normal during metoestrus. This may mean that the epidemiology of diabetes mellitus in this group of dogs parallels the epidemiology of canine mammary neoplasia to some extent. Figure 12.2 shows an overweight, middle aged, neutered female Labrador Retriever with diabetes mellitus.

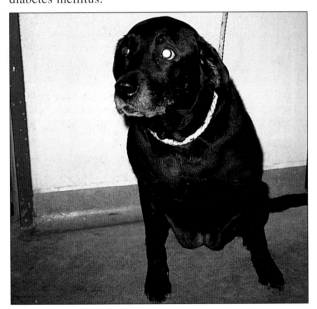

Figure 12.2: *A middle aged overweight neutered female Labrador Retriever with diabetes mellitus.*

Certain breeds appear to have a greater prevalence of diabetes mellitus than others. Doxey *et al.* (1985) found that crossbred terriers, Cairn Terriers and Poodles were over-represented when compared with a reference population. Over-represented breeds at the University of Glasgow Veterinary School include terriers (particularly the Jack Russell, Cairn and Tibetan), Miniature Poodles, English Setters, Collie crosses and Rottweilers, while underrepresented breeds include German Shepherd Dogs and Golden Retrievers (Graham, 1995). In the USA, predisposed breeds include Dachshunds, Poodles, terriers, Keeshonds, Alaskan Malamutes, Schipperkes, and Miniature Schnauzers.

Polyuria
Polydipsia
Polyphagia
Weight loss
Exercise intolerance/decreased activity
Ketotic breath
Recurrent infection (urinary tract, conjunctivitis)
Cataracts
Hepatomegaly

Table 12.2: *Clinical and historical features of canine diabetes mellitus.*

HISTORY AND CLINICAL PRESENTATION

The major clinical and historical features of canine diabetes mellitus are listed in Table 12.2.

Most diabetic dogs are alert and appear reasonably healthy apart from a history of polydipsia, polyuria and occasionally inappropriate urination. Diabetic dogs may appear less healthy if the disorder is compounded by concurrent illness such as bacterial infection. A small proportion of diabetic dogs will present in a collapsed, depressed state with a history of anorexia and vomiting in addition to previous polyuria and polydipsia. These dogs generally have ketoacidosis and require intensive care. In some rare instances, owners have failed to notice the classical features of diabetes mellitus until their dog becomes 'suddenly' blind due to cataract formation.

The classical features of polydipsia and polyuria are the result of osmotic diuresis due to hyperglycaemia. Polyphagia occurs in dogs with severe insulin deficiency. This is because the hypothalamic satiety centre requires the presence of circulating insulin to monitor blood glucose concentration and to assess the body's need for food. Weight loss occurs as a result of the mobilisation of peripheral stores of lipids (adipose tissue) and protein (muscle) for gluconeogenesis in the liver. This influx of precursors causes hepatic lipidosis which can be detected clinically as hepatomegaly.

Recurrent urinary tract infections are not uncommon

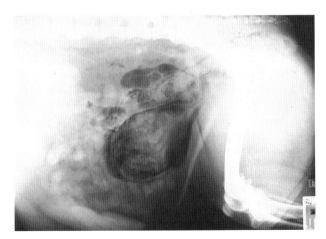

Figure 12.3: *Lateral caudal abdominal radiograph of an 11 year old neutered female Bearded Collie Dog with emphysematous cystitis. Extensive gas lying within the wall of the bladder can be clearly seen. Both diabetes mellitus and hyperadrenocorticism were present.*

Hyperglycaemia	Glucosuria

Diabetes mellitus
Diabetogenic hormonal disorders
    Hyperadrenocorticism
    Acromegaly
    Phaeochromocytoma
Iatrogenic
    Intravenous fluids containing glucose
    Glucocorticoids
    Progestogens
    α_2-Agonist sedatives e.g. xylazine, medetomidine
Stress
	Diabetes mellitus
	Stress
	Intravenous fluids containing glucose
	Renal tubular dysfunction
	    Toxicities
	    Renal failure
	    Primary renal glucosuria
	    Fanconi syndrome
	Test interference
	    Salicylates or vitamin C in urine can affect
	        glucose test strip or tablet results
	    Contamination of collecting device

Table 12.3: Causes of hyperglycaemia and/or glucosuria in the dog.

and may prompt an investigation for diabetes mellitus. The bladder of a diabetic dog provides a nutrient-rich and possibly immunologically compromised environment which favours bacterial proliferation. Occasional diabetic dogs will have emphysematous cystitis, a particularly intractable urinary tract infection associated with intramural gas-forming bacteria (Figure 12.3). Emphysematous cystitis rarely occurs in dogs that do not have diabetes mellitus and/or hyperadrenocorticism.

DIAGNOSIS AND CLINICAL PATHOLOGY

The diagnosis of diabetes mellitus is made when there is persistent fasting hyperglycaemia and glucosuria. Stress, certain other illnesses and some forms of therapy can cause moderate increases in blood glucose in animals that do not have diabetes mellitus. Generally, dogs with blood glucose concentrations exceeding 14 mmol/l are diabetic. In dogs with positive urinary glucose concentrations, hyperglycaemia should be confirmed by blood glucose analysis before embarking on insulin therapy. This ensures that the differential diagnosis of primary renal glucosuria or Fanconi syndrome is ruled out. Table 12.3 lists common reasons for erroneous diagnoses of diabetes mellitus.

Intravenous glucose tolerance test

The intravenous glucose tolerance test IVGTT (1g/kg 40% dextrose) has often been recommended for the diagnosis of diabetes mellitus in equivocal cases. In the author's experience, animals with mild hyperglycaemia (less than the renal threshold of 10–12 mmol/l) do not display the clinical signs of diabetes mellitus and are unlikely to be candidates for insulin replacement therapy, making the evaluation of impaired glucose tolerance by IVGTT academic and unnecessary. Occassionally, the IVGTT is useful in evaluating dogs in which the condition seems to have resolved. These are usually diabetic dogs who have been previously stabilised and whose insulin requirements have fallen well below 0.5 IU/kg/day. Healthy dogs can return their blood glucose concentration to baseline or below within 2 hours of the administration of 1 g/kg 40%

dextrose.

Glucagon response test

The glucagon response test may be a much more useful test for evaluating newly diagnosed diabetic dogs. Insulin concentrations are measured after the injection of 1 mg glucagon at 0, 5, 10, 15 and 30 minutes. The results can provide information on the ability of the cells to produce insulin, and may help identify those dogs with insulin insensitivity as the primary aetiology.

Other biochemical abnormalities

Other clinical chemistry abnormalities include hypercholesterolaemia and hypertriglyceridaemia resulting from increased lipid flux because of loss of hormone-sensitive lipase inhibition in adipose tissue. Lipaemia is particularly noticeable in blood samples taken following a meal when triglyceride-rich chylomicrons are at their highest concentration.

Hepatic lipidosis often causes increased plasma concentrations of alkaline phosphatase (ALP), as swelling impedes biliary flow, and hepatocellular stress may cause elevations in alanine aminotransferase (ALT). Occasionally, diabetic dogs will have elevated concentrations of plasma aspartate aminotransferase, reflecting the catabolism of peripheral tissues for gluconeogenesis in addition to any reflection of hepatocellular injury.

Measurement of ketones

Depending on the type or 'severity' of the diabetes mellitus, ketonaemia and/or ketonuria may be present. Measurement of ketones is usually semiquantitative, using test strips or powders; these are generally much more sensitive to acetoacetate or acetone than β-hydroxybutyrate. Alternatively, quantitative measurement of β-hydroxybutyrate can be performed. It is sometimes noted that ketonuria seems to worsen during early therapy for diabetic ketoacidosis. This should not cause concern as it may only reflect a shift in the principal ketone from β-hydroxybutyrate to acetoacetate to which urine test reagents are more sensitive. Therefore, such a result is an indicator of good clinical response — if there is doubt about its significance, analysis of plasma β-hydroxy-butyrate would be valuable.

Haematology

Dramatic haematological changes are rare in diabetic dogs. Dehydration may elevate haematocrit and infection may elevate the white cell count or cause a left shift. In a few cases there may be a mild non-regenerative anaemia of chronic illness. Heinz body formation or haemolysis, which occasionally arise in severely ketoacidotic cats, are not seen in dogs unless there is extreme hypophosphataemia.

Urinalysis

Urinalysis may reveal findings consistent with urinary tract infection such as haematuria, pyuria, proteinuria and bacteriuria.

TREATMENT

Oral hypoglycaemics

Sulphonylureas

The most common form of human diabetes mellitus is type II or NIDDM which tends to be associated with insulin insensitivity and normal or elevated plasma insulin concentrations. NIDDM occurs more commonly in people who are middle aged and overweight and is often controlled using dietary modification and oral hypoglycaemic medication alone. Owners of diabetic animals often enquire if their pet's disease can be controlled by diet or oral medication rather than by daily insulin injections. The most common group of hypoglycaemic agents, the sulphonylureas, are not suitable for use in dogs. Sulphonylureas exert their effects by direct stimulation of insulin secretion by the β cells, a direct hepatic effect decreasing glucose output and the potentiation of insulin action in the liver. Since it is therefore necessary for β cells to have insulin secreting capacity, sulphonylureas are of no benefit in animals without this ability. In addition, in animals with residual insulin production, the stimulation of compromised β cells to produce more insulin could hasten further deterioration. The potential toxic effects of sulphonylureas in dogs are not well defined.

Biguanides

The second group of oral hypoglycaemic agents is the biguanides; metformin is the principal agent in this group. Metformin delays gastrointestinal absorption of ingested nutrients and promotes peripheral utilisation of glucose. However, studies on the use of this drug in spontaneous canine diabetes mellitus are not currently available. In man, metformin can induce hyperlactataemia and life-threatening lactic acidosis when used at high doses, or in the presence of other diseases which predispose patients to acidosis, such as ketonaemia, renal failure and hepatic dysfunction.

α-Glucosidase inhibitors

A new therapeutic agent has been released for human type II diabetes mellitus, either alone or in combination with traditional oral hypoglycaemics. This agent delays the absorption of dietary sugars by directly inhibiting the enzymatic digestion of polysaccharides. The potential role of these α-glucosidase inhibitors in the management of canine diabetes mellitus has yet to be investigated.

Insulins

Almost all diabetic dogs are insulin dependent, or at least require insulin to manage their clinical signs.

Insulin is a large molecular weight peptide (approxi-

Insulin type	Synonym(s)	Duration	Formulation
Neutral	Soluble, regular	Rapid onset, short duration	Soluble unmodified insulin
Isophane	Neutral protamine Hagedorn (NPH)	Delayed onset, intermediate duration	Insulin in stoichiometric proportion with protamine (poorly immunogenic basic protein)
Protamine zinc		Slowly absorbed, long duration	Insulin with excess quantities of protamine and zinc which may inhibit tissue proteases
Lente	Mixed insulin–zinc suspension	Two peaks of activity, intermediate duration	30% amorphous and 70% crystalline insulin–zinc precipitate
Semilente	Amorphous insulin–zinc suspension	Rapid onset, short duration	Precipitate formed between insulin and high zinc concentrations; amorphous structure is easily absorbed to give short duration
Ultralente	Crystalline insulin–zinc suspension	Slowly absorbed, intermediate or long duration	Precipitate formed between insulin and high zinc concentrations; crystalline structure delays absorption to give extended duration
Biphasic		Rapid onset (depending on proportion of neutral insulin), intermediate duration	Mixtures of 10–50% neutral insulin with isophane insulin

Table 12.4: Types of insulin preparation.

mately 5800 kD). As peptides are digested in the intestinal tract, insulin cannot be administered orally; its large size also prevents it being administered transmucosally. Currently, the only feasible route for insulin administration is by subcutaneous injection. Oral and transmucosal delivery systems are still being investigated but so far they lack the sustained release necessary for therapeutic effect (Saffran *et al.*, 1991; Morgan, 1996). Unmodified insulin has only a very short half-life and many repeated injections or continuous infusion would be necessary for therapeutic effect. Consequently, since the purification of insulin for use as a therapeutic product, a number of pharmacological preparations have been developed which prolong the duration of action of insulin when administered subcutaneously (Table 12.4). In general, insulin preparations can be described as short, intermediate or long acting. Short-acting insulin preparations contain neutral (soluble, regular) insulin. Intermediate-acting insulins include isophane (neutral protamine Hagedorn, NPH), lente (mixed insulin–zinc suspension) and biphasic (mixed isophane and neutral) insulin. The long-acting insulin group contains protamine zinc insulin (PZI) and ultralente (crystalline insulin zinc suspension).

In human diabetic medicine there is a noticeable difference in duration of modified insulin preparations which is dependent on the species of origin of the insulin. Bovine insulin is more slowly absorbed and is more immunogenic than either porcine or genetically engineered human insulin. These differ from one another by only one amino acid residue at the end of the β chain (B30).

The choice of a porcine insulin preparation for use in dogs may have some benefits, principally because it is antigenically identical to canine insulin. In the dog, exogenous insulin therapy using purified porcine insulin preparations has induced less immunological response than those of bovine or mixed origin (Feldman *et al.*, 1983) reducing the chances of immunological interference or of unpredictable release of insulin from insulin–

antibody complexes (Bolli *et al.*, 1984). However, the presence of antibodies to exogenous insulin could prolong the duration of action of the preparation and prevent sudden fluctuations in plasma insulin concentrations by the creation of an 'insulin reservoir'. This absence of antibodies to porcine insulin preparations may explain the clinical impression of a more rapid onset and shorter duration of action of porcine insulin preparations than those of bovine or mixed origin (Feldman and Nelson, 1987).

Idealised pharmacokinetics of insulin preparations are shown in Figure 12.4. The times of onset, peak and duration of activity for insulin preparations can vary greatly between individual dogs.

There are currently four insulin preparations with British Veterinary Product Licences:

- Insuvet Neutral (Schering–Plough Animal Health)
- Insuvet Lente (Schering–Plough Animal Health)
- Insuvet PZI (Schering–Plough Animal Health)
- Caninsulin (Intervet UK, Mycofarm).

Caninsulin is an unusual lente insulin. It contains 40 IU/ml insulin while all other insulins in Britain contain 100 IU/ml. This means it must be used with specialised 40 IU syringes. Caninsulin contains porcine insulin, which is antigenically identical to canine insulin. The Insuvet range of insulins are of bovine origin and contain 100 IU/ml. At present there are no isophane insulin preparations licensed for veterinary use in Britain.

INSULIN THERAPY IN UNCOMPLICATED CASES

A relatively detailed discussion with the owners of a diabetic dog is required before action is considered. During this consultation it is necessary to establish the client's level of emotional and financial commitment to their pet, the lifestyle of the household and the owner's willingness to administer insulin every day for the rest of the dog's life. Diabetic dogs can lead an apparently healthy life but the initial cost of stabilisation is only a proportion of the overall cost. During the maintenance phase of therapy the cost of consumables, laboratory monitoring and at least 2 or 3 days of hospitalisation and/or one major laboratory and radiographic investigation per year should be included in the estimated budget.

Stabilisation
There are two distinct phases in treating diabetic dogs with insulin — the stabilisation period and maintenance period. In the stabilisation period the response to injected insulin is monitored each day or on alternate days, and insulin doses, and sometimes diet, adjusted until a satisfactory level of blood glucose control is achieved.

In the maintenance period, insulin doses and diet are not usually changed and control of blood glucose is monitored weekly or monthly. There are many published protocols for stabilisation and maintenance, and recommendations vary greatly, leading to confusion.

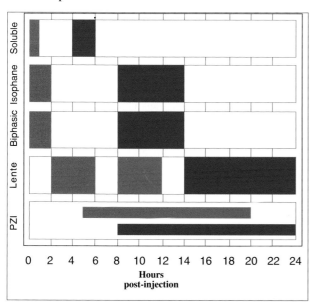

Figure 12.4: *Idealised pharmacokinetics of insulin preparations in dogs (Church, 1981; Feldman and Nelson, 1987; Goeders et al., 1987; Graham et al., 1997). Adapted from Maskell and Graham (1994).* (■ peak; ■ duration; PZI, protamine zinc insulin.)

- Starting dose 0.5–1.0 IU/kg subcutaneously
- Feed evenly divided meals 6–8 hours apart with the first at the time of injection

- **Monitor urine glucose once daily**

Measure urine glucose concentration just before the next injection and calculate insulin dose adjustments for the day.

Urine glucose concentration	Action
Negative	Reduce dose (10% or greater if clinical evidence of hypoglycaemia)
0.1–1%	Keep dose the same
>2%	Small increase in dose (10% or 0.1 IU/kg)

- **Monitor urine glucose three times daily**

Measure urine glucose three times a day and calculate insulin dose adjustment. This method should protect against insulin-induced hyperglycaemia and can be performed by owners at home.

Urine glucose result at approximately:			Dose adjustment
7 hours post–injection (e.g. 3.30 p.m.)	13-14 hours post–injection (e.g. 10.00 p.m.)	Just before insulin injection (e.g. 8.00 a.m.)	
Negative	Negative	Trace	None
Positive	Positive	Positive	Increase by 10%
Negative	Negative	Negative	Decrease by 10%
Negative	Positive	Positive	Decrease by 20% (Somogyi 'overswing')
Negative	Negative	Positive	None
Negative	Positive	Trace	None

- **Monitor single daily (nadir) blood glucose**

Requires access to in-house blood glucose analyser. A blood sample is obtained for glucose analysis when it is likely to be at its lowest (nadir) concentration. Using the single daily injection of intermediate-acting insulin and twice daily feeding schedule this is usually just before the second meal of the day.

Nadir blood glucose concentration (mmol/l)	Action
<3.5	Reduce dose
3.5–7.5	Keep dose the same
7.5–15	Small increase in dose (10% or 0.1 IU/kg)
>15	Large increase in dose (20% or 0.2 IU/kg)

- In all cases tabulate the insulin dose administered and the glucose results. Eventually, insulin doses will tend towards a mean dose which can be selected and adhered to for the first part of the maintenance period.

Table 12.5: Initial diabetic stabilisation using single daily injections of intermediate insulin preparations. Table reproduced from Caninsulin Data Sheet with the kind permission of Intervet UK.

Rigid regimens are useful but it is helpful to apply common sense and flexibility to the formulation of a diabetic management protocol. There are often limitations which prevent the institution of 'perfect' diabetic control but a lot can be achieved in many diabetic animals without extravagant effort or finance.

This section covers the treatment options for the generally bright diabetic dog which has a good appetite and is not vomiting. Dogs that are ketonuric but have a good appetite and are not vomiting can be treated as straightforward uncomplicated diabetics.

The first stage for stabilisation is to reduce the variables which affect glucose response to a particular insulin dose. Typically, this means introducing a daily dietary regimen which is consistent in composition, volume and timing of meals, and deciding on a regular exercise plan for the stabilisation period. These diabetic dogs do not need to be hospitalised if the owners can be relied upon to

adhere to the regimen. Glucose response and changes in insulin dose can be monitored either by returning the dog to the practice for daily blood glucose measurements or by its urine glucose concentrations being measured at home. If the veterinary surgeon is unsure instructions will be followed implicitly, or the dog becomes ill, then hospitalisation is the best policy.

The use of single daily injections of an intermediate-acting insulin preparation (lente or NPH) and two evenly divided meals, one fed at the time of injection and the other 6–8 hours later is a good starting point for initial stabilisation.

There are three principal strategies for adjusting insulin doses when using single daily injections of intermediate-acting insulin. These are measurements of single daily urine glucose, three times daily urine glucose or single daily blood glucose (Table 12.5).

The main disadvantage of single daily urine monitor-

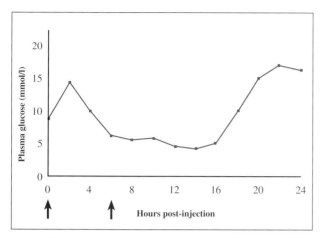

Figure 12.5: Blood glucose curve (24 hour) in a dog receiving a single daily injection of lente insulin and two evenly divided meals (arrows). Note the early morning hyperglycaemia which is comon in dogs receiving a single daily injection of intermediate-acting insulin.

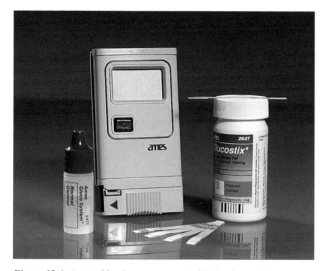

Figure 12.6: A portable glucose meter suitable for the rapid measurement of canine blood glucose.

ing is the possibility of inducing Somogyi 'overswing', i.e. insulin-induced hyperglycaemia. This phenomenon is the result of a physiological response to hypoglycaemia. An insulin-induced hypoglycaemia early in the day causes the release of potent insulin antagonists (cortisol, adrenaline and GH) in an attempt to correct this potentially life-threatening situation. This causes an 'overswing' of blood glucose to very high levels so that glucose appears in the urine and gives a high positive urine glucose result before the next injection. This result can be misinterpreted as the need for an increase in insulin dose, which will worsen the situation further. The potential for insulin-induced hyperglycaemia following single daily urine glucose monitoring may be greatest in those dogs that metabolise insulin rapidly, which are therefore always going to be significantly hyperglycaemic before the next injection.

Making daily adjustments to insulin dose during stabilisation, commonly results in the administration of a higher dose than is ultimately required. This is because it takes 1–3 days to get a consistent glucose response to a new insulin dose. For this reason, at the end of the stabilisation period, dogs should have maintained a consistent blood glucose response to a particular dose of insulin for 3 or 4 days before being considered 'stable' at that dose.

Most dogs will stabilise at 1.0-1.5 IU/kg of intermediate-duration insulin per day. Dogs requiring more than 2.0 IU/kg or that still exhibit clinical signs at or above this dose should be investigated for causes of insulin insensitivity (see Chapter 4).

Although most owners will choose morning insulin injections (8–9 a.m.) and afternoon meals (2–5 p.m.), it may suit some households better to give afternoon injections (4–6 p.m.) and bedtime meals (10 p.m. to midnight). The choice of morning *versus* evening injections has implications for blood glucose monitoring.

After the initial stabilisation period, it is often useful to create a serial blood glucose curve by repeated measurement of blood glucose over a 12–24-hour period (usually every 2 hours). Such curves help in deciding if a dog would be better managed with twice daily injections or a longer acting preparation. The curve might also be useful in deciding if the relative quantities or timing of meals should be altered. Figure 12.5 gives an example of a 24-hour glucose curve; in this example, a moderate decrease in the proportion of the daily ration fed in the first meal would be expected to smooth the glycaemic curve in the early part of the day. A portable glucose meter (Figure 12.6) is suitable for the measurement of canine blood glucose.

Twice daily insulin protocols include those in which the dose is the same at both times of day and meals are fed only at injection times or those in which the evening dose is only half of the morning dose and three equal meals are fed per day (at each injection time and 6–8 hours after the first injection). The latter protocol has two advantages: improved overnight glycaemic control; and a decrease in the risk of nocturnal hypoglycaemia, which can be associated with the equal dose strategy. Recommendations for monitoring and dose adjustments for twice daily injections are more complex than for single daily injections. The generation of 24-hour blood glucose curves provides the most useful information in formulating a monitoring strategy for dogs requiring twice daily injections of insulin.

When hospitalised, some dogs refuse meals. This need not necessarily be a concern during diabetic stabilisation, if the dog is otherwise bright and 'well'. Even in the uncommon event of the blood glucose concentration approaching subnormal range, hunger, the initial physiological response to hypoglycaemia should stimulate the dog's appetite and prevent clinical signs — providing the dog has access to food and that insulin doses are within the therapeutic range.

Diet and exercise

For dietary control, diabetic dogs that have been treated with insulin should receive a consistent ration of food at the same time each day. Diets high in soluble sugars (semi-moist diets) should be avoided. Standard complete canned and/or dry pet foods are acceptable. However, if compositional consistency is to be maintained, caution may be required with those dry diets that have a tendency to settle out leaving larger particles at the top of the container. Initial rations should be calculated as

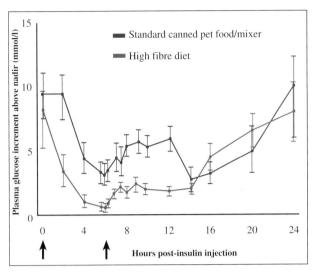

Figure 12.7: Effect of diet type on blood glucose profile in 10 dogs with naturally occurring diabetes mellitus. Blood glucose concentrations are nadir corrected (incremental plasma glucose = absolute plasma glucose minus nadir plasma glucose). Values are mean ± SEM. Evenly divided meals were fed at 0 and 6 hours post-injection (arrows). There was no statistically significant difference in the insulin doses administered between the two diets.

100–150% of normal caloric requirements, and then adjusted to maintain steady body weight once diabetic control has been achieved. Obese diabetic dogs require a weight reduction strategy while others may need to regain weight lost during their illness.

Diets containing high levels of complex carbohydrates, including fibre, can be an excellent adjunct to insulin therapy in diabetic dogs (Figure 12.7). The use of prescription forms of these diets is recommended to ensure consistency. The slow digestion and absorption of carbohydrate from these diets results in smoother glycaemic curves (Graham *et al.*, 1994). Consequently, these diets are contraindicated when rapid absorption of carbohydrate is required, e.g. the treatment of early hypoglycaemia. Although high fibre diets can be of benefit, the presence of concomitant illness with recognised dietary therapies takes priority over the diabetes mellitus. In particular, cardiac disease, renal disease, maldigestion/absorption and subnormal body weight have dietary priority over diabetes mellitus.

In treated diabetic dogs, exercise has a lowering effect on blood glucose in the presence of insulin and, consequently, the duration and timing of exercise periods should be kept reasonably consistent from day to day and should be avoided around the time of nadir (lowest concentration in the day) glucose concentration to reduce the risk of hypoglycaemia. Evening exercise may blunt postprandial increases in blood glucose concentrations in those dogs receiving single daily injections of intermediate-acting insulin in the morning.

Maintenance therapy and diabetic monitoring

Adjustments to insulin dose during the maintenance period should be made on the basis of occasional nadir, or even serial, blood glucose estimations; initially weekly, then fortnightly, and then monthly. Daily urine monitoring

should be stopped after the initial stabilisation period and only reintroduced if problems with stability are encountered. Daily urine monitoring in a clinically well diabetic dog can lead to anxiety and stress on the part of the owner and veterinary staff when spurious results are obtained. In addition, the continuous dose adjustment encouraged by daily glucose monitoring can lead to problems with diabetic stability if strict protocols or supervision are not enforced. Frequent urine (or blood) glucose monitoring is, however, indicated in dogs which are likely to have very dramatic fluctuations in insulin requirement such as diabetes associated with administration of diabetogenic therapies (e.g. long-acting progestogens), during therapy for concurrent hyperadrenocorticism, or in dogs with previously documented idiopathic fluctuating requirements. A phenomenon similar to the human diabetic 'honeymoon' phase in which there is a dramatic reduction in, or disappearance of, insulin replacement requirement during the early part of maintenance therapy, occurs occasionally in newly diagnosed diabetic dogs.

The long-term monitoring of diabetic dogs should include a monthly or two-monthly clinical examination and occasional haematological profiles and urinalyses to assist in the early identification of infections or other problems which could threaten diabetic stability.

The laboratory assessment of long-term glycaemic control can be achieved by measuring plasma fructosamine. The fructosamine concentration is a measure of plasma proteins which have undergone non-enzymatic glycation, and therefore is related to the mean blood glucose concentration over the lifetime of the proteins present (usually considered as the preceding 1–3 weeks). Fructosamine concentrations >400 µmol/l are consistent with poor diabetic control (Reusch *et al.*, 1993; Graham, 1995). Fructosamine concentrations within the canine reference range (162–310 µmol/l) in dogs on single daily injections of intermediate-acting insulin often indicate insulin overdose (Graham, 1995). One advantage of fructosamine measurement is that its concentration is not dependent on the time of day that the sample is taken (Graham, 1995) making it a particularly useful tool in dogs whose insulin protocol precludes the collection of blood for glucose analysis at the expected nadir.

Glycated haemoglobin is another useful indicator of glycaemic control, reflecting control over the preceding 1–3 months. However, few laboratories offer a valid assay for canine glycated haemoglobin and the long period of integrated blood glucose concentration that it measures compromises its clinical use. The assessment of glycated haemoglobin is useful in dogs infrequently presented for follow-up examinations, whereas fructosamine analyses can be used to follow the effects of adjustments in management more closely.

Despite the common finding of elevations in plasma concentrations of ALT and ALP in newly diagnosed and poorly controlled diabetic dogs, these are not useful measures of diabetic control. Commonly, ALT and ALP concentrations even increase during early diabetic therapy (Graham, 1995).

COMPLICATIONS AND CONSEQUENCES OF DIABETES MELLITUS

Ketoacidosis

The term 'complicated diabetes mellitus' is often applied when ketoacidosis is present. Ketoacidotic dogs which have vomited, are anorexic or collapsed require intensive care and treatment as outlined in Chapter 19.

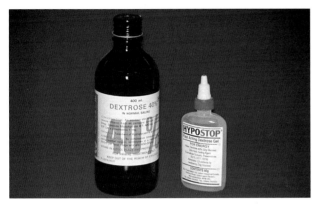

Figure 12.8: *Suitable treatments for hypoglycaemia should be available in veterinary practices.*

Hyperosmolar non-ketotic syndrome

Hyperosmolar non-ketotic syndrome is extremely rare in the diabetic dog. Clinical signs and treament are outlined in Chapter 19.

Hypoglycaemia

Hypoglycaemia becomes a potential complication once insulin therapy is initiated. Fortunately there is a low incidence of clinical hypoglycaemia in dogs treated with insulin. One possible reason for this is the presence of compensatory mechanisms in dogs of reasonable body condition, which respond to, and correct, hypoglycaemia before clinical signs develop. In this way, occasional events of modest insulin overdose can be easily tolerated by most diabetic dogs. A subset of diabetic dogs have, however, recently been identified which mount a poor endogenous response to hypoglycaemia (Duesberg *et al.,* 1995). The mechanism of this phenomenon has yet to be elucidated.

Clinical signs of hypoglycaemia progress through a series of stages depending on its severity. These signs are principally neurological, as the absence of an insulin-dependent glucose transport mechanism in neural tissue means that sufficient ambient glucose concentrations are needed for normal function. Initially, hypoglycaemic dogs will be restless and ravenous and may react unusually to common situations. Subsequently, an occasional stumble will progress to consistent staggering, ataxia and incoordination, followed by twitching and then lateral recumbency and convulsions. If untreated, coma will ensue, leading to death.

Early clinical signs of hypoglycaemia can be treated by offering regular food (but not if high fibre diets) or supplying sugar-rich foods such as sweets or biscuits. If the dog has progressed to a stage where it is unable to eat voluntarily, glucose must be provided. In the home situation, this can be achieved by applying glucose (dextrose) to the dog's gums in the form of powder, syrup, glucose solution or 40% dextrose gel (Figure 12.8). Glucose does not have to be swallowed as it can be absorbed across mucous membranes; it should be applied in this way until the dog is sufficiently coordinated to be offered a meal or until intravenous glucose can be administered.

In the veterinary clinic, 20–50% glucose can be administered intravenously followed by 4% dextrose infusion in cases of severe insulin overdose. A bolus of 1.0 ml/kg 50% dextrose is an appropriate initial dose which can be increased if there is a poor clinical response. An alternative therapy which may be transiently useful is the administration of 1–2 IU of glucagon; this is particularly effective in dogs of good body condition. Dogs in poor condition that have chronic hypoglycaemia may have insufficient mobilisable reserves of gluconeogenic precursors to respond well to glucagon administration.

Clinical hypoglycaemia is likely to occur when an excessive dose of insulin is administered, e.g. a double injection in households where more than one person is responsible for drug administration, when meals are withheld or delayed, when the dog has been inadvertently overexercised, or when insulin requirements have fallen spontaneously or in response to treatment for insulin insensitivity. Hypoglycaemic episodes will generally occur in the afternoon when single daily injections are given in the morning. Neurological signs, e.g. hepatic encephalopathy, occurring at other times of day may be unrelated to hypoglycaemia. Blood glucose estimations at the time of the neurological event will clarify the situation.

If an owner knows their dog will be receiving more exercise, e.g. a long family weekend walk, dietary ration should be increased and precautionary supplies of sweets or dextrose gel made available.

Ocular complications

Cataracts

The formation of diabetic cataracts is of concern for owners of diabetic dogs. Cataracts result from osmotic disruption of the lens due to an accumulation of sorbitol. Sorbitol is a product of the polyol pathway through which intralenticular glucose is metabolised when its concentration exceeds the capabilities of the hexokinase pathway — the first step in the metabolism of glucose by glycolysis, and the citric acid cycle. Diffusion of sorbitol out of the lens is slow; hence, it accumulates and leads to osmotic disruption. Theoretically, good glycaemic control reduces the risk of diabetic cataracts and poor control hastens their onset. However, the occurrence of cataracts is not easily predicted and there are many exceptions to the rule that good control reduces cataracts. In 64 spontaneously diabetic dogs treated with single daily injections of intermediate-acting insulin at the University of Glasgow, the median time taken to become blind due to diabetic cataract was 2.09 years (Graham and Nash, 1996). Numerous stages of development can be detected before

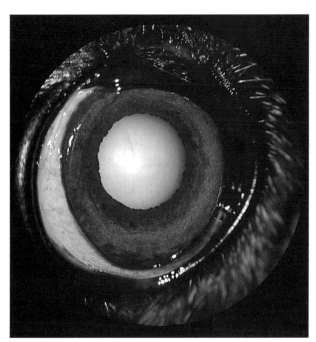

Figure 12.9: *Mature diffuse diabetic cataract in a Labrador Retriever.*

the appearance of mature dense cataracts (Figure 12.9) and blindness.

Uveitis

Another potential ocular complication of diabetes, particularly in dogs with rapid-onset diabetic cataracts, is uveitis resulting in a persistent 'red eye'. This possibility should be considered in diabetic dogs with presumed bacterial conjunctivitis.

Keratoconjunctivitis sicca

Keratoconjunctivitis sicca can occasionally accompany canine diabetes mellitus (Blaxter and Gruffydd-Jones, 1990).

Diabetic retinopathy

Diabetic retinopathy, common in human diabetics, has only rarely been reported in dogs probably due to the long natural history of the condition which exceeds the lifespan of most diabetic dogs.

Infections

Diabetic dogs appear to be susceptible to a variety of bacterial diseases. This susceptibility may result from a combination of compromised immunological function and the nutrient-rich environment which diabetic dogs provide for opportunistic bacteria. This predisposition manifests itself most commonly in the form of conjunctivitis, urinary tract infections, interdigital abscesses and small intestinal bacterial overgrowth (SIBO).

Hepatic complications

A small percentage of diabetic dogs have, or develop, hepatic cirrhosis, presumably due to chronic hepatic compromise associated with poorly controlled diabetes mellitus. The presence of cirrhosis has variable implications for insulin requirement. In some cases,

insulin dose is increased and in others it decreases.

Dermatological complications

Hepatocutaneous syndrome is a rare dermatological complication of diabetes mellitus and certain severe hepatic disorders. It can precede or follow the development of diabetes and is characterised by a severe crusting dermatopathy affecting the distal limbs, feet, face and perineum. This is a difficult skin disease to manage and treatments are palliative only. Diagnosis is made histologically on skin biopsy specimens; hyperparakeratosis with epidermal spongiosis and hyperplasia is usually present.

Neuropathies

Diabetic neuropathies have been documented in dogs. These neuropathies generally affect peripheral nerves and can sometimes resolve following extended periods of good diabetic control.

DIABETES MELLITUS IN SPECIAL SITUATIONS

Concurrent endocrinopathies

Diabetes mellitus with concurrent hyperadrenocorticism or hypothyroidism is discussed in Chapter 4.

Metoestrus

All diabetic bitches should be spayed because of the potential for significant insulin insensitivity during metoestrus. Ovariohysterectomy immediately after a metoestrus-associated occurrence of diabetes mellitus can be curative (Eigenmann, 1981; Reusch *et al.*, 1993; Graham, 1995). Bitches that have indefinite remission of diabetes following ovariohysterectomy tend to have high (>40 µIU/ml; >287 pmol/l) basal serum endogenous insulin concentrations before surgery (Graham, 1995). Bitches with low basal insulin concentrations are less likely to have their diabetes 'cured' by ovariohysterectomy. High plasma insulin concentrations attained in these bitches to compensate for progesterone/GH-induced insulin insensitivity can cause post-ovariohysterectomy hypoglycaemia. This may even occur in bitches with metoestrus-associated insulin insensitivity but without overt diabetes mellitus.

The time at which metoestrus-associated diabetes mellitus often presents after oestrus is not dissimilar to the timing of clinical signs of pyometra. In a polyuric post-oestrous bitch the diagnosis of one of these conditions should not be used to rule out the potential presence of the other.

Pancreatic disorders

Exocrine pancreatic insufficiency (EPI) is another, rare, condition which can occur with diabetes mellitus. A diagnosis is best made by measurement of serum trypsin-like immunoreactivity. The management of concurrent EPI and diabetes mellitus presents a special challenge to both owners and veterinary surgeons, and the prognosis is often poor. Successful therapy can be achieved by following recommended protocols for both conditions independently. Dietary priority is given to the EPI rather than the diabetes mellitus, and a high index of suspicion should be maintained for the potential occurrence of SIBO.

A proportion of dogs will have pancreatitis as a consequence, or a cause, of their diabetes. These dogs can be difficult to diagnose, especially in cases of ketoacidosis, and present difficulties in management. The diagnostic problem arises particularly because of the poor diagnostic efficiency of serum amylase and lipase measurements and the common elevations in the concentrations of these enzymes in azotaemic dogs because of reduced renal clearance.

Concurrent illnesses

When diabetic dogs are not eating due to illness or are being fasted as part of the management of gastrointestinal disturbance, they should still continue to receive some insulin. Withholding both insulin and food promotes ketogenesis and potentially severe illness. Administration of half the dog's normal insulin requirement is usually sufficient to control ketogenesis without significant risk of inducing hypoglycaemia. This 'half-dose' protocol should be continued over the 1 or 2 days it takes to correct gastrointestinal upset, before the dog is returned to its normal dietary management and insulin dose.

General anaesthesia

A similar dose-reduction approach is taken with animals that undergo general anaesthesia, most commonly for ovariohysterectomy or cataract surgery. A half dose of insulin is administered in the morning without food. During anaesthesia, patent intravenous access and dextrose saline infusion are maintained and regular assessment of blood glucose concentrations made throughout the surgery using a portable glucose meter or blood glucose dipsticks. Glucose infusion rate is adjusted accordingly to prevent both hypoglycaemia and significant osmotic diuresis.

Diabetogenic drugs

The use of diabetogenic drugs such as glucocorticoids or progestogens is often said to be contraindicated in diabetic dogs. In certain circumstances, a common sense 'minimal use' approach may be better than a rigid 'never use' approach. Knowledge of these agents' potential to produce insulin insensitivity enables monitoring of any increase in insulin requirement resulting from their administration. In the case of a bitch that has not been spayed, the veterinary surgeon should be aware of the potential need to increase insulin dose following the administration of a progestogen (or during the phase of endogenous progesterone release) and also of the need to decrease the dose again (in some cases very sharply) when the agent or endogenous hormone starts to disappear. In the case of glucocorticoids (e.g. in the treatment of eosinophilic or lymphocytic/plasmacytic enteritis or seasonal dermatopathies), the oral administration of minimum effective doses of prednisolone is preferred to parenteral use of long-acting preparations. In this way, the dose can be easily adjusted or therapy withdrawn if it appears to cause intolerable complications of diabetic management.

PROGNOSIS AND LONGEVITY

A common question during the initial consultation with owners of a newly diagnosed diabetic dog, is how long their dog is likely to survive if they embark on daily insulin therapy. A study of 86 diabetic dogs treated with single daily injections of intermediate-acting insulin and two meals a day revealed a median survival time of 2.71 years (Graham and Nash, 1995). However, diabetes mellitus can affect a wide age range of dogs and when survival data were corrected for age and gender using a general canine population, relative survival rates of close to, or greater than, 100% were observed for up to 4.5 years of follow up (Graham and Nash, 1995).

REFERENCES AND FURTHER READING

Alejandro R, Feldman EC, Shienvold FL and Mintz DH (1988) Advances in canine diabetes research: Etiopathology and results of islet transplantation. *Journal of the American Veterinary Medical Association* **193**, 1050–1055

Blaxter AC and Gruffydd-Jones TJ (1990) Concurrent diabetes mellitus and hyperadrenocorticism in the dog: Diagnosis and management of eight cases. *Journal of Small Animal Practice* **31**, 117–122

Bolli GB, Dimitriadis GD, Pehling GB, Baker BA, Haymond MW, Cryer PE and Gerich JE (1984) Abnormal glucose counterregulation after subcutaneous insulin in insulin-dependent diabetes mellitus. *New England Journal of Medicine* **310**, 1706–1711

Campbell KL and Latimer KS (1984) Transient diabetes mellitus associated with prednisone therapy in a dog. *Journal of the American Veterinary Medical Association* **185**, 299–301

Church DB (1981) The blood glucose response to three prolonged duration insulins in canine diabetes mellitus. *Journal of Small Animal Practice* **22**, 301-310

Doxey DL, Milne EM and MacKenzie CP (1985) Canine diabetes mellitus: a retrospective survey. *Journal of Small Animal Practice* **26**, 555–561

Duesberg CA, Havel P, Elliott D, Feldman E, Gingerich R and Nelson R (1995) Impaired counter regulatory response to insulin-induced hypoglycemia in diabetic dogs (Abstract). *Journal of Veterinary Internal Medicine* **9**, 181

Eigenmann JE (1981) Diabetes in elderly female dogs: recent findings on pathogenesis and clinical implications. *Journal of the American Animal Hospital Association* **17**, 805–812

Eigenmann JE and Venker-van Haagen AJ (1981) Progestagen-induced and spontaneous canine acromegaly due to reversible growth hormone overproduction: clinical picture and pathogenesis. *Journal of the American Animal Hospital Association* **17**, 813–822

Elie M and Hoenig M (1995) Canine immune-mediated diabetes mellitus: a case report. *Journal of the American Animal Hospital Association* **31**, 295–299

Feldman EC and Nelson RW (1987) Diabetes mellitus. In: *Canine and Feline Endocrinology and Reproduction*, pp. 229-273. WB Saunders, Philadelphia.

Feldman EC, Nelson RW and Karam JH (1983) Reduced antigenicity of pork insulin in dogs with spontaneous insulin-dependent diabetes mellitus (IDDM). *Diabetes* **32**, 153A

Goeders LA, Esposito L and Peterson ME (1987) Absorption kinetics of regular and isophane insulin in the normal dog. *Domestic Animal Endocrinology* **4**, 43–50

Graham PA (1995) *Clinical and epidemiological studies on canine diabetes mellitus*. PhD Thesis, University of Glasgow, Scotland

Graham PA, Maskell IE and Nash AS (1994) Canned high fiber diet and postprandial glycemia in dogs with naturally occurring diabetes mellitus. *Journal of Nutrition* **124**, 2712S-2715S

Graham PA, McKellar QA and Nash AS (1997) The pharmacokinetics of a highly purified porcine insulin zinc suspension (IZS-P) in dogs with naturally occurring diabetes mellitus. *Journal of Small Animal Practice* **38**, 434–438

Graham PA and Nash AS (1995) How long will my diabetic dog live? In: *Proceedings of the British Small Animal Veterinary Association Annual Congress, Birmingham.* p. 217. BSAVA, Cheltenham

Graham PA and Nash AS (1996) When will my diabetic dog become blind? In: *Proceedings of the British Small Animal Veterinary Association Annual Congress, Birmingham.* p. 224. BSAVA, Cheltenham

Haines DM and Penhale WJ (1985) Autoantibodies to pancreatic islet in canine diabetes mellitus. *Veterinary Immunology and Immunopathology* **8**,149

Krook L, Larsson S and Rooney JR (1960) The interrelationship of diabetes mellitus, obesity and pyometra in the dog. *American Journal of Veterinary Research* **21**, 120–124

Marmor M, Willeberg P, Glickman LT, Priester WA, Cypress RH and Hurvitz AI (1982) Epizootiologic patterns of diabetes mellitus in dogs. *American Journal of Veterinary Research* **43**, 465–470

Maskell IE and Graham PA (1994) Endocrine disorders. In: *The Waltham Book of Clinical Nutrition of the Dog and Cat*, ed. JM Wills and KW Simpson. Pergamon/Elsevier Science, Oxford

Mattheeuws D, Rottiers R, Baeyens D and Vermeulen A (1984a) Glucose tolerance and insulin response in obese dogs. *Journal of the American Animal Hospital Association* **20**, 287–293

Mattheeuws D, Rottiers R, Kaneko JJ and Vermeulen A (1984b) Diabetes mellitus in dogs: Relationship of obesity to glucose tolerance and insulin response. *American Journal of Veterinary Research* **45**, 98–103

Morgan RV (1996) Delivery of systemic regular insulin via the ocular route in dogs (Abstract). *Journal of Veterinary Internal Medicine* **10**, 183

Peterson ME, Nesbitt GH and Schaer M (1981) Diagnosis and management of concurrent diabetes mellitus and hyperadrenocorticism in 30 dogs. *Journal of the American Veterinary Medical Association* **178**, 66–69

Reusch CE, Liehs MR, Hoyer M and Vochezer R (1993) Fructosamine: a new parameter for diagnosis and metabolic control in diabetic dogs and cats. *Journal of Veterinary Internal Medicine* **7**, 177–182

Saffran M, Field JB, Pena J, Jones RH and Okunda Y (1991) Oral insulin in diabetic dogs. *Journal of Endocrinology* **131**, 267–278

Sai P, Debray-Sachs M, Jondet A, Gepts W and Assaw R (1984) Anti-beta-cell immunity in insulinopenic diabetic dogs. *Diabetes* **33**, 135–140

Selman PJ, Mol JA, Rutteman GR, Vangarderen E and Rijnberk A (1994) Progestin-induced growth-hormone excess in the dog originates in the mammary-gland. *Endocrinology* **134**, 287–292

Wilkinson JS (1960) Spontaneous diabetes mellitus. *Veterinary Record* **72**, 548–555

World Health Organization (1985) *Diabetes mellitus: Report of a WHO study group*. Technical Report Series 727. WHO, Geneva

CHAPTER THIRTEEN

Feline Diabetes Mellitus

Mark E. Peterson

INTRODUCTION

Diabetes mellitus is one of the most common endocrine diseases of middle-aged and old cats. In general, diabetes mellitus can be described as a heterogeneous group of disorders in which insulin secretion by pancreatic β cells is impaired, or in which tissue cells are resistant to the action of insulin, thereby compromising the body's ability to regulate glucose metabolism. Relative or absolute insulin deficiency accounts for fasting hyperglycaemia, characteristic of this disorder. In addition, some cats have marked insulin deficiency, coupled with relative or absolute glucagon excess; this results in excess delivery of fatty acids to the liver and their subsequent oxidation to ketone bodies (e.g. β-hydroxybutyrate, acetoacetate, and acetone), culminating in the clinical state of ketoacidosis.

Although the diagnosis of diabetes mellitus is often straightforward (i.e. the documentation of persistent severe hyperglycaemia), diabetes mellitus can present a true diagnostic challenge, especially in cats with equivocal clinical signs in which stress-induced hyperglycaemia has not been excluded. Treatment also can be frustrating and difficult, both for the veterinarian and the owner.

CAUSES

Efforts have been made to classify feline diabetes mellitus into categories similar to those used in human patients (Wallace and Kirk, 1990; Lutz and Rand, 1995). In devising these classification schemes, the presence or absence of ketoacidosis is of prime importance because the development of ketoacidosis generally implies absolute insulin deficiency (and therefore insulin dependence), whereas the absence of long-term ketoacidosis indicates at least some endogenous insulin secretion (and therefore lack of insulin dependence). In addition, body weight is important, because patients with absolute insulin deficiency tend to have moderate to marked weight loss, whereas those that retain some endogenous insulin secretion tend to remain either at normal weight or are obese.

Feline diabetes mellitus is classified into three types:

- Type I (insulin-dependent diabetes mellitus (IDDM))
- Type II (non-insulin-dependent diabetes mellitus (NIDDM))
- Type III (secondary diabetes).

Cats with IDDM are thin and ketoacidotic, and life-long insulin administration is absolutely crucial in order to prevent death. By contrast, cats with NIDDM are either of normal weight or obese, and ketoacidosis does not develop, even when insulin administration is withheld for prolonged periods. These cats may benefit from insulin administration but generally do not require insulin treatment in order to survive.

In cats, type III or secondary diabetes can result from a variety of factors such as primary pancreatic disease (e.g. pancreatitis), endocrinopathy (e.g. hyperadrenocorticism and acromegaly), or drug therapy (e.g. glucocorticoids and progestogens). Many cats with secondary diabetes develop moderate to marked exogenous insulin resistance and thereby require large daily doses of insulin to control severe hyperglycaemia (Peterson, 1995). Secondary diabetes may or may not be reversible after correction of the underlying disorder, and some cats require lifelong insulin administration. However, the associated state of insulin resistance generally resolves after correction of the underlying disorder.

Findings	Percentage of cats	
	Uncomplicated diabetes (*n*=66)	Ketoacidotic diabetes (*n*=38)
History		
Polyuria/polydipsia	77	79
Weight loss	68	74
Diminished activity	47	89
Anorexia or poor appetite	29	76
Weakness	20	61
Vomiting	23	45
Polyphagia	23	8
Diarrhoea	14	5
Gait change	8	8
Physical examination		
Muscle wasting	50	47
Dehydration	50	42
Unkempt haircoat	49	47
Obese body condition	38	24
Thin body condition	37	53
Hepatomegaly	21	16
Renomegaly	18	14
Hypothermia	17	45
Icterus	5	0
Plantigrade stance	3	8

Table 13.1: *Findings in 104 cats with diabetes mellitus.*

Unfortunately, most cats cannot be clearly categorised as IDDM, NIDDM, or secondary diabetes mellitus. Determination of serum insulin concentration does not reliably differentiate IDDM and NIDDM (Wallace and Kirk, 1990; Peterson *et al.*, 1994). Body condition (i.e. thin *versus* obese) and the presence or absence of keto-acidosis, appear to be the most practical and useful means of distinguishing cats with suspected IDDM from those with NIDDM.

The only clinical value of attempting such a classification is to help guide treatment, including the choice between oral hypoglycaemic drugs and insulin administration. However, most cats with diabetes mellitus, whether initially classified as IDDM, NIDDM, or secondary diabetes, ultimately require exogenous insulin to control hyperglycaemia.

CLINICAL FEATURES

Diabetes mellitus can develop in cats of any age, breed, or sex. However, the disease is seen most often in middle-aged and older cats and seems to be more common in males than females (Crenshaw and Peterson, 1996). In addition, obesity or high body weight also appear to be an important risk factor in cats.

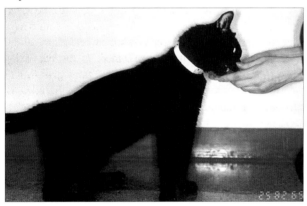

Figure 13.1: *A 10 year old male castrated cat with diabetes mellitus. Note the hindlimb weakness and plantigrade stance.*

Uncomplicated diabetes
Transient or permanent overt diabetes mellitus without acidosis, stupor, or coma is referred to as uncomplicated diabetes. In patients with diabetes, glycosuria occurs when the blood glucose concentration exceeds the renal tubular capacity for glucose resorption (i.e. blood glucose >14–15 mmol/l). The resulting osmotic diuretic effect causes an increase in urine volume. In accord with this, polyuria is one of the most classical signs associated with diabetes mellitus (Table 13.1) (Plotnick and Greco, 1995; Crenshaw and Peterson, 1996). Increased urination leads to hypovolaemia, which, coupled with hyperosmolality, results in polydipsia as the diabetic cat tries to compensate for loss of body fluids. While polyuria and polydipsia are common in cats with uncomplicated diabetes, these signs often go unnoticed by owners, and are often difficult for the veterinarian to assess accurately. Most cats with uncomplicated diabetes mellitus retain a normal appetite,

whereas polyphagia is observed in approximately 25% (see Table 13.1). Despite a normal to increased appetite, weight loss from impaired carbohydrate metabolism and increased fatty acid oxidation by peripheral tissues is common.

Physical examination of a diabetic cat may reveal muscle wasting, dehydration, a poor hair coat, and hepatomegaly (resulting from hepatic lipidosis). Cats with uncomplicated diabetes may be thin or obese. Although not common, diabetic cats may develop a plantigrade posture (i.e. walking with the hocks touching the ground), probably due to peripheral neuropathy (Figure 13.1).

Ketoacidotic diabetes mellitus
Ketoacidotic diabetes mellitus is characterised by persistent fasting hyperglycaemia, ketonaemia, and metabolic acidosis. In addition to a history consistent with previous uncomplicated diabetes mellitus, clinical signs in cats with ketoacidosis include polyuria, polydipsia, weight loss, anorexia, vomiting, diarrhoea, lethargy, weakness, and dehydration (see Table 13.1) (Plotnick and Greco, 1995; Crenshaw and Peterson, 1996; Bruskiewicz *et al.*, 1997). These clinical signs may develop in various combinations and are usually severe in the ketoacidotic cat. Without proper treatment, ketoacidosis is a major cause of death in cats with diabetes mellitus.

Non-ketotic hyperosmolar diabetic syndrome
Non-ketotic hyperosmolar diabetic syndrome is an uncommon but serious complication of diabetes mellitus in cats. The syndrome is characterised by severe hyperglycaemia (i.e. blood glucose concentration >35 mmol/l), hyperosmolality (>350 mmol/kg), extreme clinical

Findings	Percentage of cats
Complete blood count	
Haemoconcentration	50
Anaemia	6
Leucocytosis	43
Serum chemistry profile	
Hyperglycaemia	100
Elevated alkaline phosphatase	74
Elevated alanine aminotransferase	71
Hypercholesterolaemia	55
Azotaemia	41
Hyperproteinaemia	40
Hyperbilirubinaemia	36
Hypokalaemia	28
Hyponatraemia	18
Hypophosphataemia	7
Complete urinalysis	
Glucosuria	100
Proteinuria	80
Ketonuria	37
Active (inflammatory) sediment	16

Table 13.2: *Routine laboratory findings in 104 cats with diabetes mellitus.*

dehydration, and absence of ketoacidosis. Cats with non-ketotic hyperosmolar diabetes usually present with stupor or coma caused by hyperosmolarity of the plasma (Peterson et al., 1994; MacIntire, 1995). Before the development of non-ketotic hyperosmolar diabetic syndrome, classical signs of diabetes (e.g. polydipsia, polyuria, polyphagia, and weight loss) are usually observed. In cats with non-ketotic hyperosmolar diabetic syndrome, it is believed that the increasing osmolality begins to impair central nervous system (CNS) function causing mental confusion, reduced water intake, dehydration, and azotaemia. Concurrent diseases, such as cardiac or renal failure, which impair the ability to retain water and excrete sodium, may precipitate non-ketotic hyperosmolar coma. Renal excretion prevents blood glucose from exceeding 25 mmol/l, unless the glomerular filtration rate is altered by renal or prerenal factors.

DIAGNOSIS

Many abnormalities may be found during the routine laboratory testing of cats with diabetes mellitus (Table 13.2). A stress leucogram as well as a mild non-regenerative anaemia may be detected, especially in cats with ketoacidosis. Hypercholesterolaemia is common. In addition, increases in activities of serum alanine aminotransferase (ALT), alkaline phosphatase (ALP), and bilirubin may result from the hepatic lipidosis that develops in untreated diabetes. Mild to severe dehydration commonly leads to prerenal azotaemia and hyperalbuminaemia, especially in ketoacidosis. Serum electrolyte imbalances in the form of hyponatraemia, hypokalaemia, and hypophosphataemia can also occur in diabetes, most often in ketoacidosis.

The diagnosis of overt diabetes mellitus is based on the finding of persistent fasting hyperglycaemia (>10 mmol/l) together with glycosuria (see Table 13.2). However, it is not uncommon to find blood glucose concentration in excess of 10–15 mmol/l in non-diabetic cats suffering from the stress of another illness. Stress-induced adrenaline release causes hyperglycaemia by increasing hepatic glucose production and inhibiting peripheral glucose uptake. However, the vast majority of cats with untreated diabetes mellitus have marked hyperglycaemia, with blood glucose concentration increasing to >15 mmol/l and even as high as 60 mmol/l.

The use of an assay for glycosylated haemoglobin has been shown to be useful for confirming a diagnosis of diabetes mellitus (Elliot et al., 1997). The non-enzymatic and irreversible binding of glucose with haemoglobin over the lifespan of erythrocytes reflects the average blood glucose concentration over the lifespan of the red blood cells (70 days in cats). However, this test is technically difficult to perform, and therefore its availability is limited. In addition, feline haemoglobin and erythrocytes have certain peculiarities which may make the test invalid in this species.

Serum fructosamine, however, can be measured quickly, easily, and economically, and the test has been shown to be useful in differentiating long-term hyperglycaemia associated with diabetes from short-term stress hyperglycaemia (Crenshaw et al., 1996; Reusch et al., 1993; Thoresen and Bredal, 1996). Fructosamine refers to albumin and other plasma proteins which have been linked to glucose by a non-enzymatic chemical reaction known as glycation. Measuring the serum fructosamine concentration is a means of assessing the average blood glucose concentration in an individual over the preceding 1–2 weeks.

Although glycosuria is a consistent finding in cats with diabetes mellitus, the diagnosis of diabetes should never be established only on the basis of single or even multiple urine glucose determinations, since certain renal proximal tubular disorders can cause renal glycosuria. Although an unusual occurrence, even stress-induced hyperglycaemia can be severe enough to cause the renal tubular glucose threshold to be exceeded and result in transitory glucosuria in an individual cat. Trace amounts of ketone bodies can also be found in cats suffering from starvation as well as from diabetes mellitus. However, if large amounts of ketones are present, especially in a cat with concomitant hyperglycaemia (>15 mmol/l) and glucosuria, a diagnosis of diabetic ketoacidosis is strongly indicated and treatment should be initiated at once.

Overall, a diagnosis of diabetes mellitus is dependent on the finding of marked and persistent hyperglycaemia and glycosuria in a cat with clinical signs suggestive of diabetes. If marked hyperglycaemia and glycosuria are documented in a cat with concurrent ketoacidosis, a diagnosis of diabetes mellitus is indicated. If the cat lacks appropriate clinical signs or does not have glycosuria, measurement of serum fructosamine should be included as part of the initial diagnostic work-up to differentiate stress hyperglycaemia from true diabetes mellitus.

TREATMENT

After verifying the diagnosis of diabetes mellitus, proper treatment is determined by the category of the disease (i.e. uncomplicated, ketoacidotic or non-ketotic hyperosmolar). Approximately half to two thirds of diabetic cats have uncomplicated diabetes mellitus, and one third to a half are ketoacidotic (Crenshaw and Peterson, 1996). Non-ketotic hyperosmolar diabetes is very rare in cats.

The appropriate initial treatment for the three types of diabetes mellitus is different. Initial treatment of ketoacidosis and non-ketotic hyperosmolar coma requires the use of a short-acting insulin such as regular (neutral) insulin. For initial treatment of uncomplicated diabetes, the use of an intermediate-acting insulin such as lente insulin or neutral protamine Hagedorn (NPH) insulin, or a long-acting insulin such as protamine zinc insulin (PZI) is generally recommended (Nelson et al., 1992; Bertoy et al., 1995; Dowling, 1995; Greco et al., 1995). Alternatively, cats with uncomplicated diabetes that are suspected of having NIDDM can initially be managed without insulin treatment by use of dietary modification (to induce weight loss) and, possibly, oral hypoglycaemic agents (Nelson et al., 1993; Ihle, 1995; Feldman *et al.*, 1997). These cats should be monitored carefully; if they become ill or ketoacidotic, or remain persistently hyperglycaemic, then insulin administration should be initiated. It is important to remember that the presence of ketoacidosis implies an absolute lack of insulin secretion; cats that develop ketoacidosis should not under any circumstances be considered candidates for anything but insulin therapy.

Ketoacidotic diabetes mellitus

The treatment of ketoacidotic diabetes mellitus is outlined in Chapter 19.

Non-ketotic hyperosmolar diabetes

The treatment of non-ketotic hyperosmolar diabetes is outlined in Chapter 19.

Uncomplicated diabetes mellitus

The aims of treating cats with diabetes are not as stringently defined as those for humans and dogs with diabetes. In general, the aim of treatment is to achieve an acceptable concentration of blood glucose (7–14 mmol/l), to prevent ketone body formation, and to cause remission of clinical signs of the disease. Achieving strict euglycaemia throughout the day in a diabetic cat is probably not of critical importance. Cats do not generally develop the overt ophthalmological changes (e.g. cataracts) that commonly develop in dogs. Furthermore, control of polyuria and polydipsia are not as important in cats as in dogs; excessive urination is less likely to be of concern for a cat owner as most indoor cats use litter boxes.

Dietary therapy

Diabetic cats that are obese should lose weight. A gradual weight loss of no more than 1–2% of body weight weekly should be accomplished by reducing the cat's food intake to 60–70% of the caloric requirement for the cat's optimal weight, determined initially as 15% less than the current weight. Obese cats should not be allowed to undergo rapid weight loss or fast for more than 2 days because clinically symptomatic hepatic lipidosis may develop. Diabetic cats that are thin should be fed a high-calorie diet initially, and cats that are already of an acceptable body weight should be fed normally. Semi-moist foods generally should be avoided because their high sugar content may lead to postprandial hyperglycaemia.

Recently, high-fibre diets have been advocated in the management of cats with diabetes mellitus. High fibre in the diet slows the rate of glucose absorption, preventing wide fluctuations in blood glucose concentration, and this may reduce the need for insulin (Ihle, 1995). Overall, these diets may help more by promoting weight loss than by controlling postprandial hyperglycaemia.

Diabetic cats receiving insulin should have their meals spaced according to their insulin administration. With the administration of a long-acting insulin preparation once daily, the cat should be fed one half of its calorie ration at the time of insulin injection and the remainder at the time of peak insulin activity (i.e. approximately 6–12 hours later). When a cat is receiving insulin twice daily, meals should coincide with insulin administration. For cats accustomed to having dry food available at all times throughout the day, it may be unreasonable to try to adhere to a regimented feeding schedule. Indeed, cats suspected of having NIDDM that are not receiving insulin should be encouraged to eat several small meals throughout the day to minimise postprandial hyperglycaemia.

Oral hypoglycaemic agents

Hypoglycaemic agents (i.e. sulphonylureas) administered orally are often used, together with diet, to control hyperglycaemia in human patients with NIDDM. These drugs have several antidiabetic actions, including the acute stimulation of insulin secretion by β cells, chronic enhancement of muscle and adipose tissue carbohydrate transport, a direct effect on the liver to reduce hepatic glucose output, and potentiation of insulin action on the liver.

When used in conjunction with dietary therapy, oral hypoglycaemic agents seem to be effective in controlling hyperglycaemia in some cats with uncomplicated diabetes (and suspected NIDDM). Glipizide is the sulphonylurea usually used. Glipizide is administered orally at a dosage of 0.25–0.5 mg/kg every 12 hours, up to 5 mg/cat every 8–12 hours. In cats, the side effects associated with glipizide administration include vomiting, anorexia, and hepatopathy; blood dyscrasias have also been reported in humans. The efficacy of treatment with oral hypoglycaemic agents should be evaluated with home monitoring of urine glucose and ketone concentrations, as well as weekly fasting and 2-hour postprandial blood glucose concentrations. If hypoglycaemia or normoglycaemia develops, glipizide should be discontinued. Glipizide may be reinstituted if hyperglycaemia recurs, although the dose should be reduced if hypoglycaemia occurred with previous treatment. If the cat does not respond to glipizide (i.e. blood glucose concentrations are >15 mmol/l after 1–2 months of treatment), becomes ill or ketoacidotic, or develops adverse side effects, the drug should be discontinued and insulin therapy started.

Before glipizide is considered for use in a cat with NIDDM, it should be strongly suspected that the cat has residual β cell function. Although not always reliable in separating IDDM from NIDDM in cats, the best candidates for oral hypoglycaemic treatment would be cats with normal or high serum insulin concentrations, indicating the persistence of endogenous insulin secretion. It is important to remember that the use of oral hypoglycaemic agents, such as glipizide, is not the equivalent of an 'oral insulin' and that such drug treatment should be used only in cases that are properly diagnosed. Although NIDDM clearly does exist in some cats, care should be taken so as not to make it a diagnosis of convenience and an excuse to avoid insulin injections.

Insulin therapy

The value of insulin in the treatment of diabetes mellitus in cats is well established. However, there is a considerable degree of controversy regarding which type of insulin to use, how often it should be administered, and when to monitor urine and blood glucose concentrations.

In general, treatment for uncomplicated diabetes mellitus in cats should be initiated with either a long-acting insulin preparation (e.g. PZI) given once daily or an intermediate-acting insulin (e.g. lente) administered twice daily. In some diabetic cats, hyperglycaemia can be adequately controlled with the administration of PZI once daily, but others will require injections twice daily. Compared with long-acting insulin preparations, lente insulin has a more rapid onset of action and a shorter duration of action, and its administration once daily would rarely, if ever, satisfactorily control hyperglycaemia in diabetic cats. Therefore, if an intermediate-acting insulin preparation is used, it is recommended that the cats initially receive insulin injections on a split dose basis, with similar doses given at 12-hour intervals. When initiating treatment with an intermediate- or long-acting insulin, it is best to start with a relatively low dose (0.25–0.5 IU/kg/day) and to increase the dose slowly as needed.

Initial monitoring of diabetic treatment
Initial regulation of insulin dosage is best done at home by the owner, since diet and exercise are two important variables that affect insulin requirements. During the first 1–2 weeks, the owner should measure their pet's urinary glucose and ketone concentrations once to twice daily, if possible. In general, 2–3 days are required for insulin and glucose homeostasis to stabilise after initiation or adjustment of insulin dosage. Therefore, dosage adjustments should be based on recurring effects, not on the results of a single urine glucose determination. Based on the urine glucose readings and clinical response (e.g. lessening of polyuria, polydipsia, and weight gain), the daily insulin dosage should be adjusted by 0.5–1.0 unit increments (or decrements) every 3–4 days as directed by the veterinary surgeon (usually over the phone). After 7–14 days of treatment, the cat should be re-examined.

Many diabetic cats develop complications associated with underdosage or overdosage of insulin because owners are misled by urine glucose concentrations. Persistent morning glycosuria may suggest an insulin underdosage, but can also be caused by a variety of other factors. Therefore, although urine glucose measurements can help in making insulin dose adjustments, frequent blood glucose determinations are a better means of ensuring good diabetic control. Because of the remarkable variation in onset, peak, and duration of effect of both intermediate- and long-acting insulin preparations, however, checking only one or two blood glucose concentrations over a 24-hour period is of little value in assessing diabetic control and may be misleading. Multiple blood glucose determinations are required to adequately evaluate diabetic control.

Initially, the diabetic cat should be re-evaluated at intervals of 2 weeks until satisfactory glycaemic control is achieved. During these rechecks, serum fructosamine (or glycosylated haemoglobin) should be determined, and serial blood glucose concentrations monitored throughout the day, if possible (Miller, 1995). Monitoring serum fructosamine concentrations is useful in assessing the degree of glycaemic control in treated diabetic cats; fructosamine

concentrations remain very high in cats that are poorly regulated, whereas levels fall to normal or only slightly high in cats that are well regulated.

The following protocol is recommended on the day planned for evaluation of serial blood glucose concentrations:

1. In the morning, the owner should inject their cat with insulin and provide its food.
2. As soon as possible, the cat should be brought to the hospital for the first blood glucose determination.
3. Additional samples for blood glucose measurement (only a few drops of blood are needed) should be collected at 2–3-hour intervals for the first 12 hours, and additionally at 4-hour intervals for the second 12 hours if the cat is on insulin therapy once daily.
4. The evening meal should consist of the same amount and type of food that is served at home.

Based on the results of these glucose determinations, adjustments in insulin dosage or type are made as necessary. In the well controlled diabetic, circulating glucose concentrations remain between 7 and 14 mmol/l during the entire day, and serum fructosamine concentration decreases to within reference range limits.

Long-term monitoring
Once the cat is reasonably controlled, checks every few months are recommended. These rechecks should consist of a history, physical examination, review of urine glucose measurements, and blood tests to evaluate long-term glycaemic control (i.e. measurement of serum fructosamine or glycosylated haemoglobin). During long-term insulin treatment, owners should continue to monitor for recurrence of clinical signs, as well as measure urine glucose and ketone concentrations at least once or twice a week. If a cat is consistently glycosuric or if ketonuria is detected on more than 2–3 consecutive days, the cat should be brought to the hospital for re-evaluation. It is usually not necessary to perform a glucose curve on a well regulated diabetic patient. If there is ever any doubt concerning the diabetic cat's control, however, serial blood glucose determinations are recommended.

During both initial and long-term insulin treatment, owners should frequently be reminded to watch for signs of hypoglycaemia, one of the most common complications associated with insulin therapy (MacIntire, 1995). Signs of hypoglycaemia include weakness, lethargy, shaking, head tilt, ataxia, convulsions, and coma. If hypoglycaemia is prolonged, death may result from depression of the respiratory centre. If mild signs of hypoglycaemia develop, the cat should be fed its normal food. If severe signs such as convulsions or coma develop, a tablespoon of sugar water or 40% dextrose gel should be rubbed on the buccal mucosa. Food or fluids should never be forced down the mouth of a convulsing cat or fingers placed inside the cat's mouth. If no response to food or sugar is observed within a few minutes, the cat should be taken to the veterinarian and dextrose administered intravenously (see Chapter 19). Whenever signs of hypoglycaemia occur, the insulin dose needs to be decreased until the appropriate dose is determined by a serial blood glucose curve.

Some diabetic cats lose their requirements for insulin after several weeks to months of therapy (Lutz and Rand, 1995). Cats with transient diabetes usually begin to develop frequent hypoglycaemic attacks as the insulin requirements gradually decrease. Once the diabetic state has resolved, these cats may go for weeks to years without requiring insulin, although severe hyperglycaemia will again develop in some cats. Although the pathogenesis of transient diabetes in cats remains unclear, such cats must have some insulin secretory reserve (i.e. they are not totally insulin deficient), and may indeed have NIDDM. In such cats, overt diabetes could develop during periods of insulin resistance, stress, or after treatment with drugs (e.g. glucocorticoids or progestogens).

REFERENCES

Bertoy EH, Nelson RW and Feldman EC (1995) Effect of lente insulin for treatment of diabetes mellitus in 12 cats. *Journal of the American Veterinary Medical Association* **206**, 1729–1731

Bruskiewicz KA, Nelson RW, Feldman EC and Griffey SM (1997) Diabetic ketosis and ketoacidosis in cats: 42 cases (1980–1995). *Journal of the Amercan Veterinary Medical Association* **211**, 188–192

Crenshaw KL and Peterson ME (1996) Pretreatment clinical and laboratory evaluation of cats with diabetes mellitus: 104 cases (1992–1994). *Journal of the American Veterinary Medical Association* **209**, 943–949

Crenshaw KL, Peterson ME, Heeb LA, Moroff SD and Nichols R (1996) Serum fructosamine concentration as an index of glycemia in cats with diabetes mellitus and stress hyperglycemia. *Journal of Veterinary Internal Medicine* **10**, 360–364

Dowling PM (1995) Insulin therapy for dogs and cats. *Canadian Veterinary Journal* **36**, 577–579

Elliot DA, Nelson RW, Feldman EC and Neal LA (1997) Glycosylated hemoglobin concentration for assessment of glycemic control in diabetic cats. *Journal of Veterinary Internal Medicine* **11**, 161–165

Feldman EC, Nelson RW and Feldman MS (1997) Intensive 50-week evaluation of glipizide administration in 50 cats with previously untreated diabetes mellitus. *Journal of the American Veterinary Medical Association* **210**, 772–777

Greco DS, Broussard JD and Peterson ME (1995) Insulin therapy. *Veterinary Clinics of North America: Small Animal Practice* **25**, 677–689

Ihle S (1995) Nutritional therapy for diabetes mellitus. *Veterinary Clinics of North America: Small Animal Practice* **25**, 585–597

Lutz TA and Rand JS (1995) Pathophysiology of feline diabetes mellitus. *Veterinary Clinics of North America: Small Animal Practice* **25**, 553–561

MacIntire DK (1995) Emergency therapy of diabetic crises: insulin overdose, diabetic ketoacidosis, and hyperosmolar coma. *Veterinary Clinics of North America: Small Animal Practice* **25**, 639–650

Miller E (1995) Long-term monitoring of the diabetic dog and cat: Clinical signs, serial blood glucose determinations, urine glucose, and glycated blood proteins. *Veterinary Clinics of North America: Small Animal Practice* **25**, 571–584

Nelson RW, Feldman EC and DeVries SE (1992) Use of ultralente insulin in cats with diabetes mellitus. *Journal of the American Veterinary Medical Association* **200**, 1828–1829

Nelson RW, Feldman EC, Ford SL and Roemer OP (1993) Effect of an orally administered sulfonylurea, glipizide, for treatment of diabetes mellitus in cats. *Journal of the American Veterinary Medical Association* **203**, 821–827

Peterson ME (1995) Diagnosis and management of insulin resistance in dogs and cats with diabetes mellitus. *Veterinary Clinics of North America: Small Animal Practice* **25**, 691–713

Peterson ME, Randolph JF and Mooney CT (1994) Endocrine diseases. In: *The Cat: Diagnosis and Clinical Management, 2nd edn*, ed. RG Sherding, pp. 1404–1506. Churchill Livingstone, New York

Plotnick AN and Greco DS (1995) Diagnosis of diabetes mellitus in dogs and cats. Contrasts and comparisons. *Veterinary Clinics of North America: Small Animal Practice* **25**, 563–570

Reusch CE, Liehs MR, Hoyer M and Vochezer R (1993) Fructosamine: A new parameter for diagnosis and metabolic control in diabetic dogs and cats. *Journal of Veterinary Internal Medicine* **7**, 177–182

Thoresen SI and Bredal WP (1996) Clinical usefulness of fructosamine measurements in diagnosing and monitoring feline diabetes mellitus. *Journal of Small Animal Practice* **37**, 64–68

Wallace MS and Kirk CA (1990) The diagnosis and treatment of insulin-dependent and non-insulin-dependent diabetes mellitus in the dog and the cat. *Problems in Veterinary Medicine* **2**, 573–590

CHAPTER FOURTEEN

Canine Hypothyroidism

David L. Panciera

INTRODUCTION

Hypothyroidism is a common endocrinopathy in the dog, with a prevalence estimated at between 0.2% and 0.64%. A wide array of clinical signs have been attributed to hypothyroidism. Diagnosis requires specific testing, which must then be properly interpreted. An understanding of the many factors that affect thyroid function tests is necessary for establishing a correct diagnosis. Treatment is relatively straightforward and the prognosis is generally good.

AETIOLOGY AND PATHOGENESIS

Hypothyroidism may result from destruction of the thyroid gland (primary hypothyroidism), inadequate pituitary thyrotropin (thyroid stimulating hormone, TSH) secretion (secondary hypothyroidism), or decreased hypothalamic secretion of thyrotropin releasing hormone (TRH). Over 95% of cases of canine hypothyroidism are primary. Approximately 50% of these occur because of immune-mediated destruction of the thyroid gland. The remainder result from idiopathic atrophy of the thyroid gland. Thyroid neoplasia and congenital disease resulting from defects in hormone synthesis or thyroid agenesis are rare causes of primary hypothyroidism. Secondary hypothyroidism occurs when trauma, neoplasia or cyst formation destroys the TSH-secreting thyrotrophs in the anterior pituitary gland. Deficiencies of other hormones often accompany this form of hypothyroidism. Tertiary hypothyroidism (TRH deficiency) has not been confirmed in the dog.

Autoimmune thyroiditis

Anti-thyroglobulin antibodies are present in approximately 50% of hypothyroid dogs. This corresponds with a similar incidence of lymphocytic thyroiditis confirmed histologically in hypothyroid dogs. These autoantibodies have also been reported to occur in 43% of dogs with non-thyroidal endocrine diseases, and 47% of dogs closely related to hypothyroid dogs with anti-thyroglobulin autoantibodies (Haines *et al.*, 1984). Dogs with normal thyroid hormone concentrations but clinical signs consistent with hypothyroidism (Thacker *et al.*, 1992) and those without endocrine disease (Haines *et al.*, 1984) had an anti-thyroglobulin autoantibody prevalence of approximately 15%. Hypothyroidism and lymphocytic thyroiditis occur in certain breeds with a high incidence. Lymphocytic thyroiditis has been demonstrated to be inherited in laboratory Beagles and in a family of Borzois. These findings are supportive of a role of inheritance in autoimmune thyroid disease and hypothyroidism. Autoantibodies to thyroid hormones are occasionally present in dogs. The prevalence of autoantibodies to triiodothyronine (T3) is higher than that of thyroxine (T4), and estimates have varied widely from 0.3% to 33% of samples submitted for evaluation of thyroid function (Kemppainen and Young, 1992, Thacker *et al.*, 1992).

Idiopathic atrophy

Little is known about the pathogenesis of idiopathic follicular atrophy. Early in this disorder, degenerative changes occur in the follicular cells, with eventual replacement of the thyroid gland by adipose connective tissue. Inflammation is minimal if present at all. Idiopathic follicular atrophy is not associated with thyroglobulin autoantibodies and may represent a degenerative rather than an inflammatory process.

CLINICAL FEATURES

Hypothyroidism most commonly occurs in middle aged, pure bred dogs. Many breeds are seemingly predisposed, with Dobermann Pinschers and Golden Retrievers probably having the highest incidence. The prevalence of hypothyroidism among breeds is likely to vary according to country. Intact males and neutered females have been reported to have an increased risk of hypothyroidism (Panciera, 1994a), although other studies have failed to find any gender predisposition.

The clinical signs of hypothyroidism are varied (Table 14.1) because thyroid hormones act on virtually all cells in the body to cause diverse biological effects. In general, hypothyroidism causes a decrease in the metabolic rate which is manifested by lethargy, dullness, obesity, and occasionally cold intolerance. Lethargy is often overlooked by owners who comment on the increased activity level of their pet only after thyroid hormone supplementation is instituted. Hypothyroidism generally results in mild to moderate obesity, although some hypothyroid dogs are severely obese.

Dermatological features

Dermatological changes are the most common clinical

abnormalities in hypothyroid dogs. Alopecia, dry, dull hair coat, and/or seborrhoea occur in the majority of hypothyroid dogs (Table 14.1). Flaking of skin or seborrhoea may be the earliest cutaneous manifestation of hypothyroidism in many dogs. Abnormal sebum production and keratinisation lead most frequently to dry seborrhoea, although the oily form can also occur. Ceruminous otitis externa may also be present in hypothyroid dogs, and secondary *Malassezia* or bacterial pyoderma can occur. Hair loss is variable and breed dependent. Alopecia often is first noted

in areas undergoing friction, such as the neck in dogs wearing collars, and the tail, resulting in the characteristic 'rat tail' (Figure 14.1). As the disease becomes advanced, the alopecia is distributed in a bilaterally symmetrical pattern, sparing the limbs (Figure 14.2). Large breed dogs reportedly can develop alopecia on the extremities without truncal alopecia. Hyperpigmentation may or may not be present. Hypertrichosis occurs rarely in Irish Setters and possibly in other breeds due to improper shedding of hair. Alopecia occurs in hypothyroid dogs because the hair follicle fails to enter the anagen phase of hair growth in the absence of thyroid hormones. As hair is shed, new hair fails to regrow, and alopecia results. Histological findings in skin biopsies from hypothyroid dogs include follicular atrophy, epidermal hyperkeratosis, epidermal melanosis, and a predominance of hair follicles in the telogen phase.

Superficial or deep pyoderma occurs occasionally in hypothyroid dogs. Hypothyroidism may be a risk factor for development of pyoderma, since local and systemic immunity may be impaired. Studies in man and other animals have shown minimal to mild decreases in immune function in hypothyroidism. Dogs with recurrent bacterial pyoderma or *Malassezia* infection should be tested for hypothyroidism unless another underlying cause is apparent.

Myxoedema occurs when there is excessive dermal accumulation of glycosaminoglycans (hyaluronic acid), resulting in non-pitting oedema. This oedema is most

Common findings

Dermatological abnormalities:
    Seborrhoea
    Alopecia
    Pyoderma
    Myxoedema
Reduced metabolic rate:
    Obesity
    Lethargy
    Cold intolerance
Cardiovascular abnormalities:
    Low voltage ECG complexes
    Hypocontractility
    Bradycardia
Neuromuscular abnormalities:
    Weakness

Uncommon findings

Peripheral neuropathy:
    Vestibular
    Facial
    Generalised neuropathy
    Forelimb lameness
    Laryngeal paralysis
Myopathy
Megaoesophagus
Central nervous system disease
Myxoedema stupor/coma
Dwarfism
Reproductive abnormalities
Hypoadrenocorticism
Insulin-resistant diabetes mellitus
Exercise intolerance
Ocular abnormalities

***Table 14.1**: Clinical manifestations of hypothyroidism.*

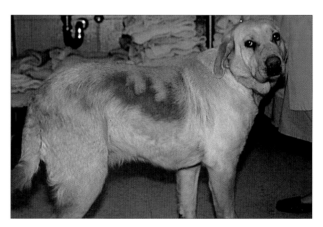

***Figure 14.2**: Truncal alopecia. Bilaterally symmetrical truncal alopecia and cutaneous hyperpigmentation are common in many breeds of dog with hypothyroidism.*

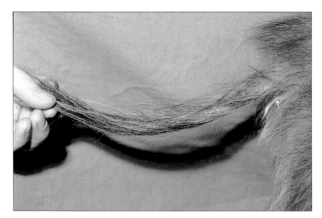

***Figure 14.1**: 'Rat tail'. Alopecia of the tail in a hypothyroid Shetland Sheepdog. Alopecia is often initially present on the tail and neck of hypothyroid dogs.*

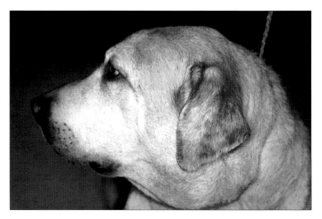

***Figure 14.3**: Myxoedema. The non-pitting oedema present in this dog causes the 'tragic' facial expression sometimes found in hypothyroid dogs. Myxoedema is rarely evident in other parts of the body.*

commonly apparent around the face, causing the 'tragic' facial expression found in some hypothyroid dogs (Figure 14.3).

Neurological features

A number of neurological abnormalities, including localised neuropathies, generalised peripheral neuropathies and central neurological disease have been reported with increasing frequency in hypothyroid dogs. Regardless of the particular neurological abnormality, other signs of hypothyroidism are usually present in affected dogs.

Generalised peripheral neuropathy has been documented in hypothyroid dogs (Jaggy et al., 1994). Signs range from mild to severe, and may include generalised weakness, exercise intolerance, proprioceptive deficits, and hyporeflexia. Although signs resulting from generalised neuropathy are uncommon, abnormalities on electromyogram occur frequently in hypothyroid dogs without signs of peripheral neuropathy (Kaelin et al., 1986), leading to the belief that subclinical neuropathy or myopathy occurs frequently. Findings on histological examination of nerve biopsies, though inconsistent, have included myelin irregularities, intercalated internodes, internodal globules and myelin degeneration. Clinical signs completely resolve within 1–3 months of initiating treatment. The cause of generalised neuropathy is unknown, but may be the result of impaired axonal transport secondary to decreased activity of the sodium–potassium ATPase pump.

A common neurological abnormality is peripheral vestibular disease (Panciera, 1994a; Jaggy et al., 1994). Dogs present with a history of acute or subacute onset of signs referrable to vestibular nerve dysfunction including head tilt, nystagmus, ataxia and circling. Many dogs will have concurrent facial nerve paralysis or paresis. It is thought that these neurological deficits occur when myxoedematous deposits in the common dural sheath of the vestibular, cochlear and facial nerves compress the nerves. Alternatively, the neuropathy could be similar in pathogenesis to that of generalised neuropathy, since some dogs with localised neuropathy have electromyographic evidence of generalised neuromuscular disease. Signs of vestibular and facial nerve dysfunction generally resolve within 2 months of initiating treatment, although the head tilt may persist for many months. Unilateral forelimb lameness has also been reported as a localised neuropathy in hypothyroid dogs (Budsberg et al., 1993). Affected dogs have pain on manipulation of the glenohumeral joint and have electromyographic abnormalities compatible with generalised peripheral neuropathy.

Laryngeal paralysis has been suggested to occur secondary to hypothyroidism (Jaggy et al., 1994). Laryngeal paralysis is often a localised manifestation of a generalised neuropathy, and a cause and effect relationship with hypothyroidism remains to be proved.

Another inadequately documented neurological or muscular abnormality that occurs in hypothyroid dogs is megaoesophagus. Although oesophageal dysfunction certainly may be present in some hypothyroid dogs, it appears to occur rarely and the megaoesophagus usually persists despite thyroid hormone supplementation (Jaggy et al., 1994; Panciera, 1994a; Dewey et al., 1995). Failure of the megaoesophagus to resolve may be more related to the prolonged duration of oesophageal dysfunction than to a lack of response to levothyroxine treatment. A recent report has described concurrent megaoesophagus, the presence of acetylcholine receptor antibody suggestive of myasthenia gravis, and subnormal thyroid function (Dewey et al., 1995).

The central nervous system (CNS) can also be affected in hypothyroidism. Central vestibular disease, strabismus, facial nerve paralysis, paresis or hemiparesis, and dysmetria are the most common findings (Bichsel et al., 1988). The cause of CNS disease is unknown, but could be due to the decreased sodium–potassium ATPase-dependent axon transport as proposed in peripheral neuropathy, or it may result from cerebrovascular atherosclerosis. Neurological signs improve gradually in most affected dogs, with partial or complete resolution within 5 months of initiating treatment.

A myopathy can also occur in hypothyroid dogs. Stiff gait, weakness, dragging of the limbs, and exercise intolerance may be manifestations of hypothyroid myopathy. However, myopathy has only been convincingly confirmed in a small number of dogs that did not have the aforementioned clinical signs. Peripheral neuropathy could account for similar clinical signs, so differentiating neuropathy from myopathy, if considered necessary, would require assessment of nerve conduction velocities and nerve or muscle biopsies.

Cardiovascular features

The cardiovascular effects of hypothyroidism are largely the opposite of those that occur during hyperthyroidism, and of a lesser magnitude. They include a weak apex beat, muffled heart sounds, poor pulse quality and bradycardia. A mild decrease in left ventricular function is often detectable using echocardiography (Panciera, 1994b). Possible mechanisms of reduced cardiac function include a change in the isoform of myosin from the V_3 form to the less active V_1 form, decreased β-adrenergic receptors, decreased myocardial adenylate cyclase activity, decreased rate of sarcoplasmal calcium uptake, coronary atherosclerosis, and changes in peripheral circulation including decreased vascular volume and increased peripheral vascular resistance. The most common electrocardiographic abnormality, a decrease in R-wave amplitude, occurs in approximately 50% of hypothyroid dogs. Some hypothyroid dogs have bradycardia (approximately 25%) and first degree atrioventricular block, while other arrhythmias, including atrial fibrillation (Gerritsen et al., 1996) and ventricular premature contractions, are less well documented. The detrimental cardiovascular effects of hypothyroidism may contribute to the development of heart failure in dogs with concurrent valvular or myocardial disease.

Reproductive features

Although reproductive abnormalities have long been considered a hallmark of canine hypothyroidism, a recent study has shown that the reproductive condition of male dogs is essentially unaffected by hypothyroidism (Johnson *et al.*, 1995). The effects of hypothyroidism on female reproductive function have not been systematically investigated in dogs, but are reported to include infertility, shortened duration of oestrus, prolonged or irregular anoestrus, and abortion (Johnson, 1994). Inappropriate galactorrhoea, defined as mammary gland development more than 60 to 90 days after oestrus, can occur in intact females with hypothyroidism. This phenomenon results from increased TRH, stimulating pituitary prolactin secretion. Given the paucity of well documented reports, it is likely that hypothyroidism is overdiagnosed as a cause of reproductive abnormalities.

Skeletal features

Dogs and cats with congenital hypothyroidism are affected with disproportionate dwarfism. This results from epiphyseal dysgenesis and delayed epiphyseal maturation. Radiographs reveal minimal epiphyseal ossification of long bones and vertebrae, as well as decreased diaphyseal length. Affected dogs frequently develop osteoarthritis despite thyroid hormone supplementation (Greco *et al.*, 1991). Hypothyroidism reduces growth hormone (GH) secretion, and therefore should be ruled out prior to investigating GH deficiency in cases of dwarfism. Adult dogs have been reported to have stiffness, joint pain and joint capsule swelling without joint effusion or radiographic evidence of articular changes. This appears to occur only rarely, and the signs of stiffness and pain may be associated with myopathy or neuropathy rather than articular disease.

Ocular features

Many ophthalmic abnormalities have been attributed to hypothyroidism, including corneal lipid dystrophy, corneal ulcers, keratoconjunctivitis sicca, anterior uveitis, and retinopathies. These abnormalities appear to occur only rarely and as a consequence of hyperlipidaemia induced by hypothyroidism, since very few documented reports exist and experimental hypothyroidism of 23 weeks' duration failed to induce any ocular abnormalities (Miller and Panciera, 1994).

Other body systems

Thyroid hormone deficiency affects virtually all body systems, in some cases resulting in mild or subclinical abnormalities. For example, gastrointestinal motility is reduced, and may result in vomiting, constipation or diarrhoea, although these signs are rarely recognised in hypothyroid dogs. Secretion of atrial natriuretic hormone is decreased in hypothyroid dogs, while arginine vasopressin secretion is increased. These abnormalities may account for the impaired water excretion that is present in severe myxoedema. Respiratory abnormalities that occur in man include central respiratory depression, respiratory muscle weakness and upper airway obstruction due to myxoedema of the tongue and pharynx, but remain to be reported in dogs.

Congenital hypothyroidism

Both dogs and cats can be affected by congenital hypothyroidism. Causes include thyroid hypoplasia or aplasia, dyshormonogenesis (abnormal thyroid hormone synthesis), decreased production or production of abnormal TSH, and decreased hypothalamic production of TRH. Affected animals typically have broad skulls, disproportionate dwarfism, macroglossia, delayed dental eruption, weakness, obtundation, hypothermia, ataxia, haircoat changes, constipation, goitre (enlarged thyroid gland) and hypercholesterolaemia (Greco *et al.*, 1991). Diagnosis is confirmed in a manner similar to that in adults, but consideration should be given to the fact that puppies have considerably higher serum T4 concentrations than adults. Treatment will fully or partially correct the abnormalities, although animals may be of short stature, develop osteoarthritis, and continue to have impaired mental function. Treatment should raise serum T4 concentrations to the normal range established for the age of the dog in order to ensure euthyroidism.

Myxoedema coma

The most severe and rare form of hypothyroidism, myxoedema coma, manifests as impairments of mental status, thermoregulation, and respiration and cardiovascular function, as well as signs typical of hypothyroidism. Most reported cases of myxoedema coma have been in Dobermann Pinschers. In addition to alopecia and cutaneous myxoedema, affected dogs have severe obtundation, stupor, or coma, hypothermia typically without shivering, bradycardia, hypotension and hypoventilation. Since myxoedema coma represents decompensation of chronic hypothyroidism, precipitating factors including infection, congestive heart failure, and administration of diuretics or respiratory or CNS depressants; or other disorders may be present in affected dogs. Hyponatraemia, hypoglycaemia, hypercholesterolaemia, hypercapnoea, and elevated serum creatine kinase activity may be present. Initial treatment in man consists of intravenous administration of a loading dose of levothyroxine at 3–5 times the standard daily dose, a loading dose of T3 or a combination of the two (Nicoloff and LoPresti, 1993). Subsequent levothyroxine treatment can be administered orally at the standard dosage. Supportive treatment consists of passive warming to relieve the hypothermia. Active warming by applying a heat source may worsen hypotension due to vasodilation of cutaneous vessels leading to circulatory collapse. Fluid therapy with normal saline should be administered judiciously, because although blood volume is decreased, cardiac function is often depressed and water excretion may be impaired secondary to inappropriate secretion of arginine vasopressin. Alternatively, water restriction is effective in correcting hyponatraemia if the patient is well hydrated. Glucose can be added to the intravenous fluids if hypoglycaemia is present. Mechanical ventilatory support may be necessary if hypoventilation and hypercapnoea are severe. Glucocorticoid supplementation is recommended because plasma cortisol concentrations may be inappropriately low for the degree of illness and glucocorticoids may relieve hypotension if present. The prognosis of dogs affected with myxoedema coma is guarded.

Hypothyroidism and other endocrinopathies

Polyglandular autoimmune disease results from auto-immune destruction of multiple endocrine glands including the thyroid, adrenal and parathyroid glands and the pancreas (see Chapter 26). The most frequently reported combination in the dog is hypoadrenocorticism and hypothyroidism. Dogs with concurrent hypoadrenocorticism and hypothyroidism are most often presented because of signs related to adrenocortical insufficiency. Hypercholesterolaemia is present in the majority of dogs with both diseases (Melendez *et al.*, 1996), and in only a small percentage of dogs without concurrent hypothyroidism and hypothyroidism. Diabetes mellitus and hypothyroidism have also been reported concurrently, but the prevalence of these diseases in the same animal appears to be low. Because hypothyroidism induces glucose intolerance and insulin resistance in dogs, adjustment in insulin dosage is frequently necessary after initiating thyroid hormone supplementation in dogs with diabetes mellitus (Ford *et al.*, 1993).

Hypothyroidism can be associated with other endocrinopathies resulting from pituitary disease. Secondary hypothyroidism apparently occurs only rarely following compression or invasion of the pituitary in dogs with neoplasia or cysts. GH deficiency, hypoadrenocorticism and hypothyroidism may occur concurrently in German Shepherd Dogs with pituitary dwarfism.

ROUTINE LABORATORY TESTS

A mild non-regenerative, normocytic, normochromic anaemia occurs commonly in hypothyroid dogs. While the cause of the anaemia is unknown, it probably results in an erythrocyte mass that is appropriate for the reduced oxygen demand present in hypothyroidism. Platelet count may be slightly increased in hypothyroidism, and platelet size is reduced (Sullivan *et al.*, 1993). Functional platelet defects have not been demonstrated in hypothyroid dogs (Avgeris *et al.*, 1990).

Hypothyroidism has been reported to be associated with bleeding tendencies. Deficiency of von Willebrand factor has been suggested to be a cause, because it is decreased in some hypothyroid human patients. Studies in dogs with spontaneous (Panciera and Johnson, 1994) and experimentally induced hypothyroidism (Panciera and Johnson, 1996) have recently shown that hypothyroidism does not induce deficiency of von Willebrand factor and that thyroid hormone supplementation in hypothyroid dogs decreases plasma von Willebrand factor. Buccal mucosal bleeding time is not altered by hypothyroidism. Thus, it appears that hypothyroidism does not result in abnormal haemostasis.

Hypercholesterolaemia is present in up to 75% of hypothyroid dogs. It results from decreased receptor-mediated clearance of cholesterol, decreased lipoprotein lipolysis, and decreased hepatic bile acid production. The elevation of serum cholesterol in hypothyroidism is frequently great, with concentrations exceeding 10 mmol/l in many hypothyroid dogs. Hypertriglyceridaemia also occurs frequently in hypothyroid dogs.

Mild elevations in creatine kinase activity may be found in hypothyroid dogs, and may result from myopathy or decreased clearance of the enzyme due to the hypothyroid state. Serum alkaline phosphatase activity is occasionally mildly elevated in hypothyroidism. The elevation may be the result of concurrent disease or could be secondary to hypothyroidism by some unknown mechanism.

THYROID HORMONE ANALYSES

The varied clinical findings and lack of specific abnormalities in routine laboratory tests make the diagnosis of hypothyroidism dependent on results of specific laboratory tests. Thyroid function tests should be utilised to confirm clinical suspicions and not as a screening test in dogs without compatible clinical abnormalities. Since many non-thyroidal illnesses (including peripheral neuropathy and megaoesophagus which may occur secondary to hypothyroidism) are associated with decreased serum T4 concentrations (Nelson *et al.*, 1991), careful patient evaluation for evidence of hypothyroidism is necessary for proper interpretation of thyroid function tests. An understanding of the control of thyroid hormone secretion is necessary for establishing a diagnosis of hypothyroidism.

Control of the hypothalamic–pituitary–thyroid axis

Circulating thyroid hormone concentrations are a result of the interactions of production, secretion, distribution, metabolism and excretion. Perturbation of any of these factors will result in altered serum thyroid hormone levels. Understanding the control of the hypothalamic–pituitary–thyroid axis has gained new importance in veterinary medicine with the recent development of assays for endogenous canine TSH. Secretion of TSH from the pars distalis of the pituitary is under the positive control of hypothalamic TRH and the negative influence of circulating thyroid hormones, particularly T4. The primary regulators of TRH secretion are the stimulatory influence of α-2 adrenergic activity in the paraventricular nucleus of the hypothalamus and the inhibitory effect of circulating thyroid hormones. TRH induces transcription and secretion of TSH, and also influences the bioactivity of TSH. TSH is a glycoprotein, composed of α and β subunits. The α subunit is identical to that of luteinising hormone and follicle-stimulating hormone, while the β subunit is unique to TSH.

Control of thyroid hormone secretion is mainly through the stimulatory effect of TSH and the negative influence of iodide. Iodide decreases the sensitivity of the thyroid gland to TSH. TSH stimulates thyroid hormone synthesis and secretion and promotes growth of thyrocytes. TSH also increases intrathyroidal deiodination of T4 to T3; so, states leading to increased TSH, such as primary hypothyroidism, are associated with proportionately greater secretion of the more biologically potent T3.

Thyroid hormone transport and metabolism are major factors influencing their serum concentration. Thyroid hormones are highly protein-bound (99.9% and 99% of T4 and T3 are protein-bound, respectively) and any perturbation of binding will have a great influence on total serum concentrations of these hormones. The high degree of protein binding contributes to the relatively long half-life of T4 (10–16 hours) in dogs, but it is short compared with that of about 7 days in human beings. This difference is due to the lower concentration of thyroxine-binding globulin, the major carrier protein in the dog. Other plasma binding proteins include thyroxine-binding prealbumin, albumin, and a high-density lipoprotein (HDL), HDL_2. The half-life of T3 is approximately 6 hours. The principal transport proteins for T3 include albumin and thyroxine-binding globulin. Because only the unbound or 'free' hormone is available to enter cells and to undergo metabolism or excretion, accurate measurements of free hormones would be expected to provide a much better estimate of thyroid status than total hormone concentrations.

The thyroid gland secretes predominantly T4, part of which is then converted intracellularly in extrathyroidal tissues to the more active T3. The primary intracellular hormone is T3, approximately 50% of which is formed by intracellular deiodination of T4 at the 5' position. The enzyme responsible for this conversion, 5'-deiodinase, is present in some form in most tissues. Deiodination can also occur at the 5 position, resulting in production of the metabolically inactive reverse T3 (rT3). Autoregulation of deiodination results in increased production of T3 in states of thyroid hormone deficiency and decreased production of T3 in hyperthyroidism. Altered production and degradation of T3 and rT3 account for many of the alterations of thyroid hormone concentrations present in nonthyroidal illness. Gastrointestinal and renal routes are significant contributors to T4 excretion in the dog.

Serum total T4 and total T3 concentrations

Thyroid function is routinely assessed by measurement of serum total thyroid hormone concentrations. Serum concentrations of total T4 and T3 are measured routinely, while rT3 and other metabolites of T4 are rarely used in the clinical setting. Total T4 concentrations are more reliable than total T3 in assessing thyroid function in most situations in the dog. Serum total T4 concentrations are infrequently normal in hypothyroid dogs, while serum total T3 concentrations have been found to be normal in 15–50% of hypothyroid dogs (Miller *et al.*, 1992; Panciera, 1994a). A likely explanation is that the thyroid gland preferentially secretes T3 in response to increases in TSH, a situation that is frequently present in hypothyroidism. Because of this, total T3 concentration should be evaluated only after considering the total T4 concentration. Serum total T4 is a reliable predictor of euthyroidism, i.e. has a high sensitivity. However, total T4 concentrations measured throughout the day fluctuate to such a degree that at least one measurement was below normal in 50% of euthyroid dogs tested in one study (Miller *et al.*, 1992), imparting a low degree of specificity to the assay. While total T4 concentrations are much more reliable than total T3 for the diagnosis of hypothyroidism, other causes of a decrease in total T4 (discussed below) should be considered.

Assay methodology is an important consideration when measuring serum total T4 concentrations in dogs since normal serum concentrations are 10–25% of those found in humans. Modifications must be introduced into many assays in order to increase the sensitivity sufficiently to detect low concentrations found in dogs. Radio-immunoassay (RIA) has been the standard and most reliable method for measurement of serum total T4 and T3 concentrations for many years. Recent developments in assay methodology have resulted in non-isotopic immunoassay techniques that are as reliable as RIA. Other immunoassay methods have recently been introduced as quantitative assays to be used for measurement of total T4 in practice, but they have not yet been critically evaluated. Enzymatic assays applicable to automated chemistry analysers are used, but their accuracy remains to be determined.

Serum free T4 concentrations

Measurement of free thyroid hormone concentrations circumvents some of the difficulties encountered in the interpretation of total T4 and T3. Because only the hormone that is not bound to plasma proteins is available for transport into cells, free T4 represents the circulating pool that is most closely related to the intracellular T4 content. Most of the non-thyroidal factors that alter protein binding of thyroid hormones have no effect on free T4 concentrations. Because total T4 concentrations are adequate for diagnosis of hypothyroidism in most cases, free T4 is most useful in dogs with non-thyroidal illness or those administered drugs that may alter total T4. Free T4 can be measured by a variety of methods, with equilibrium dialysis considered to be the 'gold standard'. In this technique, a semipermeable membrane with a pore size that allows free T4 to pass but excludes passage of proteins, is used to isolate free T4. Measurement of free T4 by equilibrium dialysis is more accurate than other methods including analogue and two-step immunoassays. Analogue assays for measurement of free T4 have been used extensively in the diagnosis of thyroid disease in veterinary medicine. Most studies have not shown a significant advantage of free T4 measured by analogue assay over measurement of total T4 (Nelson *et al.*, 1991; Beale *et al.*, 1992). Analogue assays appear to be inaccurate in circumstances where accurate measurement of free T4 is most needed — non-thyroidal illness. Although equilibrium dialysis is a relatively expensive technique, the information it provides in animals with non-thyroidal illness cannot be obtained by other methods.

Because of the difficulties inherent in interpreting thyroid hormone function on a single serum sample, it has been suggested that the combination of serum free T4 and cholesterol is the most effective method for predicting the response to thyroid hormone supplementation (Larsson, 1987). Unfortunately, any formula derived using stepwise discriminant analysis, as was used in this study, may not be applicable when other assay methods or laboratories perform the assays. Other studies attempting to develop a similar formula have not been successful.

Endogenous canine thyrotropin concentrations

With the advent of assays that accurately measure endogenous canine TSH (Nachreiner et al., 1995; Williams et al., 1995, 1996), a potentially powerful tool has been added to the diagnostic options available to the small animal practitioner. Loss of functional thyroid tissue secondary to thyroiditis or atrophy (i.e. primary hypothyroidism) leads to a lack of negative feedback of T4 and T3 on the pituitary thyrotrophs. This results in an increase in circulating TSH. The increased TSH promotes increased T4 and T3 synthesis and secretion, which then normalises serum thyroid hormone concentrations. When destruction of the thyroid gland progresses to the degree that it cannot respond to TSH sufficiently to maintain normal thyroid hormone concentrations, hypothyroidism occurs. The hormonal profile during development of primary hypothyroidism should be a progressive increase in serum TSH while serum T4 decreases. Eventually serum TSH concentrations become markedly elevated. While only a small amount of information regarding the clinical use of the canine TSH assay is available, elevated serum TSH is present in 60–80% of dogs with hypothyroidism (Dixon et al., 1996; Jensen et al., 1996; Ramsey and Herrtage, 1996; Scott-Moncrieff et al., 1996). The effects of early primary and central hypothyroidism, drug administration, and non-thyroidal illness on serum TSH in the dog are largely unknown. It does appear, however, that elevated serum TSH is present in some dogs with non-thyroidal illness.

Non-thyroidal factors affecting basal thyroid hormone tests

Age

Serum total T4 concentration at birth is similar to that of adult dogs, but rapidly increases to approximately twice normal adult values by 1 week of age. Total T4 concentrations peak at 2 to 3 weeks of age at 60–100 nmol/l, and gradually decrease to levels found in adults by 6 months of age. Total T4 and responsiveness to TSH administration decrease after middle age. Total T3 concentrations are low at birth, reaching normal adult concentrations in most pups at 5 weeks of age. Total and free T4 concentrations gradually decrease with age, while free T4 gradually increases after a nadir at 8 years. The effect of age on serum TSH concentrations in dogs is unknown, although age does not affect this hormone in humans.

Gender

Gender does not affect thyroid hormone concentrations, but bitches in dioestrus have slightly higher serum total T4 and T3 concentrations than males or females in anoestrus. Pregnant bitches have higher serum total T4 than females in anoestrus or pro-oestrus as well as males.

Breed

Small breeds of dogs have slightly higher total T4 than larger breeds. Some breeds have normal thyroid hormone concentrations that are different from the reference range established for dogs in general. Healthy pet and racing Greyhounds have serum total T4 and free T4 concentrations that are approximately 60% of those in a general pet dog population (Gaughan et al., 1996), while their T3 levels are similar to other dogs. Scottish Deerhounds also have low total T4 (Ferguson, 1994). It remains to be determined which other breeds have unique thyroid hormone concentrations.

Drugs

It is likely that, similar to man, many drugs alter serum thyroid hormone concentrations in dogs. Unfortunately, only a few drugs have been tested. Glucocorticoids are the drugs that most frequently interfere with thyroid function tests. Although the effects are variable, glucocorticoids generally decrease serum concentrations of total T4 and T3. Long-term, high-dose glucocorticoid treatment markedly suppresses total T4 and T3 concentrations. Even free T4 concentrations can be decreased in dogs with hyperadrenocorticism (Ferguson and Peterson, 1992). The mechanisms by which glucocorticoids reduce thyroid hormone concentrations in man include impaired binding to plasma carrier proteins and decreased TSH secretion. Recently, sulphonamides have been implicated in inducing hypothyroidism in dogs. Administration of sulphamethoxazole and trimethoprim (30 mg/kg every 12 hours) for 6 weeks decreased serum total T4 and T3 concentrations and impaired the thyroid hormone response to TSH administration in dogs with pyoderma (Hall et al., 1993). In contrast, a study using trimethoprim and sulphadiazine at 15 mg/kg every 12 hours for 4 weeks failed to demonstrate any effect on serum total T4 and T3, free T4 by equilibrium dialysis or thyroid hormone response to TSH (Panciera and Post, 1992). The effects of sulphonamides on the canine thyroid appear to be dependent on dosage and duration of treatment or on the specific drug used.

Other drugs implicated in reducing total T4 and/or T3 concentrations include anticonvulsants, phenylbutazone, radiocontrast agents, quinidine, mitotane and salicylates. General anaesthesia decreases serum thyroid hormone concentrations for up to 36 hours. Thyroid function testing should be undertaken prior to, or at least 48 hours after, anaesthesia. Previous thyroid hormone supplementation can also affect thyroid function tests. Administration of levothyroxine to euthyroid dogs will result in negative feedback to the pituitary gland and decreased TSH secretion. The resultant thyroid and pituitary gland atrophy will persist for at least 4 weeks after withdrawal of thyroid hormone supplementation, so TSH and thyroid hormone concentrations should be measured after withdrawing treatment for at least 8 weeks. If supplementation is withdrawn after protracted treatment, several months may be required for normalisation of the pituitary–thyroid axis.

Non-thyroidal illness

Non-thyroidal illness is a common cause of decreased total T4 and T3 concentrations, and is frequently referred to as the 'euthyroid sick syndrome'. These changes probably do not reflect a state of hypothyroidism, since free T4 concentrations are usually normal. The most common pattern of thyroid hormone concentration associated with non-thyroidal illness in the dog is a decrease in total T4 and T3, while decreased total T3 with maintenance of T4 is most frequently found in humans. The pathogenesis of the combined low T3 and low T4 in non-thyroidal illness is complex, but appears to involve: impaired deiodinase activity; increased production of sulphated and deaminated forms of thyroid hormones; reduced binding of thyroid hormones to plasma transport proteins and intracellular binding proteins; altered structure of plasma transport proteins; reduced TSH secretion; and direct inhibition of thyroid hormone secretion (Nicoloff and LoPresti, 1995). Cytokines including interleukin (IL)-1, IL-2, tumour necrosis factor-α, and interferon have been implicated in the pathogenesis of the euthyroid sick syndrome. High doses of IL-2 markedly decrease serum total T4 and T3 concentrations in dogs (Panciera et al., 1995). There is no evidence that thyroid hormone supplementation is beneficial in humans or dogs with low serum total T4 and T3 concentrations associated with non-thyroidal illness. The decrease in thyroid hormones may be an attempt by the body to reduce protein catabolism and conserve protein stores and energy.

Subnormal serum concentrations of total T4 and T3, as well as free T4 and free T3 by analogue assay, are frequently found in dogs with severe non-thyroidal illness. Decreased total T4 and/or T3 concentrations have been demonstrated in dogs with congestive heart failure, diabetes mellitus, hyperadrenocorticism, renal failure, hepatic disease, and other illnesses (Larsson, 1987; Ferguson, 1988; Vail et al., 1994). The decrease can be marked, such that serum T4 concentrations below 5 nmol/l are found. Because concurrent disease occurs commonly in hypothyroid dogs, careful assessment of the patient for clinical evidence of hypothyroidism is essential for proper interpretation of thyroid function tests.

Decreased serum total T4 concentration due to severe non-thyroidal illness is associated with a poor prognosis for survival in humans. The only study to investigate this in dogs suggested that baseline and post-TSH serum total T3 concentrations were lower in dogs that did not survive (Elliot et al., 1995). The overlap between survivors and non-survivors was considerable, making low T3 a poor tool for predicting survival in dogs with severe illness.

Two tests of thyroid function currently available for clinical use that are probably less affected by non-thyroidal illness are free T4 by equilibrium dialysis and serum TSH. In humans, free T4 by equilibrium dialysis is only rarely decreased in non-thyroidal illness, and is occasionally elevated. Dogs with a variety of non-thyroidal illnesses and decreased total T4 and T3 concentrations have normal free T4 by equilibrium dialysis (Vail et al., 1994). However, some euthyroid dogs with severe non-thyroidal illness and approximately 25% of dogs with hyperadrenocorticism will have decreased free T4 using this method. Measurement of serum TSH concentration will probably provide a valuable adjunct to free T4 by equilibrium dialysis in dogs with non-thyroidal illness. Unfortunately, little work has been done evaluating serum TSH concentrations in dogs with non-thyroidal illness. Preliminary studies comparing serum TSH concentration in euthyroid, hypothyroid, and euthyroid sick dogs demonstrated some overlap between the groups (Ramsey and Herrtage, 1996; Scott-Moncrieff et al., 1996). Approximately 10–15% of dogs with non-thyroidal illness will have elevated serum TSH concentrations. Mild elevations in serum TSH concentrations also occur in some humans with non-thyroidal illness, particularly during recovery from the illness. Thyroid function tests are best performed in the absence of non-thyroidal illness. If it is not possible to test following resolution of the non-thyroidal illness, the combination of free T4 by equilibrium dialysis and serum TSH is most likely to provide accurate results.

Anti-thyroglobulin antibodies

Antibodies to thyroglobulin, the protein in the thyroid follicle that contains T3 and T4, are present in approximately 50% of hypothyroid dogs. The presence of these antibodies is thought to be a marker for the presence of lymphocytic thyroiditis, although 13–19% of euthyroid dogs may have autoantibodies to thyroglobulin (Haines et al., 1984; Beale et al., 1990). Measurement of antithyroglobulin antibodies may prove to be useful in preventing propagation of hypothyroidism during planned mating of breeds with a high incidence of hypothyroidism, although their utility remains to be established.

Anti-thyroid hormone autoantibodies

Autoantibodies to thyroid hormones indicate the presence of autoimmune thyroid disease and, as such, affected dogs are likely to develop hypothyroidism at some time in the future. Anti-thyroid hormone autoantibodies are important because of the effect they have on measurement of serum thyroid hormones by immunoassay. Serum total thyroid hormone concentrations are falsely elevated in dogs with anti-thyroid hormone autoantibodies when measured by solid phase immunoassays, falsely lowered in assays that have a charcoal separation phase, and variably affected in double antibody techniques. The alterations in measured hormone concentrations have no bearing on the thyroid status of the individual dog, as the antibodies probably act in a manner similar to normal plasma transport proteins unless they are of unusually high affinity. While analogue assays for free T4 and free T3 are similarly affected by anti-thyroid hormone autoantibodies, free T4 measured by equilibrium dialysis is unaffected. Assessment of clinical signs, serum free T4 by equilibrium dialysis, and serum TSH concentration are the best methods by which to determine thyroid function in dogs with anti-thyroid hormone autoantibodies.

TSH response test

Dynamic tests of thyroid function are currently rarely used in clinical practice. The TSH response test, long considered the 'gold standard' for assessing thyroid function in the dog, is rarely used because of the expense and lack of availability of TSH. The TSH response test protocol most often recommended is to obtain samples for measurement of total T4 before and 6 hours after intravenous administration of 0.1 IU/kg of bovine TSH. The expected minimum response is a 6-hour post-TSH serum T4 concentration greater than 30 nmol/l. Recommendations that a doubling of the baseline serum T4 is a useful measure of thyroid function fail to take into account that there is considerable fluctuation of baseline T4 and that it is affected by many non-thyroidal factors. Given the failure of serum endogenous TSH to give an unequivocal assessment of thyroid function, the TSH response test may still be useful in some cases.

TRH response test

The TRH response test has been suggested as an alternative dynamic test of thyroid function, because of the difficulties in obtaining bovine TSH. Administration of TRH results in release of TSH from the pituitary gland, which in turn results in thyroidal secretion of T4. The increase in total T4 and free T4 is small following TRH administration, with normal values suggested to be 1.5 times the baseline or an increase in total T4 of at least 6 nmol/l. Some normal dogs fail to respond to TRH administration with an increase in total T4, while the response of free T4 to TRH appears to be more consistent (Sparkes *et al.*, 1995). The small and variable total T4 response in normal dogs limits the clinical utility of this test. Blood samples should be obtained before and 4–6 hours after intravenous administration of 500 µg of synthetic TRH. Side effects of TRH administration include transient salivation, vomiting, defecation, urination, and depression.

Serum TSH can also be measured after TRH administration. The serum TSH concentration increases by at least 0.15 ng/ml over basal concentration in normal dogs 20–30 minutes after administration of 200 µg TRH in dogs >5 kg and 100 µg in dogs <5 kg bodyweight (Ramsey and Herrtage, 1996). In preliminary studies, this test has not proven to be of use in confirming the diagnosis of primary hypothyroidism since the TSH response may be reduced, normal or exaggerated in these cases.

Recommendations for testing for hypothyroidism

Recommended tests for assessing thyroid function in a dog with classical clinical signs of hypothyroidism include serum total T4 and TSH concentrations. Dogs with uncommon or atypical signs of hypothyroidism may be best assessed by measurement of serum free T4 by equilibrium dialysis and TSH concentrations. Free T4 is preferable to total T4 since the latter is decreased in some euthyroid dogs with megaoesophagus, peripheral neuropathy, and other problems sometimes attributable to hypothyroidism. Dogs with non-thyroidal illness or those receiving drugs known to alter thyroid function tests should be tested after resolution of the illness or discontinuation of the drug if possible. If testing cannot be postponed in these circumstances, measurement of free T4 by equilibrium dialysis and serum TSH, or a TSH response test, are the most appropriate tests. The results should be interpreted cautiously and conservatively in these cases.

TREATMENT OF HYPOTHYROIDISM

The goal of thyroid hormone replacement therapy is to approximate the secretion of thyroid hormone in a normal dog and to resolve clinical signs without causing hyperthyroidism. Treatment is similar for all forms of hypothyroidism, regardless of the underlying aetiology. Treatment must be given for the remainder of the dog's life because the disease process cannot be reversed.

Thyroid hormone preparations

Thyroid extracts have been available for clinical use since hypothyroidism was first treated successfully in man using an extract from sheep thyroid gland in 1891. The amount of T4 and T3 in each preparation varies, but 60 mg of desiccated thyroid contains approximately 60 µg of T4 and 12 µg of T3 (Roti *et al.*, 1993). Thyroglobulin is another preparation available for treatment of hypothyroidism. It is similar to desiccated thyroid in composition, except that it contains approximately 30% more T3. Although preparation of these compounds has become more standardised, concerns about the consistency of hormone content make them undesirable for routine use. Other thyroid extracts include 'natural' thyroid preparations from bovine thyroid glands in the form of tablets. It has been claimed that some of these preparations have been processed to remove T4, but the process appears to be unsuccessful because hyperthyroidism can be induced by administration of these tablets.

Levothyroxine (T4) is the recommended treatment for all forms of hypothyroidism. T4 is the major secretory product of the thyroid gland, while T3 production can be accomplished in peripheral tissues. Levothyroxine administration allows tissues to autoregulate T3 production to some degree, which may be important when the dose is inadequate or excessive, or in conditions such as non-thyroidal illness, malnutrition and pregnancy where thyroid hormone concentrations can be altered in euthyroid individuals. Because the half-life of T4 in the dog is 9–15 hours, twice-daily administration most consistently normalises serum T4 concentrations (Nachreiner *et al.*, 1993). Once-daily treatment, however, is adequate to resolve clinical signs in most patients since the cellular action of thyroid hormones persists well after circulating levels decrease.

Liothyronine (T3) is rarely indicated for treatment of canine hypothyroidism. The short half-life (6 hours) necessitates administration of the drug at 4–6 µg/kg every 8 hours. In addition, thyrotoxicosis is more likely to occur with administration of T3 because it is more potent than levothyroxine, T3 levels fluctuate more after T3 than levothyroxine treatment, and autoregulation of intracellular T3 by deiodination of T4 does not occur. Liothyronine is probably more readily absorbed across the small intestine than levothyroxine and thus may be preferable for use in hypothyroid dogs with intestinal malabsorption.

Combinations of T4 and T3 may intuitively seem preferable, but are not recommended for treatment of canine hypothyroidism. The ratio of T4:T3 in commercial preparations is 4:1, while that normally secreted from the thyroid gland is 6:1. The relative overdose of T3 in combination medications is likely to result in clinical or subclinical hyperthyroidism. Sufficient T3 is produced by extrathyroidal deiodination of T4 to maintain a euthyroid state.

Principles of levothyroxine treatment

The pharmacokinetics of levothyroxine following oral administration vary considerably in individual hypothyroid dogs. Serum T4 concentrations vary as much as 4-fold among dogs on similar doses of levothyroxine (Nachreiner et al., 1993). Doses ranging from 11 to 44 μg/kg/day resulted in normal serum T4 concentrations. Doses that result in high normal to slightly elevated serum T4 concentrations frequently result in serum T3 concentrations that are still below the normal range. Only by administering levothyroxine at 44 μg/kg/day is it possible to ensure normal serum T3 (Nachreiner et al., 1993). The importance of maintaining a normal serum T3 concentration is unclear, since most dogs demonstrate resolution of clinical signs of hypothyroidism when serum T4 concentrations are in the high normal range.

Initial treatment of hypothyroidism should consist of administration of levothyroxine at a dose of 11–22 μg/kg twice daily. Administration twice daily should be continued until resolution of clinical signs because some dogs respond incompletely to once-daily treatment. Use of proprietary preparations, in particular those developed for veterinary medicine, should be strongly considered during initial treatment, as serum T4 concentrations have been reported to be higher in dogs treated with a veterinary preparation than with generic or human proprietary forms of levothyroxine (Nachreiner and Refsal, 1992). Recurrence of clinical signs after changing from a proprietary to a generic formulation has been suggested to occur (Refsal and Nachreiner, 1995). Following complete resolution of signs, treatment can be reduced to once-daily administration, if desired, to decrease cost and increase compliance.

Puppies with congenital hypothyroidism require much higher doses than adults, and close monitoring of post-pill serum total T4 concentrations should be undertaken to maintain concentrations within the normal range for the age of the dog. Dogs with concurrent illness, particularly diabetes mellitus, hypoadrenocorticism, and congestive heart failure as well as aged dogs, should have treatment instituted at 25% of the normal dose, with an increase by 25% every 2 weeks until a full dose is reached at 6 weeks. Hypothyroidism causes insulin resistance in dogs with diabetes mellitus, and the insulin dose usually has to be reduced following thyroid hormone replacement (Ford et al., 1993). Thyroid hormone treatment in dogs with cardiovascular disease will increase myocardial and peripheral tissue oxygen consumption and increase heart rate, and may increase blood pressure which may worsen the cardiac disease. On the other hand, thyroid hormones have a positive inotropic effect that may increase cardiac output and contribute to resolution of signs of heart failure. Dogs with concurrent hypoadrenocorticism and hypothyroidism should be stabilised with glucocorticoid and mineralo-corticoid treatment prior to treatment with levothyroxine to avoid precipitating a hypoadrenocortical crisis. Levothyroxine treatment may have to be increased during pregnancy, since there is an increase in protein binding of thyroid hormones and the placenta and fetus utilise some maternal T4. The dosage should be adjusted based on serum hormone concentrations, as most dogs are unlikely to require dose alteration.

Monitoring treatment

Response to treatment should be monitored by evaluating history, physical examination and serum hormone concentrations. An increase in activity and improvement in attitude usually occurs within one week of initiating treatment. Weight loss follows within 2–4 weeks, while dermatological changes including alopecia and hyperpigmentation may require months to resolve completely. Improvement in cardiovascular function is noted within 8 weeks. When present, peripheral neuropathy improves rapidly, with complete resolution in 8–12 weeks. Recovery from CNS signs may be more protracted. Failure of a dog to improve clinically within 6–8 weeks of initiating treatment should prompt investigation into owner compliance, adequacy of dosage, incorrect diagnosis, or concurrent disease.

Side effects

Thyrotoxicosis occurs occasionally during treatment of hypothyroidism. Clinical signs of hyperthyroidism include polyuria, polydipsia, polyphagia, weight loss, behavioural changes including hyperactivity and anxiousness, panting and tachycardia. Thyrotoxicosis can be confirmed by demonstrating elevated serum T4 and/or T3 concentrations. Treatment should be discontinued until signs resolve, and reinstituted at a lower dose or decreased frequencyof administration.

REFERENCES AND FURTHER READING

Avgeris S, Lothrop CD and McDonald TP (1990) Plasma von Willebrand factor concentration and thyroid function in dogs. *Journal of the American Veterinary Medical Association* **196**, 921–924

Beale KM, Halliwell REW and Chen CL (1990) Prevalence of antithyroglobulin antibodies detected by enzyme-linked immunosorbent assay of canine serum. *Journal of the American Veterinary Medical Association* **196**, 745–748.

Beale KM, Keisling K and Forster-Blouin S (1992) Serum thyroid hormone concentrations and thyrotropin responsiveness in dogs with generalized dermatologic disease *Journal of the American Veterinary Medical Association* **201**, 1715–1719

Bichsel P, Jacobs G and Oliver JE (1988) Neurologic manifestations associated with hypothyroidism in four dogs. *Journal of the American Veterinary Medical Association* **192**, 1745–1747

Budsberg SC, Moore GE and Klappenbach K (1993) Thyroxine-responsive unilateral forelimb lameness and generalized neuromuscular disease in four hypothyroid dogs. *Journal of the American Veterinary Medical Association*, 1859–1860

Dewey CW, Shelton GD, Bailey CS, Willard MD, Podell M and Collins RL (1995) Neuromuscular dysfunction in five dogs with acquired myasthenia gravis and presumptive hypothyroidism. *Progress in Veterinary Neurology* **6**, 117–123

Dixon RM, Graham PA and Mooney CT (1996) Serum thyrotropin concentrations: a new diagnostic test for canine hypothyroidism. *Veterinary Record* **138**, 594–595

Elliot DA, King LG and Zerbe CA (1995) Thyroid hormone concentrations in critically ill canine intensive care patients. *Journal of Veterinary Emergency and Critical Care* **5**, 17–23

Ferguson DC (1988) The effect of nonthyroidal factors on thyroid function tests in dogs. *Compendium of Continuing Education for the Practising Veterinarian* **10**, 1365–1377

Ferguson DC (1994) Update on diagnosis of canine hypothyroidism. *Veterinary Clinics of North America* **24**, 515-539

Ferguson DC and Peterson ME (1992) Serum free and total iodothyronine concentrations in dogs with hyperadrenocorticism. *American Journal of Veterinary Research* **53**, 1636–1640.

Ford SL, Nelson RW, Feldman EC and Niwa D (1993) Insulin resistance in three dogs with hypothyroidism and diabetes mellitus. *Journal of the American Veterinary Medical Association* **202**, 1478–1480.

Gaughan KR, Bruyette DS and Jordan FR (1996) Comparison of thyroid function testing in non-greyhound pet dogs and racing greyhounds. *Journal of Veterinary Internal Medicine* **10**, 186

Gerritsen RJ, van den Brom WE and Stokhof AA (1996) Relationship between atrial fibrillation and primary hypothyroidism in the dog. *Veterinary Quarterly* **18**, 49–51

Greco DS, Feldman EC, Peterson ME, Turner JL, Hodges CM and Shipman LW (1991) Congenital hypothyroidism and dwarfism in a family of Giant Schnauzers. *Journal of Veterinary Internal Medicine* **5**, 57–65

Haines DM, Lording PM and Penhale WJ (1984) Survey of thyroglobulin autoantibodies in dogs. *American Journal of Veterinary Research* **45**, 1493–1497

Hall IA, Campbell KL, Chambers MD and Davis CN (1993) Effect of trimethoprim/sulfamethoxazole on thyroid function in dogs with pyoderma. *Journal of the American Veterinary Medical Association* **202**, 1959-1962

Jaggy A, Oliver JE, Ferguson DC, Mahaffey EA and Glaus jun T (1994) Neurological manifestations of hypothyroidism: a retrospective study of 29 dogs. *Journal of Veterinary Internal Medicine* **8**, 328–336

Jensen AL, Iversen L, Hoier R, Kristensen F, and Henriksen P (1996) Evaluation of an immunoradiometric assay for thyrotropin in serum and plasma samples of dogs with primary hypothyroidism. *Journal of Comparative Pathology* **114**, 339–346

Johnson CA (1994) Reproductive manifestations of thyroid disease. *Veterinary Clinics of North America* **23**, 509–514

Johnson CA, Nachreiner RF and Mullaney TP (1995) Effects of hypothyroidism on canine reproduction. *Journal of Veterinary Internal Medicine* **9**, 184.

Kaelin S, Watson ADJ and Church DB (1986) Hypothyroidism in the dog: a retrospective study of sixteen cases. *Journal of Small Animal Practice* **27**, 533–539

Kemppainen RJ and Young DW (1992) Canine triiodothyronine antibodies. In: *Kirk's Current Veterinary Therapy* IX, ed. RW Kirk and JD Bonagura, pp. 327–330. WB Saunders, Philadelphia

Larsson M (1987) *Diagnostic methods in canine hypothyroidism and influence of nonthyroidal illness on thyroid hormones and thyroxine-binding proteins.* PhD thesis, Uppsala, Sweden

Melendez LD, Greco DS, Turner JL, Hay DA and van Liew CH (1996) Concurrent hypoadrenocorticism and hypothyroidism in 10 dogs. *Journal of Veterinary Internal Medicine* **10**, 182

Miller AB, Nelson RW, Scott-Moncrieff, Neal L and Bottoms GD (1992) Serial thyroid hormone concentrations in healthy euthyroid dogs, dogs with hypothyroidism, and euthyroid dogs with atopic dermatitis. *British Veterinary Journal* **148**, 451–458

Miller PE and Panciera DL (1994) Effects of experimental hypothyroidism on the eye and ocular adnexa of dogs. *American Journal of Veterinary Research* **55**, 692–697.

Nachreiner RF, Forsber M, Johnson CA and Refsal KR (1995) Validation of an assay for canine TSH (cTSH). *Journal of Veterinary Internal Medicine* **9**, 184

Nachreiner RF and Refsal KR (1992) Radioimmunoassay monitoring of thyroid hormone concentrations in dogs on thyroid replacement therapy: 2,674 cases (1985-1987). *Journal of the American Veterinary Medical Association* **201**, 623–629

Nachreiner RF, Refsal KR, Ravis WR, Hauptman J, Rosser EJ and Pedersoli WM (1993) Pharmacokinetics of L-thyroxine after its oral administration in dogs. *American Journal of Veterinary Research* **54**, 2091–2098

Nelson RW, Ihle SL, Feldman EC and Bottoms GD (1991) Serum free thyroxine concentration in healthy dogs, dogs with hypothyroidism, and euthyroid dogs with concurrent illness. *Journal of the American Veterinary Medical Association* **198**, 1401–1407

Nicoloff JT and LoPresti JS (1993) Myxoedema coma, a form of decompensated hypothyroidism. *Endocrinology and Metabolism Clinics of North America* **22**, 279–290

Nicoloff JT and LoPresti JS (1995) Nonthyroidal illness. In: *Endocrinology, 3rd edn*, ed. LJ DeGroot, pp. 665–675. WB Saunders, Philadelphia

Panciera DL (1994a) A retrospective study of 66 cases of canine hypothyroidism. *Journal of the American Veterinary Medical Association* **204**, 761–767

Panciera DL (1994b) An echocardiographic and electrocardiographic study of cardiovascular function in hypothyroid dogs. *Journal of the American Veterinary Medical Association* **205**, 996–1000

Panciera DL, Helfand SC and Soergel SA (1995) Acute effects of continuous infusions of human recombinant interleukin-2 on serum thyroid hormone concentrations in dogs. *Research in Veterinary Science* **58**, 96–97

Panciera DL and Johnson GS (1994) Plasma von Willebrand factor antigen concentrations in hypothyroid dogs. *Journal of the American Veterinary Medical Association* **205**, 1550–1553

Panciera DL and Johnson GS (1996) Plasma von Willebrand factor antigen concentration and buccal mucosal bleeding time in dogs with experimental hypothyroidism. *Journal of Veterinary Internal Medicine* **10**, 60–64

Panciera DL and Post K (1992) Effect of oral administration of sulfadiazine and trimethoprim in combination on thyroid function in dogs. *Canadian Journal of Veterinary Research* **56**, 349–352

Ramsey I and Herrtage M (1996) Distinguishing normal, sick and hypothyroid dogs using total thyroxine and thyrotropin concentrations. *Proceedings of the International Symposium on Canine Hypothyroidism*, Davis, California, pp. 50–51

Refsal KR and Nachreiner RF (1995) Monitoring thyroid hormone replacement therapy. In: *Kirk's Current Veterinary Therapy*, XI, ed. JD Bonagura, pp. 364–368. WB Saunders, Philadelphia

Roti E, Minelli R, Gardini E and Braverman LE (1993) The use and misuse of thyroid hormone. *Endocrine Reviews* **14**, 401–423

Scott-Moncrieff JC, Nelson RW, Bruner JM and Williams DA (1996) Serum canine thyrotropin concentration (cTSH) in euthyroid, hypothyroid, and sick euthyroid dogs. *Journal of Veterinary Internal Medicine* **10**, 186

Sparkes AH, Gruffydd Jones TJ, Wotton PR, Gleadhill A, Evans H and Walker MJ (1995) Assessment of dose and time responses to TRH and thyrotropin in healthy dogs. *Journal of Small Animal Practice* **36**, 245–251

Sullivan P, Gompf R, Schmeitzel L, Clift R, Cottrell M and McDonald TP (1993) Altered platelet indices in dogs with hypothyroidism and cats with hyperthyroidism. *American Journal of Veterinary Research* **54**, 2004–2009

Thacker EL, Refsal KR and Bull RW (1992) Prevalence of autoantibodies to thyroglobulin, thyroxine, or triiodothyronine and relationship of autoantibodies and serum concentrations of iodothyronines in dogs. *American Journal of Veterinary Research* **53**, 449--453

Vail DM, Panciera DL and Ogilvie GK (1994) Thyroid hormone concentrations in dogs with chronic weight loss, with special reference to cancer cachexia. *Journal of Veterinary Internal Medicine* **8**, 122–127

Williams DA, Scott-Moncrieff JC and Bruner J (1995) Canine serum thyroid-stimulating hormone following induction of hypothyroidism. *Journal of Veterinary Internal Medicine* **9**, 184

Williams DA, Scott-Moncrieff JC, Bruner J, Sustarsic D, Panosian-Sahakian N, Unver E and El Shami ES (1996) Validation of an immunoassay for canine thyroid-stimulating hormone and changes in serum concentration following induction of hypothyroidism in dogs. *Journal of the American Veterinary Medical Association* **209**, 1730–1732

CHAPTER FIFTEEN

Feline Hyperthyroidism

Carmel T. Mooney

INTRODUCTION

Hyperthyroidism (thyrotoxicosis) is a multisystemic disorder resulting from excessive circulating concentrations of the active thyroid hormones triiodothyronine (T3) and/or thyroxine (T4). First described in cats in 1979, hyperthyroidism has emerged as the most common endocrine disorder of this species, and a disease frequently diagnosed in small animal practice. It is unclear if this represents a true increase in the incidence of the disease, an increased awareness of the condition by practitioners and clients, an increased longevity for cats, or a combination of these.

AETIOLOGY

Benign adenomatous hyperplasia (adenoma) of one or, more usually, both thyroid lobes is the most common pathological abnormality in feline hyperthyroidism, and the disease has been likened to toxic multinodular goitre in humans. Microscopically, the normal thyroid follicular architecture is replaced by one or more readily discernible foci of hyperplastic tissue forming nodules ranging from <1 mm to >2 cm in diameter. Thyroid carcinoma is a rare cause of hyperthyroidism in cats.

To date, the underlying aetiology of feline hyperthyroidism remains obscure. Thyroid stimulating immunoglobulins, responsible for Graves' thyrotoxicosis in humans, have not been identified. An early epidemiological study suggested that the feeding of canned cat foods, living strictly indoors, being a non-Siamese breed, and having reported exposure to flea sprays, fertilisers, insecticides, and herbicides increased the risk of developing hyperthyroidism (Scarlett *et al.*, 1988). However, the significance of these factors is unclear.

SIGNALMENT

Hyperthyroidism is a disease of middle-aged and old cats, with an average age at onset of 12–13 years. Almost all cats with hyperthyroidism are over 6 years of age, but only 5% are under 10 years of age at the time of diagnosis. There is no apparent breed or sex predisposition.

HISTORICAL AND CLINICAL FEATURES

Thyroid hormones are responsible for a variety of actions

Finding	Number of cats affected (%)
Weight loss	119 (94.4)
Polyphagia	98 (77.8)
Polyuria/polydipsia	90 (71.4)
Tachycardia	78 (61.9)
Hyperactivity	70 (55.6)
Diarrhoea (increased frequency or volume, steatorrhoea)	64 (50.8)
Respiratory abnormalities (tachypnoea, dyspnoea, coughing, sneezing)	48 (38.1)
Other cardiac abnormalities (powerful apex beat, murmurs, gallop rhythm, arrhythmias)	43 (34.1)
Skin lesions (patchy or regional alopecia, matting, harsh dry coat, dry or greasy seborrhoea, thin skin)	40 (31.8)
Vomiting	38 (30.2)
Moderate temperature elevation	24 (19.1)
Decreased activity	13 (10.3)
Decreased appetite	13 (10.3)
Congestive cardiac failure	4 (3.2)
Haematuria	4 (3.2)
Intermittent decreased appetite	3 (2.4)
Ventral neck flexion	1 (0.8)
Palpable goitre	129 (97.6)

Table 15.1: Major historical and clinical findings in 126 hyperthyroid cats. (Reproduced with permission from Thoday and Mooney, 1992.)

including the regulation of heat production, and carbohydrate, protein, and lipid metabolism. They also appear to interact with the central nervous system by increasing overall sympathetic drive. When thyroid hormones are in excess, virtually every organ system is affected. Most cats present with a variety of clinical signs reflecting multiple organ dysfunction, although in some cats one clinical sign may predominate. The signs vary from mild to severe depending on the duration of the condition, the ability of the cat to cope with the thyroid hormone excess, and the presence or absence of concomitant abnormalities in other organ systems. The disease is insidiously progressive, and the signs, when mild, are often considered part of the

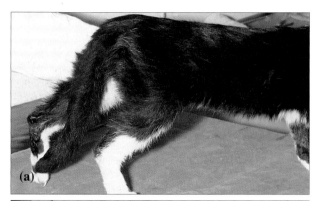

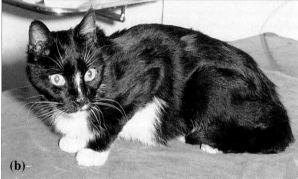

Figure 15.1: *Hyperthyroid 11 year old domestic shorthaired cat showing (a) evidence of weight loss and (b) an anxious facial expression. (Reproduced with permission from Thoday and Mooney, 1992.)*

generalised ageing process. For this reason, several months may elapse before veterinary attention is sought. However, because of the current increased awareness of the condition, a diagnosis may be made in cats less symptomatic than 10 or 15 years ago, and often before the owners realise their pets are ill (Peterson *et al.*, 1981; Broussard and Peterson, 1995). Table 15.1 outlines the historical and clinical features of the largest group (*n*=126) of hyperthyroid British cats reported (Thoday and Mooney, 1992).

General features

Almost all hyperthyroid animals exhibit signs of mild to severe weight loss, despite a normal or increased appetite, reflecting an overall increase in the metabolic rate (Figure 15.1a). Occasionally, affected cats exhibit intermittent periods of anorexia alternating with periods of normal or increased appetite. Muscle weakness, muscle wasting, heat intolerance, and intermittent mild pyrexia may occur.

Polyuria and polydipsia

Polyuria and polydipsia are frequent complaints of hyperthyroidism. Various mechanisms may be responsible, including concurrent primary renal dysfunction, decreased renal medullary solute concentration because of increased renal blood flow, electrolyte abnormalities (e.g. hypokalaemia), and primary polydipsia because of a hypothalamic disturbance associated with thyroid hormone excess. Haematuria is a rare presenting sign — the exact mechanism is unclear and while its occurrence may be coincidental, in human thyrotoxicosis thrombocytopenia or clotting factor deficiencies have been recorded.

Hyperactivity

Hyperactivity, exhibited particularly as nervousness, restlessness, and aggressive behaviour, is common in hyperthyroidism. In extreme cases tremor may be apparent and the cats are often described as having an anxious facial expression (Figure 15.1b). There is impaired tolerance to stress which can result in severe respiratory distress,

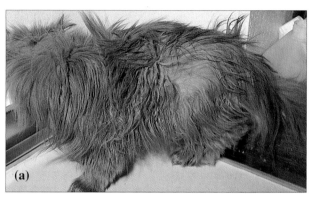

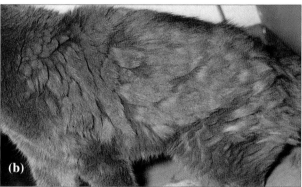

Figure 15.2: *(a) Hyperthyroid 14 year old pedigree longhaired cat showing evidence of alopecia. (b) Hyperthyroid 13 year old Russian Blue cat with extensive matting.*

cardiac arrhythmias, and extreme weakness. Aimless pacing and easily interrupted sleep patterns may be apparent. Recently, although rare, focal or generalized seizures characteristic of epilepsy have been described. In such cases, there is a reduction in the severity of the seizures or complete resolution after treatment of the hyperthyroidism (Joseph and Peterson, 1992).

Skin changes

Skin changes are common in hyperthyroid cats although usually less of an owner concern. Unkempt matted hair results from a failure to groom, and alopecia—bilaterally symmetrical or patchy—may be related to excessive grooming (Figures 15.2a and b); the latter is usually seen in longhaired cats and presumably reflects heat intolerance. Excessive nail growth with increased fragility may also be noted.

Gastrointestinal features

Gastrointestinal signs are common in hyperthyroid cats. Vomiting may result from a direct action of thyroid hormones on the chemoreceptor trigger zone, or from gastric stasis. Vomiting seems to be more common in cats from multicat households, and usually occurs shortly after feeding so may simply be related to rapid overeating. In humans, rapid gastrointestinal transit contributes to the increased frequency of defecation and diarrhoea. In addition, malabsorption and steatorrhoea may result from excess fat intake associated with polyphagia, rapid gastric emptying and intestinal transit, and/or a reversible reduction in pancreatic trypsin secretion. Many of these mechanisms have not been investigated in cats. However, orocaecal transit time, as assessed by breath hydrogen measurements, seems to be accelerated in hyperthyroid cats (Papasouliotis *et al.*, 1993; Schlesinger *et al.*, 1993).

Cardiorespiratory features

Tachycardia (heart rate >240 beats per minute), a powerful apex beat, and systolic murmurs are the most common cardiovascular abnormalities encountered in hyperthyroid cats. These abnormalities are related to direct effects of thyroid hormone on cardiac muscle and indirect effects mediated through the interaction of thyroid hormone with the adrenergic nervous system, or occur to compensate for altered peripheral tissue perfusion. Less commonly, arrhythmias, particularly ectopic atrial and ventricular arrhythmias, may be audible. Gallop rhythms and signs associated with pleural effusion and pulmonary oedema (coughing, dyspnoea, muffled heart sounds, ascites) are suggestive of heart failure. Hypertension has been documented (Kobayashi *et al.*, 1990). This may be manifested clinically as hyperaemia of the pinnae and mucous membranes or by the ocular findings of retinal haemorrhage, oedema, or partial or complete retinal detachment (Stiles *et al.*, 1994). Sudden onset blindness or cerebrovascular accidents are possible, but rare complications of hyper-tension.

Respiratory abnormalities, chiefly tachypnoea and dyspnoea at rest, are also common but tend to occur most frequently during periods of stress. In the absence of cardiac failure, respiratory muscle weakness due to chronic thyrotoxic myopathy and decreased compliance of the lungs are the most likely explanations.

Apathetic hyperthyroidism

Approximately 10% of cats with hyperthyroidism present with apathy or depression and anorexia. Affected human patients usually have severe cardiac complications induced by thyroid hormone excess. In cats, apathetic hyperthyroidism has been associated with congestive cardiac failure. However, concurrent severe non-thyroidal illness may also be a complicating factor requiring further investigation. A small number of these cats have pronounced ventroflexion of the head and neck; this may result from thiamin deficiency, hypokalaemia, or severe muscle weakness.

Palpable goitre

In healthy individuals, the thyroid lobes are positioned just below the cricoid cartilage, extend ventrally over the first five or six tracheal rings, and are not palpable. In hyperthyroid cats, either unilateral or bilateral thyroid enlargement (goitre) is invariably present. Thyroid lobes are loosely attached to the surrounding tissues and tend to migrate ventrally, occasionally through the thoracic inlet into the anterior mediastinum.

Sometimes goitre is visible but, more commonly, palpation is required. To palpate for goitre, the cat is restrained by holding its front legs in a sitting position. With the cat's neck gently extended, the thumb and forefinger are placed on either side of the trachea and swept carefully downwards from the larynx to the manubrium. Visualisation of small nodules may be aided by clipping the ventrocervical area and moistening the skin with alcohol. Intrathoracic goitre may become palpable by holding the animal vertically with the head pointing downward. Rarely, ectopic thyroid tissue, found anywhere from the larynx to the base of the heart, may be involved in the pathogenesis of the condition.

The presence of a cervical mass is not always associated with hyperthyroidism. However, if found in an apparently euthyroid individual, it is possible that hyperthyroidism eventually results as the thyroid nodule continues to grow and secrete excessive thyroid hormone.

In conclusion, a variety of clinical signs are associated with hyperthyroidism, and the presence or absence of any one sign does not confirm or exclude the diagnosis. Hyperthyroidism should be part of the differential diagnosis in old cats, regardless of presenting signs, and therefore palpation for goitre should form part of a routine physical examination.

INVESTIGATIVE PROCEDURES

A variety of procedures have been recommended for investigation of hyperthyroidism. Often these simply lend support to the diagnosis but may be useful, particularly if concurrent disorders are suspected and an accurate prognosis is required. Specific thyroid function tests are necessary to confirm the diagnosis.

Supportive diagnostic tests

Haematological features

Haematological changes are of limited diagnostic value in hyperthyroidism, although mild to moderate erythrocytosis (increased packed cell volume, red blood cell count, and haemoglobin concentration) and macrocytosis have been described (Peterson *et al.*, 1981). These changes presumably result from a direct effect of thyroid hormone on erythroid precursors, and increased production of erythropoietin. Anaemia is a rare complication of hyperthyroidism which, in humans, is related to bone marrow exhaustion or a deficiency of iron or other micronutrients. Heinz body formation may be a complicating factor in cats (Christopher, 1989). Not surprisingly, a stress leucogram, as evidenced by mature neutrophilia usually accompanied by lymphopenia and eosinopenia, is common. Occasionally, there is a lymphocytosis and eosinophilia which is thought to be due to a relative lack of cortisol. Platelet size may be increased (Sullivan *et al.*, 1993).

Serum biochemical features

Mild to marked elevations in the serum concentrations of

alanine aminotransferase (ALT), aspartate aminotransferase (AST), alkaline phosphatase (ALP), and lactate dehydrogenase (LDH) are the most common biochemical abnormalities in feline hyperthyroidism. Hepatic damage, caused by malnutrition, congestive cardiac failure, hepatic hypoxia, infections, and direct toxic effects of thyroid hormones on the liver, is a plausible explanation. Histopathological examination of the liver usually reveals only modest and non-specific changes including centrilobular fatty infiltration (Peterson *et al.*, 1981). Part of the increase in serum ALP concentrations is related to the bone isoenzyme (Horney *et al.*, 1994; Archer and Taylor, 1996). Approximately 90% of affected cats have an elevation in at least one of these enzymes. In some severely thyrotoxic cats, the elevations may be only mild or moderate. However, concurrent hepatic disease should be suspected if there are marked elevations in either ALT, ALP, AST, or LDH, but only mildly elevated serum thyroid hormone concentrations.

Mild to moderate increases in serum concentrations of urea and creatinine may be found in over 25% of hyperthyroid cats. This may represent pre-existing renal dysfunction which is not unexpected in a group of aged cats. Thyrotoxicosis may also play a role by increasing protein catabolism and, possibly in some cases, by reducing renal perfusion because of decreased cardiac output. However, increased glomerular filtration rate is associated with hyperthyroidism, and the decrease in glomerular filtration rate upon successful management of the thyrotoxicosis may unmask occult renal disease (Graves *et al.*, 1994; DiBartola *et al.*, 1996). If serum urea and creatinine concentrations are elevated, the choice of treatment for hyperthyroidism may be limited.

Increased phosphate concentration without evidence of azotaemia occurs in approximately 20–40% of hyperthyroid cats. In thyrotoxic humans, there is increased bone metabolism attributed to the direct effects of thyroid hormones on bone cells, which can lead to osteopenia and pathological fractures. This is associated with increased serum concentrations of the bone isoenzyme of ALP, osteocalcin, and phosphorus, and a tendency towards increased serum calcium and decreased parathormone and active vitamin D (1,25 dihydroxy cholecalciferol) concentrations. In hyperthyroid cats, serum total calcium concentration is unaffected but ionized calcium is decreased and circulating parathormone concentration increased. In addition, elevated osteocalcin and 1,25 dihydroxy cholecalciferol concentrations have been found in a small number of thyrotoxic cats (Archer and Taylor, 1996; Barber and Elliott, 1996). The reasons for the differences between humans and cats is unclear, but the hyperparathyroidism noted in feline patients may have implications for skeletal integrity.

Blood glucose concentrations may be mildly increased in hyperthyroid cats presumably reflecting a stress response. In cases with pre-existing diabetes mellitus, accelerated insulin catabolism increases requirements for exogenous insulin (Feldman and Nelson, 1996).

Hypokalaemia has occasionally been associated with hyperthyroidism and should be suspected in any cat with

| **Haematology** |
| Erythrocytosis |
| Macrocytosis |
| Leucocytosis |
| Neutrophilia |
| Eosinopenia |
| **Serum biochemistry** |
| Elevated alanine aminotransferase |
| Elevated alkaline phosphatase |
| Elevated aspartate aminotransferase |
| Elevated lactate dehydrogenase |
| Azotaemia |
| Hyperphosphataemia |
| Mild hyperglycaemia |

Table 15.2: *Common haematological and biochemical abnormalities associated with hyperthyroidism.*

evidence of severe muscle weakness (Nemzek *et al.*, 1994).

Other biochemical parameters such as cholesterol, sodium, chloride, bilirubin, albumin, and globulin are largely unaffected by the hyperthyroid state (Table 15.2).

Urinalysis

Urinalysis is generally unremarkable in hyperthyroidism but useful in differentiating other diseases with similar clinical signs such as diabetes mellitus. Urine specific gravity is variable.

Diagnostic imaging

Hyperthyroidism is associated with a largely reversible hypertrophic cardiomyopathy. In approximately 50% of affected cats, there is evidence of mild to severe cardiac enlargement on thoracic radiography. The most common abnormalities on cardiac ultrasound include left ventricular hypertrophy, increased left atrial and ventricular diameter, interventricular septum hypertrophy, and enhanced contractility, as evidenced by increased shortening fraction and velocity of circumferential fibre shortening (Bond *et al.*, 1988). These changes resolve or improve following successful treatment of the hyperthyroidism.

Occasionally, hyperthyroid cats may show evidence of congestive cardiac failure (pleural effusion or pulmonary oedema) indicating irreversible structural damage to the heart induced by the thyrotoxicosis, or a co-existing cardiomyopathy. Rarely, hyperthyroidism is associated with a dilatative form of cardiomyopathy which is usually accompanied by evidence of severe congestive cardiac failure (Jacobs *et al.*, 1986).

Electrocardiography

The most frequent electrocardiographic abnormalities recorded in hyperthyroidism are tachycardia (heart rate >240 beats per minute) and increased R-wave amplitude in lead II (> 0.9 mV). Other less common abnormalities include prolonged QRS duration, shortened Q–T interval, intraventricular conduction disturbances, and a variety of atrial and ventricular arrhythmias (Peterson *et al.*, 1981, 1982). In more recent reports the prevalence of these abnormalities has decreased, presumably reflecting earlier diagnosis and a less severely affected thyrotoxic population (Broussard and Peterson, 1995).

Confirmatory diagnostic tests

Pathophysiology

In cats, T4 is the main secretory product of the thyroid gland. T3 is three to five times more potent than T4 but approximately 60% of circulating T3 is produced by extrathyroidal 5'-deiodination of T4. T4 is therefore often considered to be a prohormone, and activation to T3 a step autoregulated by peripheral tissues. Over 99% of circulating T4 is protein bound while approximately 0.1% is free and considered active. Overall control of thyroid hormone production is provided by a negative feedback mechanism of circulating T4 and T3 on thyrotropin releasing hormone (TRH) from the hypothalamus, and thyrotropin (thyroid stimulating hormone, TSH) from the anterior pituitary. In hyperthyroid cats, there is autonomous and excessive secretion of thyroid hormones from the abnormally functioning thyroid gland.

Thyroidal radioisotope uptake

Quantitative thyroidal uptake of radioactive iodine (^{123}I or ^{131}I) or technetium-99M as pertechnetate (^{99}mTcO$_4^-$) tends to be increased in hyperthyroidism (Mooney *et al.*, 1992a). Sophisticated computerised medical equipment is required.

Basal total thyroid hormone concentrations

Elevated circulating concentrations of total T4 and T3 are the biochemical hallmarks of hyperthyroidism, and methods for their measurement are easily accessible. Radioimmunoassay (RIA) is the preferred method, but non-isotopic and automated techniques are becoming increasingly popular and could prove valuable providing there is good correlation with the results of RIA. Semiquantitative assays for total T4 measurement, suitable for in-house use, appear to be useful in the diagnosis of overt hyperthyroidism in cats, but studies of large numbers of cases have not been reported (Eckersall *et al.*, 1991). Assays intended for human serum are acceptable but must be fully validated for use with cat serum and, as in the dog, modified to allow for measurement of the lower circulating concentrations of hormone in this species.

Serum total T4 and T3 concentrations are highly correlated in hyperthyroid cats. However, in up to 30% of cases, serum total T3 concentration remains within the reference range (Broussard and Peterson, 1995). In such cases, serum total T4 concentration is usually only mildly elevated and it is likely that the T3 would increase into the thyrotoxic range if the disorder was allowed to progress untreated. It is likely that as T4 production begins to increase, there is a compensatory decrease in peripheral conversion of T4 to the more active T3. Thus, measurement of serum total T4 concentration alone is preferred.

	T3 suppression	TSH stimulation	TRH stimulation
Drug	Tertroxin	Bovine TSH	TRH
Dose	20 µg 8-hourly for 7 doses	0.5 IU/kg	0.1 mg/kg
Route	Oral	Intravenous	Intravenous
Sampling times	0 and 2–4 hours after last dose	0 and 6 hours	0 and 4 hours
Assay	Total T$_4$	Total T$_4$	Total T$_4$
Interpretation: Euthyroidism	<20 nmol/l with >50% suppression	>100% increase	>60% increase
Hyperthyroidism	>20 nmol/l ± <50% suppression	Minimal/no increase	<50% increase
Reference	Peterson *et al.* (1990)	Mooney *et al.* (1996b)	Peterson *et al.* (1994)

Table 15.3: *Commonly used protocols for dynamic thyroid function tests in cats. Values quoted for interpretation are guidelines only. Each individual laboratory should furnish its own reference range. T3, triiodothyronine; T4, thyroxine; TRH, thyrotropin releasing hormone; TSH, thyroid stimulating hormone.*

A serum total T4 concentration exceeding 3 standard deviations from the reference range is useful in differentiating hyperthyroid animals from the small number of healthy animals with values above the reference range. While this is exceeded in most affected cats, with serum total T4 concentrations up to 20 times the upper limit of the reference range, a small number of hyperthyroid cats (approximately 5–10%) have serum total T4 concentrations below this or within the mid to high end of the reference range. In such cases, the disease may be in the early stages or, in mildly affected cases, serum total T4 concentrations can randomly fluctuate to within the reference range (Peterson *et al.*, 1987). In addition, severe non-thyroidal illness is capable of significantly suppressing serum total T4 concentrations to the low end or below the reference range (Peterson and Gamble, 1990; Mooney *et al.*, 1996a). Thus, marginally elevated serum total T4 concentrations may be suppressed to within the mid to high end of the reference range in cats with concurrent mild hyperthyroidism and severe non-thyroidal disease (McLoughlin *et al.*, 1993).

In early or mildly hyperthyroid cats, serum total T4 concentrations will eventually increase into the diagnostic thyrotoxic range upon retesting 3–6 weeks later. Concurrent hyperthyroidism should always be suspected in severely ill cats with mid to high reference range serum total T4 concentrations. Thus, further diagnostic tests for equivocal cases are rarely required. Protocols for some of these tests are outlined in Table 15.3.

T3 suppression test

In healthy individuals, T3 has a suppressive effect on pituitary TSH secretion and subsequently on T4 production by the thyroid gland. In hyperthyroidism, because of autonomous production of thyroid hormones and chronic

Considerations	Radioactive iodine therapy	Surgical thyroidectomy	Long-term medical management
Persistent/recurrent hyperthyroidism	Rare	Possible (if appropriate technique used)	Common (dependent on owner/cat compliance)
Time to achieve euthyroidism	1–20 weeks	Prior treatment recommended	3–15 days
Hospitalisation	30 days	1–10 days (dependent on post-operative complications)	Not required
Adverse reactions	None	Hypoparathyroidism common	Possible
Availability	Limited	Skilled surgeon required	Always available
Cost	High	Intermediate	Low

Table 15.4: *Advantages and disadvantages of the three different treatment modalities for hyperthyroidism in cats.*

suppression of TSH, this suppressive effect is lost. Thus, serum total T4 concentrations show minimal or no decrease in hyperthyroid cats following T3 administration. Simultaneous measurement of serum total T3 concentrations is required to ensure adequate administration and absorption of the drug and thus avoid false positive results.

TSH stimulation test
Exogenous TSH is a potent stimulator of thyroid hormone secretion. However, serum total T4 concentrations show little or no increase following TSH administration in hyperthyroid cats. This is presumably because the thyroid gland of affected cats secretes thyroid hormones independently of TSH control or that T4 is already being produced at a near maximal rate with limited reserve capacity. Apart from the expense and difficulty in obtaining TSH, cats with equivocally elevated serum total T4 concentrations tend to exhibit results which are indistinguishable from healthy animals. Therefore this test is not recommended.

TRH stimulation test
TRH is less expensive and easier to obtain than TSH. Serum total T4 concentrations increase minimally after TRH administration in mildly hyperthyroid cats. Compared with the T3 suppression test, this test is faster and avoids the administration of tablets. However, TRH is associated with transient adverse reactions such as salivation, vomiting, tachypnoea, and inappropriate defecation.

Serum free T4 concentration
Serum free and total T4 concentrations are highly correlated in hyperthyroidism. However, serum free T4 concentrations, as measured by equilibrium dialysis, are more consistently elevated in mildly hyperthyroid cases (Peterson *et al.*, 1995). Apart from the expense, caution is advised in using serum free T4 measurements by equilibrium dialysis as the sole diagnostic test for hyperthyroidism, because cats with non-thyroidal illness occasionally have elevated values (Mooney *et al.*, 1996a). Controversy surrounds the validity of other methods, particularly those involving analogues, for accurately measuring free T4 concentrations, and therefore they are unlikely to provide any additional information over total T4 estimations alone.

TREATMENT

The treatment of hyperthyroidism is aimed at controlling the excessive secretion of the thyroid hormones from the abnormally functioning gland by medical inhibition of thyroid hormone synthesis, surgical removal of the thyroid tissue, or destruction through radioablation. Currently, the last two are the only curative methods available. The major advantages and disadvantages of the three forms of therapy are outlined in Table 15.4. Treatment is tailored to each individual cat considering the factors outlined in Table 15.5.

Severity of clinical thyrotoxicosis
Presence/absence of concurrent illness
Age of cat
Access to, waiting list for, radioactive iodine therapy
Availability of skilled surgeon
Adequate post-thyroidectomy care facilities
Owner/cat compliance for drug administration
Potential complications
Cost

Table 15.5: *Factors to consider before selecting a treatment modality for hyperthyroidism in cats.*

Medical management
Chronic medical management is a practical treatment option for many hyperthyroid cats. It requires no special licensing, is readily available, and reasonably inexpensive. There is a rapid return to euthyroidism, which may be desirable in severely affected cases. Anaesthesia is avoided, as are the peri- and postoperative complications associated with surgical thyroidectomy, and the prolonged hospitalisation necessary after radioactive iodine administration. However, medical management is not curative, is highly dependent on adequate owner and cat compliance, and requires regular biochemical monitoring to ensure the efficacy of treatment. It is therefore often reserved for cats of advanced age or for those with concurrent diseases, and for when owners refuse, or facilities are not available for, either surgery or radioactive iodine. Of all the treatment options, however, medical management is the only one with no long-term effects and therefore is the best option for trial therapy when deterioration of renal function is a possibility once euthyroidism is restored.

Medical management is also necessary before surgical

Drug	Mode of action	Formulations	Indications	Dosage	Contraindications
Carbimazole	Inhibition of thyroid peroxidase-catalysed reactions ?Alteration to thyroglobulin structure	5 mg tablets	Before surgery Chronic management	5 mg tid 5 mg bid	Immediately before ^{131}I therapy
Stable iodine	Inhibition of thyroid peroxidase-catalysed reactions Inhibition of hormone release	SSKI (50 mg iodide per drop) Lugol's solution (6 mg iodine per drop) 85 mg potassium iodate tablets (50 mg free iodine)	Before surgery	30–100 mg sid or÷ bid	Alone, before surgery Before ^{131}I therapy Chronic management
Propranalol	β_1/β_2–adrenoceptor blocking agent	10 mg tablets	Before sugery Symptomatic control	2.5–5 mg tid	Alone, before surgery Chronic management
Atenolol	β_1-adrenoceptor blocking agent	25 mg tablets 25 mg/5 ml syrup	Before surgery Symptomatic control	6.25–12.5 mg sid	Alone, before surgery Chronic management
Calcium ipodate	Inhibits peripheral T4 to T3 conversion Releases iodine	500 mg capsules	Before surgery	15 mg/kg bid	Before ^{131}I therapy Chronic management

Table 15.6: *Drugs used in the medical management of feline hyperthyroidism. T3, triiodothyronine; T4, thyroxine; bid, twice daily; sid, once daily; tid, three times daily.*

thyroidectomy to decrease the metabolic and cardiac complications associated with hyperthyroidism, and may be desirable in providing symptomatic control while awaiting radioactive iodine therapy.

Table 15.6 details the variety of drugs, mode of action, dosage regimens, indications, and contraindications of medical management of feline hyperthyroidism.

Thioureylene antithyroid drugs

Thioureylene antithyroid drugs (propylthiouracil, methimazole, and carbimazole) are used for the preoperative control of hyperthyroidism because of their consistent reliable suppression of hormone production. They are the only drugs currently available for chronic management of hyperthyroidism. Propylthiouracil is associated with a high incidence of adverse reactions (immune-mediated

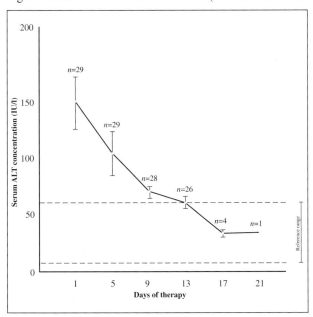

Figure 15.3: *The progressive decline in serum alanine aminotransferase (ALT) concentrations in a series of hyperthyroid cats which became euthyroid with carbimazole at a dose of 5 mg three times daily. (Reproduced and modified with permission from Mooney et al., 1992b.)*

haemolytic anaemia and thrombocytopenia) and is no longer recommended. Methimazole is unavailable in the UK. Carbimazole exerts its antithyroid effect through immediate conversion to methimazole such that a 5 mg dose of carbimazole is approximately equal to 3 mg of methimazole; this may explain, at least in part, the differences in recommended dosages between the two agents and the apparent lower incidence of adverse reactions associated with carbimazole compared with methimazole (Peterson *et al.*, 1988; Mooney *et al.*, 1992a; Peterson and Aucoin, 1993). An additional advantage of carbimazole is that it is tasteless whereas methimazole is bitter. These drugs are actively concentrated by the thyroid gland where they inhibit thyroid hormone synthesis but not iodide trapping or release of preformed hormone.

Initial therapy: Carbimazole is initially administered at a dose of 5 mg, strictly every 8 hours. The length of time to achieve biochemical euthyroidism is correlated with the basal serum total T4 concentration but usually occurs within a mean of 5.7 days (range 3–15 days). Clinical evidence of euthyroidism tends to lag but is usually present after 2 weeks and thus for practical reasons a 2-week course is prescribed initially. At that time, if the serum total T4 concentration is within or below the reference range, surgical thyroidectomy can be carried out, with administration of the last pill on the morning of surgery. For severely affected cats, a longer period of treatment may be required before being considered good surgical candidates, and these cases should subsequently be managed chronically until surgery is performed. In a small number of cases, euthyroidism is not achieved at 2 weeks and a longer treatment course is necessary. Increasing the daily dosage (in increments of 2.5–5 mg) is rarely required as therapeutic failure is invariably related to poor owner/cat compliance.

Elevated serum concentrations of ALT and ALP decline progressively as euthyroidism is achieved (Figure 15.3). Thus, their measurement can be used as a non-specific indicator of therapeutic efficacy.

Chronic management: Once euthyroidism has been achieved, the dosage is decreased to 5 mg administered twice daily and continued for life. A serum total T4 concentration is measured 2 weeks after each dose adjustment and once stability has been attained, every 3–6 months or as indicated clinically.

Adverse reactions: Most adverse reactions occur within the first 3 months of therapy for hyperthyroidism. Mild clinical side effects of vomiting, with or without anorexia and depression, occur in approximately 10% of affected cats, usually within the first 3 weeks of therapy. In most cases, these reactions are transient and do not require withdrawal of the drug. Early in the course of therapy, mild and transient haematological abnormalities including lymphocytosis, eosinophilia, or leucopenia occur in approximately 5% of cases but without any apparent clinical effect. Self-induced excoriations of the head and neck have been rarely described, usually within the first 6 weeks of therapy. Permanent withdrawal of the drug together with symptomatic therapy is required. More serious adverse reactions have not yet been documented with carbimazole. Agranulocytosis and/or thrombocytopenia, which have been reported in less than 5% of cats treated with methimazole, remain a possibility. For this reason, fortnightly complete blood and platelet counts have been recommended, at least for the first 3 months of therapy, in order to detect such reactions. However, because of their rarity and unpredictability, assessment of a complete blood count if clinical signs indicate may be a more cost-effective way of dealing with such reactions. Hepatopathy and development of serum antinuclear antibodies without systemic signs of a lupus-like syndrome have also been described with methimazole therapy but not yet with carbimazole.

Serum total T4 concentrations are frequently depressed below the reference range in cats treated with carbimazole. Clinical signs suggestive of hypothyroidism do not develop. This is presumably because corresponding serum total T3 concentrations tend to remain within the reference range due to increased extrathyroidal conversion from T4 or preferential thyroidal production of T3.

All treatments for hyperthyroidism have been associated with a decrease in glomerular filtration rate capable of unmasking latent renal disease. Therefore renal dysfunction should always be considered a potential adverse reaction of treatment, and assessed if clinical signs develop. Antithyroid medication offers the optimum treatment when there is evidence of pre-existing renal disease. If there is no discernible deterioration of renal function after euthyroidism has been achieved medically, other more permanent treatment options (surgery, radioactive iodine) may be considered. If renal function deteriorates, the effects of carbimazole will dissipate within 48 hours of withdrawal. The decision whether to continue treatment for hyperthyroidism depends on which of the two diseases is more severe.

Alternative medical therapies

Occasionally alternative medical therapies are required in cats intolerant of carbimazole. For the most part, these therapies are short term and only recommended before surgical thyroidectomy. Carbimazole therapy immediately before radioactive iodine therapy is controversial as it may increase the radioresistance of thyroid tissue, although this has never been objectively addressed. It is therefore usual to recommend withdrawal at least 2–6 weeks before therapy. In the interim, symptomatic control of the clinical signs of thyrotoxicosis may be desirable.

Stable iodine: Large doses of stable iodine acutely decrease the rate of thyroid hormone synthesis (Wolff–Chaikoff effect) and release, although these effects are erratic, inconsistent, short lived, and escape from inhibition can occur. Thus, it is rarely used as sole therapy but usually in association with β-adrenoceptor blocking agents before surgery. A reported advantage of stable iodine is its apparent effect on decreasing the vascularity and friability of the thyroid gland. Potassium iodide can cause excessive salivation and partial to complete anorexia in some cats. This can be avoided by dilution, by placing the dose in a gelatin capsule, or by using potassium iodate tablets. Stable iodine is obviously contraindicated before the administration of radioactive iodine.

β-adrenoceptor blocking agents: β-adrenoceptor blocking agents have no discernible effect on serum thyroid hormone concentrations but are useful in controlling the tachycardia, tachypnoea, hypertension, and hyperexcitability associated with hyperthyroidism. Propranolol is most frequently used. It is recommended when rapid control of clinical signs is desirable, and may be used in combination with stable iodine or carbimazole. Alone, propranolol is a useful treatment option for cats awaiting radiotherapy or in those cases in which there is a delayed return to euthyroidism after treatment. Propranolol is a non-selective β-adrenoceptor blocker and is contra-indicated in cats with pre-existing uncontrolled asthma or congestive cardiac failure. Atenolol is a useful alternative because of its selective $β_1$-adrenoceptor blocking effect, longer duration of action, and availability in syrup form.

Iodinated radiographic contrast agents: A number of oral cholecystographic agents (e.g. calcium ipodate) decrease T4 production, an effect presumably mediated by release of iodine as the drug is metabolised, and also acutely inhibit peripheral T4 conversion to T3. The latter effect has been clearly demonstrated in hyperthyroid cats where administration of the drug was associated with clinical improvement and normalisation of serum total T3 concentrations in over 60% of cases (Murray and Peterson, 1997). Waning of the effect is possible after 3 months of therapy. Therefore calcium ipodate is only likely to serve as an alternative to stable iodine in the short-term preparation for surgery. Calcium ipodate is currently unavailable in the UK, but there are no restrictions to its import.

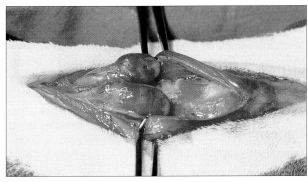

Figure 15.4: Appearance of bilateral thyroid lobe enlargement at the time of surgery. The external parathyroid glands are easily visualised as small spherical pale glands at the cranial pole of each thyroid lobe.

Surgical thyroidectomy

Surgical thyroidectomy is an extremely effective treatment for feline hyperthyroidism, and in many cats is the treatment of choice particularly if radioactive iodine is unavailable.

Preoperative stabilisation

Anaesthetising hyperthyroid cats carries a significant risk of cardiac and metabolic complications serious enough to cause death and it is therefore necessary to control the production or effects of excess thyroid hormone as outlined above.

Anaesthetic management

Once hyperthyroidism is well controlled, a variety of routine anaesthetic regimens can be used with a few exceptions. Drugs which stimulate or potentiate adrenergic activity capable of inducing tachycardia and arrhythmias should be avoided while drugs capable of preventing such arrhythmias are preferred. Thus, acepromazine is considered a useful premedicant, and glycopyrrolate is usually used in place of atropine. Xylazine and ketamine are avoided while isoflurane, if available, is preferred over halothane. Minimal anaesthetic time and continual monitoring are essential. Ventricular arrhythmia is a possible complication particularly if hyperthyroidism is not adequately pre-controlled. If such arrhythmias persist despite routine anaesthetic management, propranolol (0.1 mg intravenously) may restore normal sinus rhythm.

Surgical technique

A ventral skin incision is made from the larynx to the manubrium. The sternohyoideus and sternothyroideus muscles are separated by blunt dissection in the midline, and gently retracted. Both thyroid lobes and the external parathyroid glands can then be visualised before excision (Figure 15.4). In addition, the right recurrent laryngeal nerve which lies in close proximity to the right thyroid gland can be identified and avoided.

Unilateral versus bilateral involvement: Bilateral lobe involvement occurs in over 70% of cases of feline hyperthyroidism and thus the majority of cats require bilateral thyroidectomy. In many of these cases, lobe enlargement is not symmetrical and the smaller lobe may not be clearly palpable. The decision whether to perform a unilateral or bilateral thyroidectomy is therefore often taken at the

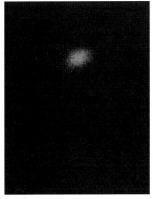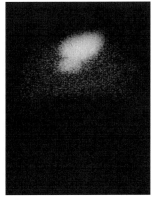

Figure 15.5: (a) Unilateral and (b) bilateral thyroid lobe involvement as detected by thyroid imaging using pertechnetate.

time of surgery. However, in up to 15% of bilateral cases, one thyroid lobe may appear grossly normal and if left *in situ* will result in recurrence of the condition. In unilateral cases, there is atrophy of the contralateral lobe but the distinction between what is considered normal and atrophic is not clearly defined.

Thyroid imaging, if available, is an extremely useful procedure to determine unilateral or bilateral lobe involvement, alterations in position, and the site of hyperfunctioning ectopic/accessory tissue (Peterson and Becker, 1984). This can be carried out using ^{123}I, ^{131}I, or $^{99}mTcO_4^-$; the last is usually preferred because of its short half-life and imaging time, relative inexpense, low radiation dose, and consistent image quality (Figure 15.5); access to a gamma camera is required. High resolution ultrasonography, in experienced hands, may be an alternative to thyroid imaging, but larger studies are required for its evaluation (Wisner *et al.*, 1994).

In the absence of thyroid imaging, both thyroid lobes should be carefully identified and, if abnormal in any way, removed. If a unilateral thyroidectomy is carried out, future monitoring for recurrence of the condition is required. Routine bilateral thyroidectomy, while increasing the risk of postoperative complications, obviates the need for decision making at the time of surgery.

Intracapsular versus extracapsular thyroidectomy: Two techniques have been described for thyroidectomy, both of which attempt to preserve the cranial (external) parathyroid gland (Figures 15.6 and 15.7). The original intracapsular technique involved incision through the thyroid capsule and blunt dissection of the thyroid lobe, leaving the capsule *in situ*. This technique was designed to minimise damage to the external parathyroid gland but was associated with a high rate of recurrence due to regrowth of tissue adherent to the capsule. The original extracapsular technique involved removal of the intact thyroid lobe and capsule with ligation of the cranial thyroid artery, while attempting to preserve blood supply to the cranial parathyroid gland. This technique decreases the rate of recurrence but increases the risk of postoperative hypoparathyroidism. Both techniques have therefore been successfully modified; the intracapsular technique by removal of the majority of the capsule after thyroid lobe removal and the extracapsular technique by using bipolar

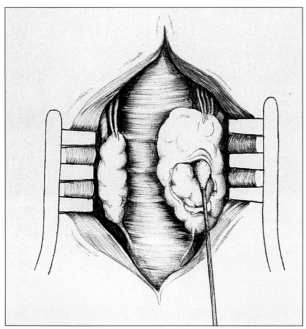

Figure 15.6: Intracapsular thyroidectomy. The thyroid capsule is incised and the thyroid lobe removed. (For the modified intracapsular technique the capsule is subsequently excised.) Reproduced from Mooney (1990).

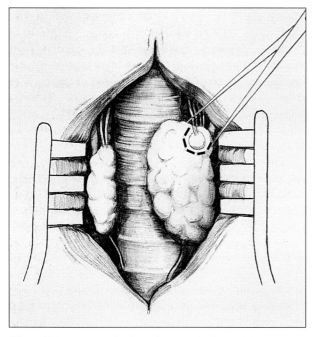

Figure 15.7: Extracapsular thyroidectomy. The thyroid lobe and capsule are removed while preserving vascular supply to the external parathyroid glands. (For the modified technique, bipolar cautery is used instead of ligatures.) Reproduced from Mooney (1990).

cautery instead of ligatures which minimises blunt dissection around the cranial parathyroid glands (Welches *et al.*, 1989). Haemorrhage obscuring the surgical field is a significant problem with the modified intracapsular technique, and for this reason, and because of its quickness, the modified extracapsular technique is usually preferred. Staging bilateral thyroidectomies, while recommended by some authors, does not sufficiently reduce the risk of postoperative complications to justify the risk and expense of two surgical procedures (Flanders *et al.*, 1987). Repeat thyroidectomies, following recurrence after bilateral thyroidectomy, are not recommended because of a higher incidence of severe life-threatening complications.

Following removal of the thyroid gland, the surgical field is carefully examined for haemostasis before closing the incision routinely.

Postoperative complications
The most significant postoperative complication of thyroidectomy is hypocalcaemia which occurs if the parathyroid glands are injured, devascularised, or inadvertently removed during the course of surgery. Since only one parathyroid gland is required to maintain function, hypoparathyroidism only develops after bilateral thyroidectomy. If removal of the cranial parathyroid glands is noted at the time of surgery, small pieces can be transplanted into a muscular pouch in the neck where revascularisation and return of function may occur. Hypocalcaemia occurs within 1–5 days of surgery. Biochemical hypocalcaemia alone does not warrant treatment but it should be instituted if clinical signs develop. These signs include anorexia, vocalisation, irritability, muscle twitching, tetany, and generalised convulsions. The treatment of postoperative hypocalcaemia is outlined in more detail in Chapter 17.

Other rarer but potential complications of thyroidectomy include haemorrhage, Horner's syndrome, laryngeal oedema or paralysis, and voice change. These can be avoided by a meticulous surgical technique. Serum total T4 concentrations are usually low for weeks to months after surgical thyroidectomy, but eventually increase into the reference range. Treatment with exogenous T4 is not indicated as permanent hypothyroidism is a rare sequel.

Radioactive iodine
Treatment with radioactive iodine is simple, safe, and effective, and is the best treatment for most hyperthyroid cats. The radioisotope most commonly used is ^{131}I, which, like stable iodine, is concentrated by the thyroid gland. It has a half-life of approximately 8 days and emits both β particles and γ radiation. The β particles, which cause 80% of tissue damage, travel a maximum of 2 mm and have an average path length of 400 µm. The particles are therefore locally destructive but spare adjacent atrophic thyroid tissue and other cervical structures. [131]I can be administered intravenously or orally but the subcutaneous route is preferred; this route is equally effective, not associated with gastrointestinal side effects, safer for personnel, and can be performed under light sedation thereby avoiding anaesthesia.

The principle of treatment with radioactive iodine is to administer a dose which will restore euthyroidism while avoiding the onset of hypothyroidism. Traditionally, this involved the administration of a small tracer dose of ^{131}I to determine various parameters of iodine kinetics before calculation of a therapeutic dose. While successful, access to nuclear medicine equipment is required. Use of fixed high or low doses may result in over- or undertreatment of a significant number of animals. The estimation of a dose based on a scoring system which includes the severity of the clinical thyrotoxicosis, elevation of circulating total T4

Score	Severity of clinical signs	Serum total T4 concentration (nmol/l)	Size of goitre
1	Mild	<80	Palpable with difficulty
2	Mild–moderate	<100	1.0 × 0.5 cm
3	Moderate	100–150	1.5 × 0.5 cm
4	Moderate–severe	150–400	>1.5 × 0.5 cm
5	Severe	>400	Visible to naked eye

Table 15.7: *Scoring system for estimation of a dose of radioactive iodine (^{131}I) for treatment of hyperthyroid cats. Scores of 3–9 obtain a dose of less than or equal to 120 MBq, scores of 9–12, 120 to 150 MBq, and scores >12, 160 MBq or more, with greater weighting in each group being given to the size of the goitre. (Reproduced with permission from Mooney, 1994).*

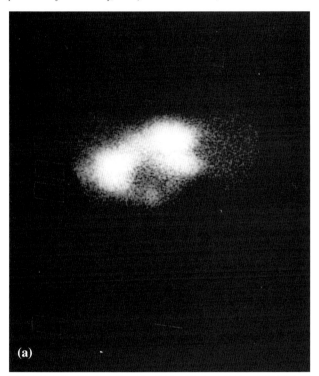

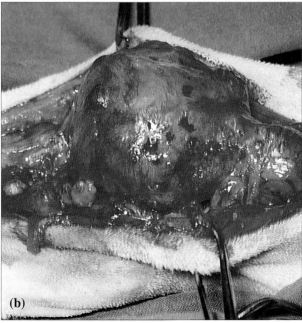

Figure 15.8: *(a) Appearance of a pertechnetate scan in thyroid carcinoma with multiple areas of uptake.*
(b) The same gland as visualised at the time of surgery.

concentration, and the size of the goitre as estimated by palpation, is currently the most popular method and is successful in over 90% of cases (Mooney, 1994; Peterson and Becker, 1995) (Table 15.7).

There are few complications from ^{131}I therapy. Persistent hyperthyroidism, more common in severely affected cats with large goitres and extreme elevations in serum total T4 concentration, can be successfully managed with a repeat injection. Permanent hypothyroidism is rare as is recurrence after successful treatment. Several drawbacks do exist. Facilities for ^{131}I are only available in the UK at the universities of Glasgow and Bristol and post-treatment hospitalisation is approximately 4–8 weeks. Due to the popularity of the treatment, waiting lists may be lengthy; this, and a possible delay in the return to euthyroidism for up to 6 months in a small number of cats, may necessitate interim symptomatic control of the thyrotoxicosis.

THYROID CARCINOMA

Functional thyroid carcinoma accounts for less than 2% of cases of hyperthyroidism and, in the author's experience, approximately 50% of all cases of feline thyroid carcinoma. Affected cats present with similar clinical signs to those with benign adenomatous hyperplasia. Evidence of thyroid carcinoma includes palpable large multilobulated masses in the neck, signs of distant metastases (usually pulmonary), locally invasive appearance at the time of surgery, or rapid recurrence following routine bilateral thyroidectomy or radioactive iodine therapy (Turrel *et al.*, 1988). Thyroid imaging usually reveals multifocal areas of increased uptake (Figure 15.8).

Cats presenting with distant metastatic disease carry a poor prognosis. In other cases, stabilisation of the clinical signs can be achieved using carbimazole although as this drug is not cytotoxic the prognosis remains guarded. Removal of all affected tissue is often difficult at the time of surgery, and routine radioactive iodine therapy may not be effective because malignant tissue appears to concentrate and retain iodine less efficiently than normal or adenomatous cells. Therefore the optimum choice appears to be surgical debulking followed by high dose (>1000 MBq) [131]I therapy. With such treatment, survival time may be increased by up to 41 months (Guptill *et al.*, 1995).

REFERENCES AND FURTHER READING

Archer FJ and Taylor SM (1996) Alkaline phosphatase bone isoenzyme and osteocalcin in the serum of hyperthyroid cats. *Canadian Veterinary Journal* **37**, 735–739

Barber PJ and Elliott J (1996) Study of calcium homeostasis in feline hyperthyroidism. *Journal of Small Animal Practice* **37**, 575–582

Bond BR, Fox PR, Peterson ME and Skavaril RV (1988) Echocardiographic findings in 103 cats with hyperthyroidism. *Journal of the American Veterinary Medical Association* **192**, 1546–1549

Broussard JD and Peterson ME (1995) Changes in clinical and laboratory findings in cats with hyperthyroidism from 1983 to 1993. *Journal of the American Veterinary Medical Association* **206**, 302–305

Christopher MM (1989) Relation of endogenous Heinz bodies to disease and anemia in cats: 120 cases (1978–1987). *Journal of the American*

Veterinary Medical Association **194**, 1089–1095

DiBartola SP, Broome MR, Stein BS and Nixon M (1996) Effect of treatment of hyperthyroidism on renal function in cats. *Journal of the American Veterinary Medical Association* **208**, 875–878

Eckersall PD, McEwan NA and Mooney CT (1991) An assessment of the cite T$_4$ immunoassay. *Veterinary Record* **129**, 532–533

Feldman EC and Nelson RW (1996) Feline hyperthyroidism (thyrotoxicosis). In: *Canine and Feline Endocrinology and Reproduction, 2nd edn*, ed. EC Feldman and RW Nelson, pp. 118–166. WB Saunders, Philadelphia

Flanders JA, Harvey HJ and Erb HN (1987) Feline thyroidectomy. A comparison of postoperative hypocalcemia associated with three different surgical techniques. *Veterinary Surgery* **16**, 362–366

Graves TK, Olivier B, Nachreiner RF, Kruger JM, Walshaw R and Stickle RL (1994) Changes in renal function associated with treatment of hyperthyroidism in cats. *American Journal of Veterinary Research* **55**, 1745–1749

Guptill L, Scott-Moncrieff JCR, Janovitz EB, Blevins WE, Yohn SE and DeNicola DB (1995) Response to high-dose radioactive iodine administration in cats with thyroid carcinoma that had previously undergone surgery. *Journal of the American Veterinary Medical Association* **207**, 1055–1058

Horney BS, Farmer AJ, Honor DJ, MacKenzie A and Burton S (1994) Agarose gel electrophoresis of alkaline phosphatase isoenzymes in the serum of hyperthyroid cats. *Veterinary Clinical Pathology* **23**, 98–102

Jacobs G, Hutson C, Dougherty J and Kirmayer A (1986) Congestive heart failure associated with hyperthyroidism in cats. *Journal of the American Veterinary Medical Association* **188**, 52–56

Joseph RJ and Peterson ME (1992) Review and comparison of neuromuscular and central nervous system manifestations of hyperthyroidism in cats and humans. *Progress in Veterinary Neurology* **3**, 114–119

Kobayashi DL, Peterson ME, Graves TK, Lesser M and Nichols CE (1990) Hypertension in cats with chronic renal failure or hyperthyroidism. *Journal of Veterinary Internal Medicine* **4**, 58–62

McLoughlin MA, DiBartola SP, Birchard SJ and Day DG (1993) Influence of systemic nonthyroidal illness on serum concentration of thyroxine in hyperthyroid cats. *Journal of the American Animal Hospital Association* **29**, 227–234

Mooney CT (1990) Hyperthyroidism in cats. *Veterinary Practice* **22**, 1–3

Mooney CT (1994) Radioactive iodine therapy for feline hyperthyroidism: Efficacy and administration routes. *Journal of Small Animal Practice* **35**, 289–294

Mooney CT, Little CJL and Macrae AW (1996a) Effect of illness not associated with the thyroid gland on serum total and free thyroxine concentrations in cats. *Journal of the American Veterinary Medical Association* **208**, 2004–2008

Mooney CT, Thoday KL and Doxey DL (1992a) Carbimazole therapy of feline hyperthyroidism. *Journal of Small Animal Practice* **33**, 228–235

Mooney CT, Thoday KL and Doxey DL (1996b) Serum thyroxine and triiodothyronine responses of hyperthyroid cats to thyrotropin. *American Journal of Veterinary Research* **57**, 987–991

Mooney CT, Thoday KL, Nicoll JJ and Doxey D (1992b) Qualitative and quantitative thyroid imaging in feline hyperthyroidism using technetium-99m as pertechnetate. *Veterinary Radiology and Ultrasound* **33**, 313–320

Murray LAS and Peterson ME (1997) Ipodate as medical treatment in 12 cats with hyperthyroidism. *Journal of the American Veterinary Medical Association* **211**, 63–67

Nemzek JA, Kruger JM, Walshaw R and Hauptman JG (1994) Acute onset of hypokalaemia and muscular weakness in four hyperthyroid cats. *Journal of the American Veterinary Medical Association* **205**, 65–68

Papasouliotis K, Muir P, Gruffydd-Jones TJ, Galloway P, Smerdon T and

Cripps PJ (1993) Decreased orocaecal transit time, as measured by the exhalation of hydrogen in hyperthyroid cats. *Research in Veterinary Science* **55**, 115–118

Peterson ME and Aucoin DP (1993) Comparison of the disposition of carbimazole and methimazole in clinically normal cats. *Research in Veterinary Science* **54**, 351–355

Peterson ME and Becker DV (1984) Radionuclide thyroid imaging in 135 cats with hyperthyroidism. *Veterinary Radiology* **25**, 23–27

Peterson ME and Becker DV (1995) Radioiodine treatment of 524 cats with hyperthyroidism. *Journal of the American Veterinary Medical Association* **207**, 1422–1428

Peterson ME, Broussard JD and Gamble DA (1994) Use of the thyrotropin releasing hormone stimulation test to diagnose mild hyperthyroidism in cats. *Journal of Veterinary Internal Medicine* **8**, 279–286

Peterson ME and Gamble DA (1990) Effect of nonthyroidal illness on serum thyroxine concentrations in cats: 494 cases (1988). *Journal of the American Veterinary Medical Association* **197**, 1203–1211

Peterson ME, Graves TK and Cavanagh I (1987) Serum thyroid hormone concentrations fluctuate in cats with hyperthyroidism. *Journal of Veterinary Internal Medicine* **1**, 142–146

Peterson ME, Graves TK and Gamble DA (1990) Triiodothyronine (T$_3$) suppression test. An aid in the diagnosis of mild hyperthyroidism in cats. *Journal of Veterinary Internal Medicine* **4**, 233–238

Peterson ME, Keene B, Ferguson DC and Pipers FS (1982) Electrocardiographic findings in 45 cats with hyperthyroidism. *Journal of the American Veterinary Medical Association* **180**, 934–937

Peterson ME, Kintzer PP, Cavanagh PG, Fox PR, Ferguson DC, Johnson GF and Becker DV (1981) Feline hyperthyroidism: pretreatment clinical and laboratory evaluation of 131 cases. *Journal of the American Veterinary Medical Association* **183**, 103–110

Peterson ME, Kintzer PP and Hurvitz AI (1988) Methimazole treatment of 262 cats with hyperthyroidism. *Journal of Veterinary Internal Medicine* **2**, 150–157

Peterson ME, Liminana CM and Nichols CE (1995) Determination of free T4 by dialysis as an aid in diagnosis of mild hyperthyroidism in cats. *Journal of Veterinary Internal Medicine* **9**, 183

Scarlett, JM, Sydney Moise N and Rayl J (1988) Feline hyperthyroidism: a descriptive and case-control study. *Preventive Veterinary Medicine* **6**, 295–309

Schlesinger DP, Rubin SI, Papich MG and Hamilton DL (1993) Use of breath hydrogen measurement to evaluate orocecal transit time in cats before and after treatment for hyperthyroidism. *Canadian Veterinary Journal* **57**, 89–94

Stiles J, Polzin DJ and Bistner SI (1994) The prevalence of retinopathy in cats with systemic hypertension and chronic renal failure or hyperthyroidism. *Journal of the American Animal Hospital Association* **30**, 564–572

Sullivan P, Gompf R, Schmeitzel L, Clift R, Cottrell M and McDonald TP (1993) Altered platelet indices in dogs with hypothyroidism and cats with hyperthyroidism. *American Journal of Veterinary Research* **54**, 2004–2009

Thoday KL and Mooney CT (1992) Historical, clinical and laboratory features of 126 hyperthyroid cats. *Veterinary Record* **131**, 257–264

Turrel JM, Feldman EC, Nelson RW and Cain GR (1988) Thyroid carcinoma causing hyperthyroidism in cats: 14 cases (1981–1986). *Journal of the American Veterinary Medical Association* **193**, 359–364

Welches CD, Scavelli TD, Matthiesen DT and Peterson ME (1989) Occurrence of problems after three techniques of bilateral thyroidectomy in cats. *Veterinary Surgery* **18**, 392–396

Wisner ER, Theon AP, Nyland TG and Hornof WJ (1994) Ultrasonographic examination of the thyroid gland of hyperthyroid cats: Comparison to ^{99}mTcO$_4^-$ scintigraphy. *Veterinary Radiology and Ultrasound* **35**, 53–58

PART THREE

Complex Endocrine Disorders

CHAPTER SIXTEEN

Disorders of Calcium Metabolism

Andrew G. Torrance

INTRODUCTION

The concentration of serum ionised calcium is normally maintained within very narrow limits by the actions of parathyroid hormone (PTH) on bone resorption, renal calcium excretion, and the metabolism of vitamin D. The four parathyroid glands (two in association with each thyroid lobe) respond immediately to a fall in serum ionised calcium by secreting PTH which rapidly induces increased calcium release from bone, coupled with increased calcium resorption and phosphorus excretion by the distal renal tubule. At the same time PTH stimulates the activity of α-hydroxylase in the renal tubule cells which increases the synthesis of the active form of vitamin D, 1,25-dihydroxycholecalciferol (calcitriol). This causes a more long-term (24–48 hours) increase in calcium and phosphorus absorption from the gastrointestinal tract. Thus, PTH controls the concentration of two potent serum components, ionised calcium and calcitriol. To ensure that neither product accumulates in excess, the parathyroid glands are exquisitely sensitive to negative feedback from both. Abnormalities of calcium metabolism in small animals result in hypercalcaemia, hypocalcaemia, and normocalcaemia with excessive bone resorption.

HYPERCALCAEMIA

Hypercalcaemia is the most common abnormality of calcium metabolism in dogs, and has a limited differential diagnosis (Table 16.1). Hypercalcaemia is less common in cats but the differential diagnosis is similar.

Hypercalcaemia has three primary nephrotoxic actions:
- Acute vasoconstriction of renal vasculature, and renal ischaemic injury
- Antagonism of antidiuretic hormone (ADH) in the distal tubule, and nephrogenic diabetes insipidus
- Nephrocalcinosis, i.e. the precipitation of calcium phosphate in renal tissue.

The severity of the nephrocalcinosis is dependent upon the serum calcium (mmol/l) × phosphate (mmol/l) product. Therefore, vitamin D toxicosis, which causes simultaneous elevations of calcium and phosphate, induces renal damage more rapidly than excessive PTH and substances which mimic the actions of PTH. Animals which present with a calcium × phosphate product >5.0–6.0 require urgent treatment to prevent irreversible renal damage.

Hypercalcaemia of malignancy:
Lymphoma
Apocrine cell adenocarcinoma of the anal sac (dogs only)
Multiple myeloma
Hypoadrenocorticism
Chronic renal failure
Primary hyperparathyroidism
Hypervitaminosis D

Table 16.1: Differential diagnosis of hypercalcaemia in dogs and cats.

Hypercalcaemia of malignancy

Tumours that cause hypercalcaemia either secrete humoral factors which mimic PTH, or local osteoclast activating factors. Lymphoma is the most common cause of hypercalcaemia of malignancy in dogs and cats. Approximately 20% of dogs with lymphoma have hypercalcaemia. Anterior mediastinal lymphoma, in particular, has a strong association with hypercalcaemia, which occurs in approximately 40% of cases. Lymphomas release a humoral factor which mimics PTH, and invasion of bone by the tumour is not necessary for hypercalcaemia to develop. Current research indicates that PTH-related protein (PTH-RP) is the cause of humoral hypercalcaemia of malignancy (Broadus *et al.*, 1988). Increased concentrations of this peptide have been discovered in a significant number of cases of hypercalcaemic lymphoma in dogs (Weir *et al.*, 1988a,b,c). The PTH-RP is a much larger molecule than intact PTH and only shares structural similarities in the first 13 N-terminal amino acids. Functional similarities exist in the first 34 amino acids, which readily bind to the PTH receptor activating PTH responses in the cell; the remaining 107 amino acid sequence bears no resemblance to PTH. The PTH-RP can induce bone resorption and renal calcium conservation but appears not to stimulate synthesis of calcitriol. The molecule is sufficiently different from PTH not to react with valid, two site PTH assays (Feldman, 1995).

Apocrine cell adenocarcinomas of the anal sac also cause humoral hypercalcaemia of malignancy by secreting PTH-RP (Rosol *et al.*, 1990). These tumours are quite uncommon and occur most frequently in aged bitches. The primary mass in the anal sac is often quite small but the tumour metastasises readily, usually via the route of the sublumbar nodes, to the lungs or to bone. On palpation, secondary tumour in the sublumbar nodes can be more obvious than the primary in the anal sac. Complete resection of these tumours results in normocalcaemia. There have been occasional reports of humoral hypercalcaemia of malignancy associated with thymomas, squamous cell carcinomas, and adenocarcinomas.

Multiple myelomas (disseminated plasma cell tumours) can cause hypercalcaemia depending upon the extent of bone invasion. This tumour causes bone lysis through production of local osteoclast activating factors. Occasionally, other types of tumour, e.g. carcinomas with very extensive, disseminated bone metastases, can cause hypercalcaemia by a similar mechanism.

Hypoadrenocorticism

Dogs presenting with addisonian crises frequently have mild hypercalcaemia. This is a biochemical finding of academic interest only, since it has little or no effect on the course and outcome of Addison's disease. The mechanism is obscure, but the magnitude of hypercalcaemia does appear to parallel the severity of hyperkalaemia and hypovolaemia. Hypercalcaemia resolves when Addison's disease is successfully treated.

Chronic renal failure

Chronic renal failure usually causes increased renal calcium loss with normo- or hypocalcaemia, and elevation of PTH. Hypercalcaemia develops in rare cases, especially when renal failure is particularly longstanding, e.g. in congenital renal disease. In many of these cases total serum calcium is elevated, but ionised calcium is normal to low and the 'hypercalcaemia' has no pathophysiological significance. The elevation of total calcium in such cases is probably due to increased serum binding of calcium by retained anions. There are rare cases of renal disease accompanied by ionised hypercalcaemia. Presumably the parathyroid gland has been stimulated continuously for so long, that the calcium set point for autoregulation becomes elevated, or the parathyroid glands become insensitive to calcium feedback and begin to secrete PTH autonomously. The mechanism of secondary renal hyperparathyroidism will be reviewed in more detail below.

Primary hyperparathyroidism

This syndrome is usually due to a solitary parathyroid adenoma (Figures 16.1 and 16.2). It occurs in middle-aged to elderly dogs, with no sex predilection. Cases in cats are much less frequent but do occur (Kallet *et al.*, 1991). An interesting clinical difference between the species is that parathyroid adenomas in dogs are not palpable, whereas approximately half of those documented in cats have presented as unilateral palpable masses in the neck. Keeshonds are particularly susceptible to parathyroid adenomas, and accounted for 36% of the cases in a survey of 72 dogs with primary hyperparathyroidism (Feldman, 1995). Whereas most causes of hypercalcaemia are associated with a rapid onset of serious illness and severe signs including polyuria and polydipsia, incontinence, muscle weakness, gastrointestinal signs, depression, and even coma, the majority of cases of primary hyperpara-

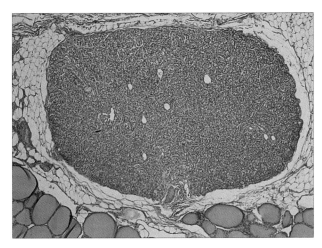

Figure 16.1: Histological section of normal parathyroid gland. Haematoxylin and eosin. Reproduced from the Veterinary Annual, *with the permission of Blackwell Science.*

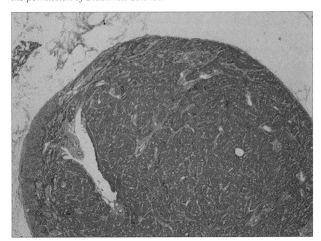

Figure 16.2: Histological section of a parathyroid adenoma. Haematoxylin and eosin.

thyroidism have long-term histories of mild or minimal signs. The most common finding is polyuria/polydipsia with more infrequent evidence of weakness, lethargy, dysuria, and inappetance. Calcium-containing urinary calculi were found in 22 of 72 dogs with primary hyperparathyroidism, and investigations of the urinary tract should be carried out whenever this primary diagnosis is suspected. Surgical removal of parathyroid adenomas may result in a complete cure.

Vitamin D toxicosis

When house plants such as *Cestrum diurnum* were the only potential source of high concentrations of vitamin D available to pets, this was a minor differential diagnosis limited to pets with peculiar appetites. The recent inclusion of massive doses of vitamin D2 in rat poisons has made this a significant household threat. Early studies in dogs and cats indicated that vitamin D causes a florid toxicosis, with severe gastrointestinal signs, haematemesis, collapse, and death within 60–70 hours (Gunther *et al.*, 1988). Naturally occurring cases show a spectrum of severity ranging from acute death to prolonged bouts of hypercalcaemia and hyperphosphataemia with subsequent renal compromise. Vitamin D2 is cleared very slowly from the body because it is fat-soluble; consequently hypercalcaemia tends to be very persistent. The prolonged

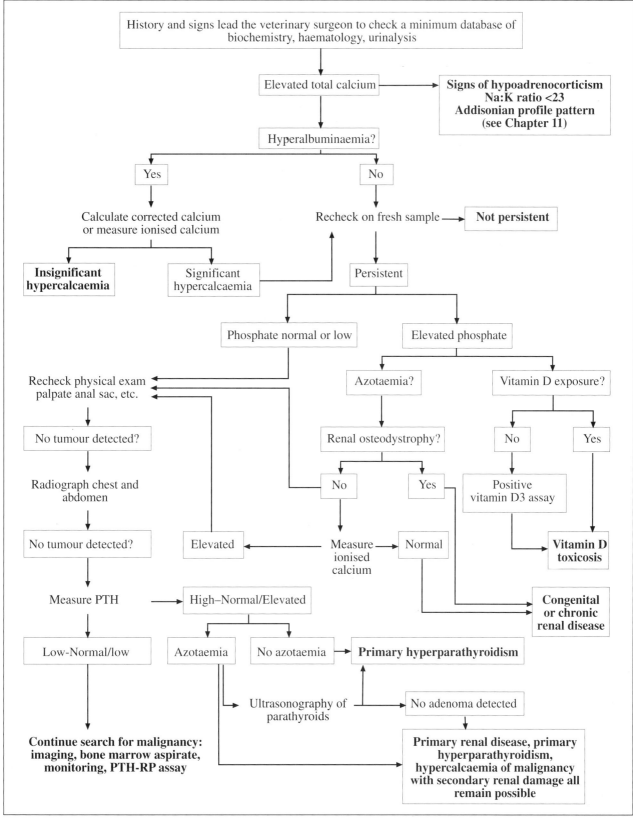

Figure 16.3: *Algorithm of the diagnostic investigation of hypercalcaemia.*

intensive therapy needed to prevent renal complications is expensive.

Diagnosis of vitamin D toxicosis is usually dependent upon a history of exposure. Assays for vitamin D3 exist and do show elevations in vitamin D toxicosis, but further investigation is required before such assays become widely available to practising veterinary surgeons. Serumphosphate is a useful parameter for differentiating

the causes of hypercalcaemia. Vitamin D toxicosis, hypoadrenocorticism, and chronic renal disease are associated with elevations of serum phosphate, but primary hyperparathyroidism and hypercalcaemia of malignancy more often induce normal or low serum phosphate, unless they are accompanied by secondary renal failure. Unfortunately, phosphate is one of the most labile biochemical parameters included in profiles, and tends to increase when samples are lipaemic, haemolysed, or aged (e.g. in transit to a reference laboratory). Careful evaluation of the validity of elevated phosphate values is important when interpreting a biochemical profile. Corticosteroids directly antagonise the hypercalcaemic actions of vitamin D3 and are useful in the specific therapy of vitamin D toxicosis.

Miscellaneous causes of hypercalcaemia

Young dogs and cats (<1 year of age) have higher serum calcium concentrations than adults. These are mild elevations of calcium, and are usually accompanied by similar age-related elevations of serum alkaline phosphatase and phosphate. Elevations of serum albumin cause increases in total serum calcium without affecting ionised calcium. Such elevations are of no pathophysiological significance and must be ruled out before any further clinical investigation of hypercalcaemia is attempted. The total calcium concentration can be corrected against the albumin concentration:

Corrected Ca (mmol/l) = [(Ca (mmol/l) × 4) – (albumin (g/l) × 0.1) + 3.5] × 0.25

Since ionised calcium assays are now becoming commercially available, this rather crude mathematical correction is likely to become obsolete. Spurious hypercalcaemia can result from serum lipaemia or haemolysis and it is always advisable to check for the persistence of hypercalcaemia on a second serum sample before embarking on a systematic diagnostic investigation. Other infrequent causes of hypercalcaemia include the diuretic phase of acute renal failure, a small percentage of cases of nutritional hyperparathyroidism, disseminated fungal osteomyelitis, and severe hypothermia. Acidosis decreases the binding affinity of calcium for albumin and causes mild ionised hypercalcaemia. Alkalosis has the opposite effect and causes mild ionised hypocalcaemia. These changes may also be reflected in mild changes of total serum calcium.

Investigating hypercalcaemia

Hypercalcaemia is usually discovered when history and clinical signs lead the veterinary surgeon to request a data base of haematology, biochemistry, and urinalysis. Several of the differential diagnoses, e.g. hypoadrenocorticism and vitamin D toxicosis, can often be excluded simply by evaluating the existing information carefully (Figure 16.3). Problems arise when hypercalcaemia is complicated by renal failure, and when occult malignancy or primary hyperparathyroidism are suspected. Malignancy searches usually involve imaging (radiography and ultrasonography), and sampling organs and bone marrow for cytology. Surgical exploration of the neck for a parathyroid adenoma has even been recommended. The recent validation of PTH assays for canine and feline patients, and the increasing availability of valid ionised calcium measurements, provide less invasive diagnostic approaches to assist with these difficult cases.

PTH assays

PTH exists in circulation as a mixture of very small quantities (pmol/l) of intact hormone with a very short half-life (<4 minutes) which are biologically active, and large numbers of C-terminal fragments of the molecule (ng/l) which are not biologically active and have a 10–20-fold longer half-life. The concentration of C-terminal fragments changes very slowly in response to changes in ionised calcium, whereas the changes in intact hormone are almost instantaneous. In addition, C-terminal fragments are excreted by the kidney and accumulate in renal failure. The first PTH assays were single site, C-terminal or mid-molecule, radioimmunoassays which crossreacted with the inactive fragments and therefore gave little insight into parathyroid gland function. The development of two site assays which bound both ends of the molecule, thus trapping intact PTH in a sandwich with two antibodies, enabled accurate detection of the active PTH moiety without C-terminal fragment interference. The first of these human PTH assays to be validated for the dog was an immunoradiometric assay (Torrance and Nachreiner, 1989a). This assay was subsequently also validated for the cat (Barber *et al.*, 1993). The assay is best interpreted in conjunction with either an ionised or total calcium

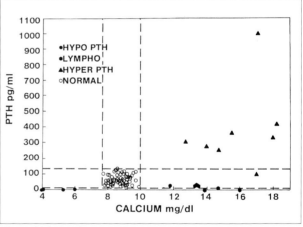

Figure 16.4: *Graph comparing intact parathyroid hormone (PTH) concentration with total serum calcium concentration in dogs with primary hyperparathyroidism (Hyper PTH), hypoparathyroidism (Hypo PTH), hypercalcaemic lymphoma, and in 85 normal samples. Horizontal and vertical lines show the normal ranges of intact PTH and total serum calcium concentration, respectively. (Reprinted with permission from Torrance and Nachreiner, 1989b.)*

measurement (Figure 16.4), and is clinically useful for distinguishing hypercalcaemia due to an occult malignancy from primary hyperparathyroidism (Torrance and Nachreiner, 1989b). Hypercalcaemia of malignancy is characterised by an elevated calcium concentration with an appropriately suppressed PTH (usually undetectable). Primary hyperparathyroidism is associated with an elevated calcium and an inappropriately elevated PTH (often markedly elevated), indicating autonomous PTH secretion and insensitivity to calcium feedback. The assay is less easy to interpret if moderate to marked azotaemia is present since reduced renal clearance will result in an elevated PTH concentration, regardless of the original cause of hypercalcaemia.

However, if the PTH concentration is normal or low in the presence of hypercalcaemia and renal failure, it is still consistent with hypercalcaemia of malignancy. An elevated PTH concentration in this situation is uninterpretable. The PTH assay is also useful for confirming primary hypoparathyroidism which is characterised by low serum calcium and inappropriately low PTH. Parathyroid hormone is quite a labile peptide and samples must be handled carefully to avoid proteolysis and loss of hormone during shipment and storage. Both heparin and serum samples can be used. Serum or plasma should be separated at room temperature within 1–2 hours, and then chilled in a refrigerator before assay, or frozen to –10 to –20 ºC before shipment in an insulated container or with ice packs (see Chapter 33).

Ionised calcium

The value of this measurement for identifying physiologically relevant changes in serum calcium has already been discussed. Ionised calcium measurements are superior to total serum calcium in detecting genuine abnormalities of calcium metabolism. They have not been widely available because studies investigating the optimal handling of blood samples to prevent spurious changes in the concentration of ions were lacking. With the widespread use of ion-sensitive electrodes, and some recent findings on sample handling, the measurement of ionised calcium by commercial and inhouse laboratories will become commonplace (Feldman, 1995). If kept anaerobic, samples for ionised calcium can be handled at room temperature for 72 hours without significantly altering the ionised calcium concentration (Schenck *et al.*, 1995). Blood must be collected in an evacuated tube, separated by centrifugation, and the serum extracted into a plastic syringe, which is immediately capped. Any air bubbles in the serum should be removed by gentle tapping before the syringe is sealed. Serum-separator tubes should not be used because the silicon gel contains calcium.

PTH-RP

The significance of PTH-RP in hypercalcaemia of malignancy has already been discussed. Assays valid for PTH-RP (from canine and feline tumours) are anticipated, and will offer a further diagnostic tool for identifying the presence of an occult malignancy. It is known, however, that PTH-RP will be increased in renal insufficiency even in the absence of an underlying malignancy (Burtis *et al.*, 1990).

Imaging

Radiographs of the thorax, abdomen, and skeleton are used at an early stage in the investigation to detect, for example, anterior mediastinal lymphoma. Ultrasonography is also used for assessing the internal structure of organs, and for guided biopsy and aspirate procedures. Recent studies have shown that 80–95% of parathyroid adenomas can be identified by an experienced ultrasonographer using a 10 MHz transducer (Feldman *et al.*, 1997).

Treatment of hypercalcaemia

Controlling hypercalcaemia

The emergency treatment of hypercalcaemia is discussed in Chapter 19. The decision to implement symptomatic therapy of hypercalcaemia depends upon the clinical condition and stability of the patient. A calcium phosphorus product >5–6 indicates a significant risk of nephrocalcinosis and the need for rapid intervention to reduce hypercalcaemia. Renal function should be monitored closely in any persistently hypercalcaemic patient. It is important to remember that use of corticosteroids to combat hypercalcaemia, before the underlying diagnosis has been established, is likely to interfere with the diagnostic investigation. All causes of hypercalcaemia will respond partially to the renal calciuretic effects of corticosteroids. The lympholytic effects of these drugs will temporarily remove all evidence of lymphoma. When the neoplasm recurs it will be more resistant to other forms of chemotherapy. Salmon calcitonin can be very useful for rapid correction of severe hypercalcaemia but its actions are short lived. Drugs not discussed in Chapter 19 are the bisphosphonates. These osteoclast inhibitors are widely used in human medicine for the treatment of osteoporosis and for controlling intractable hypercalcaemia. First generation bisphosphonates, such as etidronate, have limited potency. More recent generations of these drugs, such as pamidronate and clodronate, have superior efficacy in humans. A single infusion of pamidronate (human dose, 1 mg/kg intravenously over 3–24 hours) can control hypercalcaemia for a week or more, thus giving the clinician ample time to discover the underlying cause of hypercalcaemia while minimising the risk of nephrocalcinosis. Clodronate (human dose, 25 mg/kg intravenously in 500 ml normal saline, over 4 hours) has better gastrointestinal absorption than previous bisphosphonates, and can therefore be used for both acute (intravenous infusion) and more chronic (oral dosage) cases of hypercalcaemia. Both drugs are associated with significant risk of inducing hypocalcaemia. Veterinary use of these drugs has been very limited but the author is aware of a study in which normocalcaemia was restored in five of six hypercalcaemic dogs within 72 hours of infusing intravenous clodronate (G. Petrie, personal communication).

Specific therapy

Treatment of lymphoma, myeloma, and other malignancies is described elsewhere. Apocrine cell adenocarcinoma of the anal sac responds poorly to chemotherapy but, even in cases with metastatic disease, surgical debulking or removal of tumour tissue will alleviate the hypercalcaemia to some extent and prolong life. Long-term use of the new generation bisphosphonates or corticosteroids are also considerations when the bulk of the tumour is inoperable. Primary hyperparathyroidism is usually associated with a solitary parathyroid adenoma in the neck. These are readily identifiable at surgery either on the ventral surface of the thyroid gland or within the substance of the gland visible from the dorsal surface (Figures 16.5 and 16.6). Removal of the mass is usually quite straightforward.

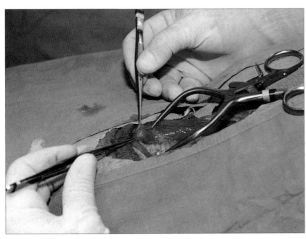

Figure 16.5: Surgical identification of a parathyroid adenoma of the external parathyroid of a dog. Reproduced from the Veterinary Annual *with the permission of Blackwell Science.*

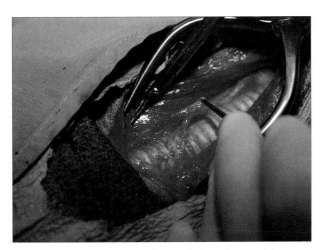

Figure 16.6: Blunt dissection and removal of an adenoma of the external parathyroid gland of a dog. Reproduced from the Veterinary Annual *with the permission of Blackwell Science.*

Cases involving the internal parathyroid may require removal of the whole thyroid/parathyroid unit on the affected side. There are some descriptions of unexpected findings (Feldman and Nelson, 1996). Occasional dogs have hyperplasia of all four glands not attributable to secondary causes of hyperparathyroidism. Parathyroid adenomas have been known to recur, particularly in Keeshonds. The source of excessive PTH can be ectopic parathyroid tissue located in the mediastinum. In addition, hyperparathyroidism resolved acutely in two dogs after infarction of the adenoma. These dogs presented with spontaneous hypocalcaemia following a prolonged history of hypercalcaemia.

The histopathology of parathyroid masses must be interpreted cautiously because the morphological features of the cells may belie their behaviour. Generally, a single parathyroid mass accompanied by atrophy of the other parathyroid glands is described as an adenoma, while enlargement of all four parathyroids is described as hyperplasia, even if the cellular morphology is the same in both cases. Parathyroid carcinomas are defined by both behavioural and morphological characteristics. Carcinomas are more

invasive, adherent structures and may be palpable in dogs. In one series of cases, two masses which were described as carcinomas on histopathology had the gross appearance and overall behaviour of adenomas (Feldman and Nelson, 1996). Parathyroid carcinomas are very rare in dogs and cats.

Hypocalcaemia frequently occurs following the removal of a solitary parathyroid adenoma due to the hypercalcaemia-induced atrophy of the remaining parathyroid glands. The risk of clinically significant post-surgical hypocalcaemia increases depending upon the magnitude of the calcium elevation. Presurgical calcium values <3.5 mmol/l are unlikely to be associated with significant post-surgical hypo-calcaemia. Such patients should be hospitalised with cage rest (minimal activity) and their serum calcium closely monitored for at least 5 days after surgery. Presurgical calcium values >3.5 mmol/l have a significant risk of post-surgical hypocalcaemia. The higher the calcium value, the greater the risk. In such cases, vitamin D preparations with a rapid onset of activity (within 24 hours), such as calcitriol, should be on hand for rapid post-surgical intervention. Alternatively, a slower acting vitamin D preparation, such as dihydro-tachysterol onset of action 3–5 days), may be started prophylactically, immediately after surgery. The time of onset of hypocalcaemia following surgery is unpredictable, but in most cases will be within the first 5–6 days. Withdrawal of vitamin D supplementation should be undertaken gradually, over 3–4 months, as vitamin D itself will have a suppressive effect on parathyroid function, and delays parathyroid recovery. Emergency treatment of hypocalcaemia is discussed further in Chapter 19.

Both calcitonin and corticosteroids are of use as specific therapy for vitamin D toxicosis: calcitonin for management of acute hypercalcaemia in the short term, and corticosteroids for long-term control. Bisphosphonate drugs are also potentially useful for long-term control of vitamin D toxicosis. Strategic use of these drugs may serve to reduce the costs of intensive fluid therapy and hospitalisation.

Prognosis for hypercalcaemia

Hypercalcaemia generally worsens the prognosis for chemotherapy of malignant lymphoma and multiple myeloma. Apocrine cell adenocarcinomas of the anal sac can be managed surgically, but the prognosis is guarded since these tumours readily metastasise. Addison's disease has a good prognosis when managed correctly. Primary hyperparathyroidism is a curable disease but the complications of post-surgical hypo-calcaemia and renal damage may be significant. Vitamin D toxicosis has a guarded to poor prognosis. A major prognostic factor for all causes of hypercalcaemia is the presence or absence of accompanying renal damage. Nephrocalcinosis can be halted by appropriate therapy, but the damage incurred by the kidneys may lead to an inexorable progression to chronic, end stage renal failure.

Primary hypoparathyroidism:
        Immune destruction of the gland
        Idiopathic atrophy
        Damage induced by a locally invasive
        disease process
Iatrogenic (post-surgical) hypoparathyroidism
Puerperal tetany (eclampsia)
Chronic renal failure
Ethylene glycol toxicosis
Acute renal failure
Phosphate-containing enemas
Citrate-containing blood transfusions
Acute pancreatitis
Medullary carcinoma of the thyroid

Table 16.2: Differential diagnosis of ionised hypocalcaemia in dogs and cats.

HYPOCALCAEMIA

Naturally occurring hypocalcaemia (low serum ionised calcium) is a rare finding in dogs and cats, and presents with a specific spectrum of signs. The differential diagnosis of ionised hypocalcaemia is limited (Table 16.2). There are numerous causes of mild reductions in serum total calcium which are rarely of clinical significance. The signs of ionised hypocalcaemia are primarily neuromuscular and intermittent, and reflect hyperexcitability of both motor and sensory nerves. Dogs tend to show a stiff gait, muscle fasciculations, tremor, cramps, and tonic spasms of the limbs which are often exacerbated by exercise or excitement (latent tetany). There is increased anxiety and aggression, and often reluctance to be handled. The last may be due to the fact that handling can precipitate painful muscle cramps. These abnormalities may precipitate a grand mal convulsion, but seizures also occur spontaneously with little advanced warning. Seizures may mimic grand mal epilepsy or may be atypical with maintained consciousness and continence. Seizures usually resolve spontaneously, but can be very prolonged. Sensory signs include intense pruritus, facial rubbing, and self-mutilation. Non-specific signs such as vomiting, diarrhoea, listlessness, inappetance, and depression may also be present.

Cats show predominantly intermittent motor signs, similar to those described, in addition to non-specific feline signs of illness such as raised nictitans membranes and ptyalism. Long-standing causes of hypocalcaemia, e.g. primary hypoparathyroidism, induce lenticular cataract formation. These are small, punctate to linear, white opacities in the anterior and posterior cortical, subcapsular region of the lens.

Primary hypoparathyroidism
This is an uncommon syndrome which has been recorded in both dogs and cats. It occurs in a broad age range from under 1 year to the elderly, but the majority of cases occur in young adults. Breed associations include Miniature Poodles, Miniature Schnauzers, terriers, Labrador Retrievers and German Shepherd Dogs. The pathogenesis is lymphoplasmacytic destruction of the parathyroid glands, which pass through a phase of nodular hyperplasia before the gland is replaced by lymphocytes and fibrous tissue. The diseased glands are difficult to locate, but biopsies either contain evidence of lymphocytic infiltration or replacement of the gland with fibrous tissue. The latter is described as idiopathic atrophy, but is probably the end stage of lymphoid destruction. Signs of hypocalcaemia may present abruptly, forcing rapid veterinary attention, or may be present in a less acute form for many months before presentation. The first opinion diagnosis is frequently idiopathic epilepsy, and a large proportion of cases will be treated with anticonvulsants before the definitive diagnosis is established. Hypocalcaemia should always be considered in the differential diagnosis of epilepsy, and is easily ruled out by performing an appropriate data base including a biochemical profile. Primary hypoparathyroidism is characterised by a very low calcium concentration (<1.6 mmol/l) and a normal or elevated serum phosphate concentration. Valid PTH assays will show an inappropriately low/normal or low PTH concentration and this is sufficient to confirm the diagnosis. A presumptive diagnosis of hypoparathyroidism can generally be made in any non-lactating, non-azotaemic patient presenting with appropriate signs, severe hypocalcaemia, and hyperphosphataemia. The role of magnesium deficiency has been questioned in dogs (Feldman, 1995). In humans, hypomagnesaemia causes functional hypoparathyroidism by suppressing PTH secretion and inducing PTH resistance. This causes a syndrome which mimics the signs and biochemical findings of primary hypoparathyroidism. An equivalent syndrome has not been documented in the dog and cat, and the majority of cases of canine hypoparathyroidism, in which magnesium has been measured, have had a normal serum concentration. Another human syndrome which mimics primary hypoparathyroidism is pseudohypoparathyroidism. This is a rare familial syndrome caused by resistance of peripheral tissues to PTH. This syndrome has not been definitively identified in the dog or cat to date.

Iatrogenic (post-surgical) hypoparathyroidism
Parathyroid glands may be inadvertently removed, damaged, or deprived of their blood supply during surgery of the neck. The resulting hypoparathyroidism varies in severity depending upon the nature of the injury. Patients with severe post-surgical hypoparathyroidism will develop signs of hypocalcaemia unless treated. Others may suffer transient subclinical hypoparathyroidism. Permanent hypoparathyroidism following neck surgery is rare. Post-surgical hypoparathyroidism is the most common abnormality of calcium metabolism in cats because surgery for hyperthyroidism is widely practised. The modified thyroidectomy techniques described in Chapter 15 have reduced the incidence of post-surgical hypoparathyroidism, but a significant risk (20–30% of all cats undergoing bilateral thyroidectomy) still exists.

Puerperal tetany (eclampsia)

This is an acute onset of life-threatening hypocalcaemia in the lactating bitch or queen. It is most common in small dogs. Hypocalcaemia is always severe and associated with the typical signs. Most cases occur during the first 3 weeks of nursing a litter, although ante-natal and late onset cases have occurred. The pathogenesis is poorly understood. Under normal circumstances the mechanisms of calcium homeostasis compensate for the heavy drain of calcium into fetal skeletons and maternal milk, by ensuring avid gastrointestinal calcium absorption and controlling minute to minute fluctuations in the drain of calcium from serum, through renal conservation and bone resorptive mechanisms. The stores of calcium in maternal bone are enormous, and an absolute calcium deficiency is most unlikely. Presumably, the rapidity of calcium utilisation simply overwhelms the ability of homeostatic mechanisms to maintain the serum ionised calcium concentration. Parathyroid atrophy and temporary hypoparathyroidism due to the inappropriate, ante-natal supplementation of calcium may be important. Respiratory alkalosis due to panting during whelping will decrease serum ionised calcium and may precipitate eclampsia. The diagnosis of eclampsia is usually made on the grounds of history and clinical signs alone, and calcium treatment instituted without delay. Measurement of serum calcium is rarely necessary.

Renal failure

Most cases of chronic renal failure in dogs and cats will have elevations of serum phosphate and PTH concentrations, with normal serum ionised calcium. A few cases demonstrate a mild ionised hypocalcaemia, but this is rarely severe enough to be of clinical significance and does not cause signs of hypocalcaemia. The severity of ionised hypocalcaemia may be ameliorated by the presence of acidosis, which will increase the ionised fraction relative to albumin bound calcium.

Acute, post-renal renal failure which occurs in tom cats with urethral obstruction, causes a very rapid increase in serum phosphorus which will bind calcium and may cause acute hypocalcaemia. In such cases, signs of hypocalcaemia may develop simultaneously with the presence of life-threatening hyperkalaemia and acid–base abnormalities. Acute renal failure induced by ethylene glycol intoxication can be complicated by hypocalcaemia resulting from calcium chelation by metabolites of the toxin.

Acute pancreatitis

An association between acute pancreatitis and hypocalcaemia has been recognised but the hypocalcaemia tends to be mild and of little clinical significance. Signs of hypocalcaemia are unlikely. The mechanism of hypocalcaemia is thought to be saponification of peripancreatic fat following the leakage of lipase.

Miscellaneous causes of hypocalcaemia

Signs of hypocalcaemia have been induced by administration of phosphate-containing enemas to dehydrat-ed cats with colonic atony. The ionised hypocalcaemia is due to calcium binding by the rapidly escalating serum phosphate concentration. A similar effect is seen when donor blood containing excessive citrate anti-coagulant is administered to small dogs or cats. Typically, this occurs when the volume of donor blood is insufficient to fill a blood bag containing a fixed quantity of citrate. The citrate chelates calcium causing a rapid decline in serum ionised calcium in the recipient. Functional carcinomas of the medullary c-cells of the thyroid, which secrete calcitonin, are a very rare cause of hypocalcaemia in dogs and cats. Alkalosis increases calcium binding to albumin and reduces serum ionised calcium. In extreme cases, for example, alkalosis induced by a large bicarbonate infusion, ionised hypocalcaemia may be severe enough to induce signs.

Ionised hypocalcaemia is a rare clinical finding, however, mild reductions of total serum calcium concentration are frequently seen on biochemical profiles. Syndromes which cause hypoalbuminaemia such as malabsorption, protein-losing enteropathy, protein-losing nephropathy, and hepatic dysfunction will lower the total serum calcium, leaving the ionised fraction unchanged. The 'corrected' calcium concentration should be calculated before hypocalcaemia is investigated any further. Sample ageing artefacts may cause spurious hypocalcaemia, so low calcium values should always be rechecked on a fresh sample. Contamination of serum samples with EDTA or citrate, causes chelation of calcium and spurious hypocalcaemia.

Investigating hypocalcaemia

Hypocalcaemia is detected when clinical signs and history lead to further investigation with a biochemical profile. The cause of hypocalcaemia can usually be established by careful consideration of an appropriate minimum data base of biochemistry, haematology, and urinalysis (Figure 16.7). All routine profile parameters contribute to the diagnosis, but parameters which are particularly important are albumin, urea, creatinine, phosphate, amylase, lipase, urine specific gravity, and complete blood counts. Significant hypocalcaemia induces bradycardia and specific ECG findings, which may be useful both diagnostically and for monitoring the response to therapy. Prolongation of the S-T segment correlates with the severity of hypocalcaemia. Additional findings include deep, wide T waves, prolonged Q-T intervals, and tall R waves. Intact PTH assay is useful for confirming the presence of primary hypoparathyroidism.

Treatment of hypocalcaemia

This is described in Chapter 19. Therapeutic PTH preparations are not available and, therefore, treatment of primary hypoparathyroidism relies upon administration of vitamin D preparations for life. Although the prognosis for therapy of primary hypoparathyroidism is generally considered good, the need for life-long medication and the severity of signs

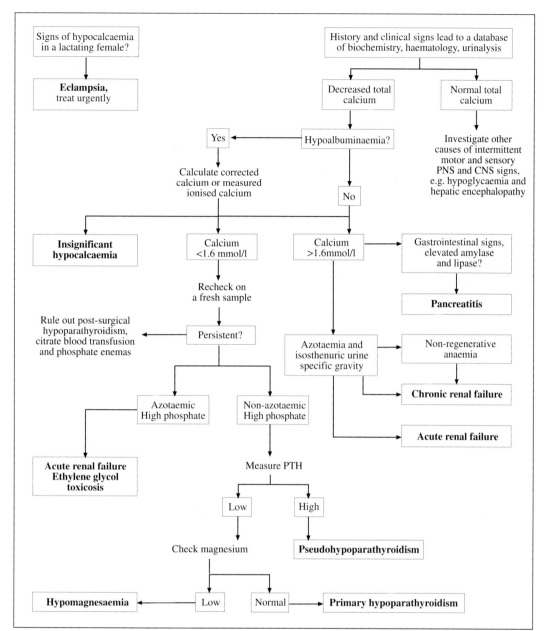

Figure 16.7: The diagnostic investigation of hypocalcaemia. The significance of hypomagnesaemia and pseudohypopara-thyroidism in dogs and cats is unclear.

associated with failure to administer medication, may be discouraging to owners in the long term. Careful monitoring of therapy is essential since vitamin D administration readily leads to hypercalcaemia and hyperphosphataemia with associated irreversible renal damage.

NORMOCALCAEMIA WITH EXCESSIVE BONE RESORPTION

Renal secondary hyperparathyroidism

This syndrome contributes to the complicated pathogenesis of chronic renal failure, and is the subject of significant research effort in dogs and cats. The pathogenesis of renal secondary hyperparathyroidism (RSHPTH), its contribution to the inexorable progression of chronic renal failure, and the role of PTH as a uraemic toxin, are all under debate. The most obvious manifestation of RSH-PTH is renal osteodystrophy. Persistently high PTH

concentrations and the progressive reduction in renal tubule cells capable of manufacturing calcitriol, result in excessive calcium resorption from bone, and reduced gastrointestinal calcium uptake. This causes a progressive demineralisation of bone which is particularly evident in the bones of the head. The mandible and maxilla become pliable and swollen with loosening of the teeth (Figures 16.8 and 16.9). There may also be generalised skeletal pain and bowing of long bones, with occasional pathological fractures. In humans on long-term dialysis, this syndrome is a particular threat, but dogs and cats with acquired renal failure rarely live long enough to develop significant skeletal signs. Renal osteodystrophy occurs primarily in young, growing cats and dogs with long-standing congenital or juvenile renal disease.

Evidence from the human field suggests that RSHPTH contributes to the progression of renal failure through the toxic effects of PTH on renal cells (Massry, 1989). These effects are manifested by intracellular calcium accumulation followed by cellular disruption and death. Parathyroid hormone is regarded as a serious uraemic

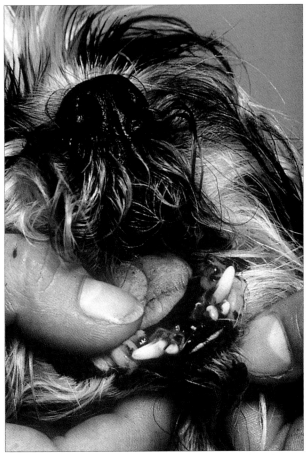

Figure 16.8: *Renal osteodystrophy in a dog with longstanding chronic renal failure: 'Rubber jaw'. Reproduced from the* Veterinary Annual *with the permission of Blackwell Science.*

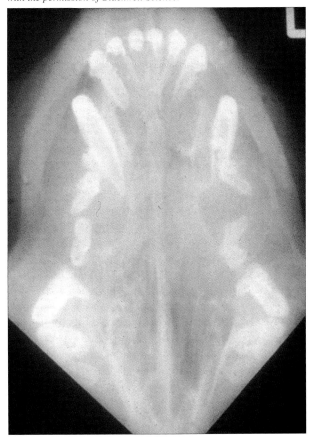

Figure 16.9: *Renal osteodystrophy in a dog with longstanding chronic renal failure: The radiograph shows marked demineralisation of the jaw.*

toxin contributing to neurological signs, glucose intolerance, anaemia, leucocyte dysfunction, and acidosis. Combined with the problems of osteodystrophy and soft tissue calcification, these adverse effects of PTH provide a strong argument for therapeutic control of RSHPTH.

Data from the dog and cat are less convincing. Nephrectomy models of chronic renal failure in the dog have shown that renal failure remains stable until extreme reductions of renal mass, such as the 15/16 nephrectomy, are used (Bovee, 1992; Finco *et al.*, 1992). Only then does progressive renal failure ensue. Complete removal of PTH by parathyroidectomy before induction of renal failure by nephrectomy, resulted in no demonstrable beneficial effects on either the uraemic syndrome or progression of renal failure in dogs (Finco *et al.*, 1994). While the rationale for close control of RSHPTH in canine and feline chronic renal failure remains debatable, there is good evidence to suggest that control of hyperphosphataemia has a beneficial effect (Finco *et al.*, 1992). The mechanism of this effect is not fully understood, but it does not appear to be mediated, simply, by the secondary reduction of RSHPTH.

Two major feedback systems interact in the pathogenesis of RSHPTH. The first is triggered by the failure of renal phosphorus excretion which results in hyperphosphataemia. This causes a reduction in serum ionised calcium which stimulates PTH secretion. Calcium phosphate is deposited in soft tissues, and more calcium is resorbed from bone. The parathyroid glands become hyperplastic and chronic stimulation of PTH secretion causes RSHPTH. At the same time, the decreasing population of viable renal tubular cells synthesise less calcitriol. The reduction in calcitriol has a direct feedback effect on the parathyroid gland, causing increased PTH secretion. The increased PTH is permissive to the activity of 1α-hydroxylase in the renal tubule cells and allows increased calcitriol synthesis. This feedback mechanism fails when the loss of renal mass is sufficient to prevent the increase in calcitriol concentration in response to PTH. Reduced calcitriol then leads to reduced calcium absorption from the gastrointestinal tract, and the cycle of bone resorption is perpetuated. Different authors make different claims about the relative importance of hyperphosphataemia and vitamin D deficiency in the pathogenesis of RSHPTH in dogs and cats (Feldman, 1995; Barber and Elliot, 1998). Proponents of vitamin D therapy claim that the decrease in calcitriol precedes the increase in phosphate, and the latter only develops in the later stages of RSHPTH. Hyperphosphataemia itself inhibits the production of calcitriol by its suppressive action on 1α-hydroxylase. Recent data from cats with naturally occurring chronic renal failure suggest that significant decreases in vitamin D occur only in end stage renal failure, and are preceded by elevations in phosphate (Barber and Elliot, 1998). In this study, only phosphate concentration was significantly correlated with that of PTH. Control of hyperphosphataemia alone provided adequate control of RSHPTH, and therapy with calcitriol was deemed unnecessary.

Treatment of RSHPTH

At present, strong indications for treatment of RSHPTH in dogs and cats only exist in rare cases of renal osteodystrophy. However, phosphorus restriction appears to be beneficial in all cases of chronic renal failure. Coincidentally, phosphorus restriction also appears to be an effective method for controlling RSHPTH. The extent of RSHPTH should be documented by PTH assay. Then a staged approach of intervention and monitoring used to bring the PTH concentration back into the normal range.

Phosphate restriction

Phosphate intake is reduced by combining a phosphate-restricted diet with phosphorus binders. Sources of dietary phosphorus are proteins, amino acids, bone meal, and additives. The bioavailability of phosphorus depends upon the source of protein. Various levels of protein restriction are available in commercial veterinary diets, the percentage dry matter of phosphate ranging from 0.5% to 0.13%. Selection of diet depends upon the individual patient and the severity of hyperphosphataemia and uraemia. In most patients this level of phosphate restriction will not induce normophosphataemia, and phosphate binders will also be required. Aluminium- and calcium-containing binders are available and should be administered with meals. Aluminium salts (carbonate, hydroxide, and acetate) are preferred because calcium-containing binders may induce hypercalcaemia, particularly if administered in conjunction with calcitriol. Concerns about the toxicity of aluminium in human patients were not found to be of significance in three dogs (Finco *et al.*, 1985). The dose should be individualised for each patient by monitoring, but an appropriate starting dose is 100 mg/kg/day. The most common limiting factor for the dose of binders is poor palatability.

The goal of therapy is to maintain normophosphataemia. Regular monitoring is necessary and samples for serum phosphate should be taken at the same time of day, after a 12 hour fast, to minimise feeding-related and diurnal variations. Plasma intact PTH concentration should be measured simultaneously to ascertain whether phosphate restriction has successfully controlled RSHPTH. In some cases, normophosphataemia will not be achieved for several weeks.

Vitamin D therapy

Calcitriol can be used if phosphate has normalised but PTH is still elevated. The recommended doses range from 1.5 to 6.5 ng/kg/day. Hypercalcaemia is the main limiting factor for the use of vitamin D in renal failure. Using low doses reduces the likelihood of hypercalcaemia, and the choice of calcitriol ensures that, should hypercalcaemia occur, it can be rapidly reversed (within 4 days) by discontinuation of the drug. This is a great improvement over other vitamin D analogues (ergocalciferol) which induce persistent hypercalcaemia for several weeks. The low doses of calcitriol cause problems for prescription because the calcitriol doses in capsules manufactured for human patients are too large (250–500 ng). This problem can be solved by requesting a customised preparation from a pharmacist. Alternatively, small volumes of drug can be aspirated from the human capsules and suspended in olive oil or injected into gelatin capsules. Calcitriol is readily absorbed through the skin, so the preparations must be handled carefully. A potential alternative to calcitriol is α-calcidiol, which requires hepatic metabolism to calcitriol for a therapeutic effect. This drug is available in the UK in a suspension at 200 ng/ml. After starting the calcitriol therapy, repeat measures of phosphate should be made at 1 week and then monthly. Re-evaluation of the PTH concentration at 1, 3, and 6 months is appropriate.

Newly recognised secondary hyperparathyroid syndromes in cats

Recent studies have identified two previously undescribed hyperparathyroid states in cats.

A group of 30 hyperthyroid cats were found to have significantly lower blood ionised calcium and plasma creatinine concentrations and significantly higher plasma phosphate and parathyroid hormone concentrations than age-matched controls. Hyperparathyroidism occurred in 77% of the hyperthyroid cats. The aetiology and significance of this finding have not been established as yet, but concurrent hyperparathyroidism could have important implications for both bone strength and renal function in hyperthyroid cats (Barber and Elliot, 1996).

A series of five cats which presented with osteopenia was recently described (Barber *et al.*, 1997). Three of the cats had 'rubber jaw'. On investigation, none of these cats had evidence of hypercalcaemia, renal disease, vitamin D deficiency, or a dietary history suggestive of nutritional secondary hyperparathyroidism. All had massive elevations of PTH, and three had parathyroid hyperplasia on histopathology. Two of the cats were related. The syndrome has been called atypical hyperparathyroidism, but further investigation is required to discover the pathogenesis.

Nutritional secondary hyperparathyroidism (NSH)

This disease is characterised by excessive bone resorption and osteopenia which are induced by persistent feeding of diets with excessive phosphate or inadequate calcium. These are usually pure meat or offal diets with calcium:phosphate ratios of 1:16–1:35, far removed from the recommended ratios of 1.2:1 for dogs and 1:1 for cats. The calcium phosphate imbalance causes ionised hypocalcaemia which stimulates PTH secretion. The compensatory mechanisms induced by hyperparathyroidism are unable to restore calcium homeostasis in the face of continued challenge from the unbalanced diet, and skeletal demineralisation ensues. Clinical signs include bone pain, pathological fractures, reluctance to move, lameness, swelling of costochondral junctions and metaphyses, and limb deformity. Collapse of the axial skeleton may lead to neurological signs. The disease usually affects young, growing animals but can also occasionally be seen in adults. The latter may show less florid signs including generalised osteopenia, bone pain, and loss of teeth.

Investigation

The data base is usually non-specific. Total serum calcium will be normal or slightly low. Phosphate and serum alkaline phosphatase are likely to be elevated but these are common findings in normal growing dogs and cats and so must be interpreted conservatively. Radiographic signs include reduced bone density, thin cortices, pathological fractures, and loss of alveolar bone. Long bone metaphyses may be mushroom-shaped, and an area of relative radiodensity, representing the area of primary mineralisation, may be present adjacent to the growth plate. These changes are best appreciated in the distal radius and ulna. The diagnosis is made on the basis of history, clinical signs, and radiographic findings.

Treatment

Absolute cage rest for several weeks is a necessity. The diet must be changed to a good quality, balanced ration. Calcium should be supplemented in the diet to achieve a calcium:phosphate ratio of 2:1 for the first 2–3 months of treatment, after which the additional calcium is withdrawn. Severely affected patients can be treated with intravenous calcium gluconate (1.0–1.5 ml/kg, 10% calcium gluconate by slow intravenous infusion over 10–20 minutes) for the first 2–3 days, to reduce bone pain and lameness. This will do little to correct the calcium deficit. Skeletal mineralisation is restored slowly over several months, and this process can be monitored periodically using radiographs as a crude estimate of skeletal mineralisation. Non-steroidal anti-inflammatory drugs can be used for short-term analgesia. The prognosis is generally good unless the case is complicated by severe pathological fractures and skeletal deformity.

REFERENCES

Barber PJ and Elliott J (1996) Study of calcium homeostasis in feline hyperthyroidism. *Journal of Small Animal Practice* **37**, 575–582

Barber PJ and Elliot J (1998) Feline chronic renal failure: calcium homeostasis in 80 cases diagnosed between 1992 and 1995. *Journal of Small Animal Practice* **38**, 78–85

Barber PJ, Arthur JA, Hartley NJW, Troughton CG, Elliot J (1997) Atypical hyperparathyroidism in five cats. *Proceedings of the World Small Animal Veterinary Association Congress* p. 221

Barber PJ, Elliot J, Torrance AG (1993) Measurement of feline intact parathyroid hormone: Assay validation and sample handling studies. *Journal of Small Animal Practice* **34**, 614–619

Bovee K (1992) High dietary protein intake does not cause progressive renal failure in dogs after 75% nephrectomy or aging. *Seminars in Veterinary Medicine and Surgery* **7**, 227–232

Broadus AE, Mangin M, Ikeda K, Insogna KL, Weir EC, Burtis WJ, Stewart AF (1988) Humoral hypercalcemia of cancer. Identification

of a novel parathyroid hormone-like peptide. *New England Journal of Medicine* **319**, 556–563

Burtis WJ, Brady TG, Orloff JJ, Ersbak JB, Warrell RP Jr, Olson BR, Wu TL, Mitnick ME, Broadus AE, Stewart AF (1990) Immunochemical characterization of circulating parathyroid hormone-related protein in patients with humoral hypercalcemia of cancer. *New England Journal of Medicine* **322**, 1106–1112

Feldman EC (1995) Disorders of the parathyroid glands. In: *Textbook of Veterinary Internal Medicine*, eds SJ Ettinger and EC Feldman, pp. 1437–1465. WB Saunders, Philadelphia

Feldman EC and Nelson RW (1996) Hypercalcaemia and primary hyperparathyroidism. In: *Canine and Feline Endocrinology and Reproduction*, pp. 488–489. WB Saunders, Philadelphia

Feldman EC, Wisner ER, Nelson RW, Feldman MS, Kennedy PC (1997) Comparison of results of hormonal analysis of samples obtained from selected venous sites versus cervical ultrasonography for localizing parathyroid masses in dogs. *Journal of the American Veterinary Medical Association* **211**, 54–56

Finco DR, Brown SA, Cooper T, Crowell WA, Hoenig M, Barsanti JA (1994) Effects of parathyroid hormone depletion in dogs with induced renal failure. *American Journal of Veterinary Research* **55**, 867–873

Finco DR, Brown SA, Crowell WA, Groves CA, Duncan JR, Barsanti JA (1992) Effects of phosphorus/calcium-restricted and phosphorus/calcium-replete 32% protein diets in dogs with chronic renal failure. *American Journal of Veterinary Research* **53**, 157–163

Finco DR, Crowell WA, Barsanti JA (1985) Effects of 3 diets on dogs with induced chronic renal failure. *American Journal of Veterinary Research* **46**, 646–651

Gunther R, Felice LJ, Nelson RK, Franson AM (1988) Toxicity of a vitamin D3 rodenticide to dogs. *Journal of the American Veterinary Medical Association* **193**, 211–214

Kallet AJ, Richter KP, Feldman EC, Brum DE (1991) Primary hyperparathyroidism in cats: seven cases (1984–1989). *Journal of the American Veterinary Medical Association* **199**, 1767–1771

Massry SG (1989) Pathogenesis of uremic toxicity. Part 1. Parathyroid hormone as a uremic toxin. In: *Textbook of Nephrology*, ed SG Massry and RJ Glassock, pp. 1126–1144. Williams and Wilkins, Baltimore

Rosol TJ, Capen CC, Danks JA, Suva LJ, Steinmeyer CL, Hayman J, Ebeling PR, Martin TJ (1990) Identification of parathyroid hormone-related protein in canine apocrine adenocarcinoma of the anal sac. *Veterinary Pathology* **27**, 89–95

Schenck PA, Chew DJ, Brooks CL (1995) Effects of storage on serum ionized calcium and pH values in clinically normal dogs. *American Journal of Veterinary Research* **56**, 304–307

Torrance AG (1992) Parathyroid diseases in the adult dog. *Veterinary Annual* **32**, 143–153

Torrance AG (1994) Control of parathyroid hormone in chronic renal failure in small animals *Veterinary Annual* **34**, 165–173

Torrance AG and Nachreiner R (1989a) Human-parathormone assay for use in dogs: Validation, sample handling studies, and parathyroid function testing. *American Journal of Veterinary Research* **50**, 1123–1127

Torrance AG and Nachreiner R (1989b) Intact parathyroid hormone assay and total calcium concentration in the diagnosis of disorders of calcium metabolism in dogs. *Journal of Veterinary Internal Medicine* **3**, 86–89

Weir EC, Burtis WJ, Morris CA, Brady TG, Insogna KL (1988a) Isolation of 16,000-dalton parathyroid hormone-like proteins from two animal tumors causing humoral hypercalcemia of malignancy. *Endocrinology* **123**, 2744–2751

Weir EC, Centrella M, Matus RE, Brooks ML, Wu T, Insogna KL (1988b) Adenylate cyclase-stimulating, bone-resorbing and β TGF-like activities in canine apocrine cell adenocarcinoma of the anal sac. *Calcified Tissue International* **43**, 359–365

Weir EC, Norrdin RW, Matus RE, Brooks MB, Broadus AE, Mitnick M, Johnston SD (1988c) Humoral hypercalcemia of malignancy in canine lymphosarcoma. *Endocrinology* **122**, 602–608

CHAPTER SEVENTEEN

Hypoglycaemia

Kenneth W. Simpson and Audrey Cook

INTRODUCTION

Hypoglycaemia is a relatively uncommon but potentially life-threatening problem in small animal practice. The list of differential diagnoses is quite short, and the cause is often evident after review of the signalment, physical examination, history and initial investigations (complete blood count, serum chemistry profile, urinalysis). This chapter presents an overview of the aetiology, pathophysiology and diagnosis of hypoglycaemia in dogs and cats. The treatment of insulinoma is discussed in detail. The reader is referred elsewhere for detailed discussion of the management of hypoadrenocorticism (see Chapter 11), sepsis (Kirby, 1995) and hepatic disease (Johnson, 1995; Madison, 1995).

AETIOLOGY AND PATHOPHYSIOLOGY

Blood glucose homeostasis is a complex balance between energy utilisation, mobilisation and storage, and is achieved by hormonal regulation of intermediary metabolism. In general, hypoglycaemia can be explained by decreased glucose production, increased glucose utilisation, or a combination of the two processes (Table 17.1). Weakness, collapse, seizures and altered consciousness are the most common signs associated with hypoglycaemia. A diagnosis of hypoglycaemia is achieved by documenting a subnormal concentration of blood glucose.

Cause	Comments
Decreased glucose production:	
Endocrine	Hypoadrenocorticism (Addison's disease — primary and secondary)
	Panhypopituitarism (cortisol and growth hormone deficiency)
Hepatic	Portosystemic shunt
	• congenital vascular anomalies
	• acquired shunts in cirrhotic patients
	Hepatocyte loss
	• acute necrosis (infection, toxin)
	• chronic fibrosis
	Abnormal hepatocyte metabolism
	• glycogen storage diseases:
	Type I = glucose-6-phosphatase deficiency suspected in young toy breeds
	Type II = lysosomal α-1,4-glucosidase deficiency in young Lapland dogs
	Type III = amylo-1,6-glucosidase deficiency in young German Shepherd Dogs
Increased glucose utilisation:	
Excessive insulin/insulin-like factors	Insulinoma
	Extrapancreatic neoplasms
	Exogenous insulin overdose
Consumption of glucose	Sepsis
	Large tumour burden
	Polycythaemia
Miscellaneous	Hunting dog hypoglycaemia
Erroneous	Delayed separation of serum/plasma
	Laboratory error

Table 17.1: Principal causes of fasting hypoglycaemia.

Decreased glucose production

During a brief fast, blood glucose levels are maintained by the breakdown of hepatic glycogen stores (glycogenolysis). Decreased glucose production can be the result of hormone, substrate or enzyme deficiency.

Inadequate release of insulin-antagonising hormones, particularly cortisol and growth hormone (GH), can result in hypoglycaemia. In general however, blood sugar levels are just below normal in patients with these disorders, and other signs of hormone deficiency will dominate the clinical picture, e.g. dwarfism in panhypopituitarism, hyperkalaemia and hyponatraemia in hypoadrenocorticism.

Liver disease and malnutrition are important causes of hypoglycaemia resulting from a deficiency of substrate. Dogs with congenital portal vascular anomalies and acute or chronic liver failure are commonly hypoglycaemic, as there is insufficient functioning hepatic mass. In addition, poor hepatic function and diminished portal blood flow result in impaired insulin catabolism, which may exacerbate hypoglycaemia.

Enzyme deficiencies are the least common causes of decreased glucose production. Dogs with glycogen storage diseases are unable to release glucose due to specific enzymatic defects in the glycogenolysis pathway (see Figure 17.1). Large amounts of glycogen accumulate in the liver and other tissues, with subsequent hepatomegaly and organ dysfunction. Other potential enzyme deficiencies which may result in hypoglycaemia are abnormalities of the gluconeogenic enzymes phosphoenolpyruvate carboxykinase, fructose-1,6-bisphosphatase and pyruvate carboxylase.

Increased glucose utilisation

A number of hormones are involved in the regulation of blood glucose, through modification of enzymatic pathways or changes in the uptake of glucose by target tissues. The most common endocrine cause of hypoglycaemia is excessive insulin release by insulinoma (Figure 17.1). Insulinomas are malignant tumours of the pancreatic islet ß cells, which produce and secrete insulin or proinsulin (Kruth *et al.*, 1982; Mehlhaff *et al.*, 1985; Leifer *et al.*, 1986; Caywood *et al.*, 1988; Dunn *et al.*, 1992; Nelson, 1995). Although immunohistochemical studies have indicated that these tumours may produce a number of other peptide hormones (pancreatic polypeptide, glucagon, serotonin, gastrin) (Hawkins *et al.*, 1987), the clinical signs observed in patients with insulinoma reflect the excessive and inappropriate secretion of insulin. Hyperinsulinaemia drives glucose out of the circulation and into cells, while inhibiting the mobilisation of energy stored as amino acids, triglycerides or glycogen. Profound hypoglycaemia can ensue. Because glucose is the primary substrate for generation of energy in the central nervous system (CNS), the most obvious manifestation of inadequate circulating glucose is neurological dysfunction. The cerebral cortex has the highest energy requirements, and is therefore affected first (depression, seizures). The neoplastic ß cells may spontaneously secrete insulin in an autonomous manner or release excessive amounts of insulin in response to the usual stimuli (i.e. postprandially; Figure 17.2, dog 1). These episodes of neurological impairment are generally transient (often a matter of minutes), as the drop in blood glucose concentration triggers the release of counter-regulatory hormones (catecholamines, glucagon, cortisol). Stimulation of the sympatheticoadrenal system results in minor signs such as muscle tremors, agitation and hunger, which may in fact precede an episode of collapse.

Other tumours may also cause hypoglycaemia (Leifer *et al.*, 1981; Beaudry *et al.*, 1995). These non-islet cell tumours are often of hepatic origin (e.g. hepatocellular carcinoma, hepatoma), although a number of different types have been described (e.g. intestinal leiomyoma, melanoma, salivary gland adenocarcinoma, haemangiosarcoma). Initially, hypoglycaemia was attributed to excessive glucose consumption by the tumour, but studies in humans suggest that hypoglycaemia is related to production of insulin-like substances. The high glucose turnover, high peripheral glucose utilisation and hepatic glycogen abundance documented in people with tumour-associated hypoglycaemia can be explained by secretion of insulin-like substances by neoplastic tissue. Research

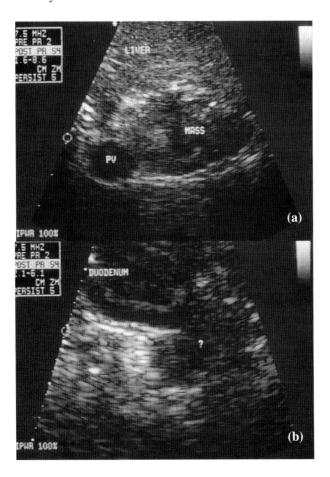

Figure 17.1: Ultrasound images of pancreatic neoplasms. (a) An oblong, approximately 4 cm, hypoechoic mass is visible adjacent to the portal vein (PV) and caudal aspect of the liver in an oblique ultrasound image. The histological diagnosis was insulinoma. (b) A focal, approximately 1 cm, hypoechoic lesion is visible in the right pancreatic lobe adjacent to the duodenum in a sagittal ultrasound image. The small size and lack of distinct margins of the lesion led to an ultrasonographic diagnosis of 'probable pancreatic nodule'. A tumour of the same size was found in this location at laparotomy. The histological diagnosis was insulinoma. Reproduced from Lamb et al., (1995) with permission of The Veterinary Record.

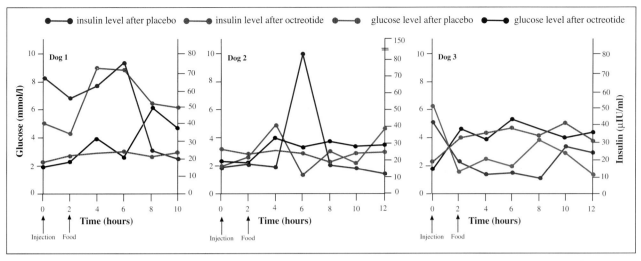

Figure 17.2: *Plasma concentrations of glucose and insulin after the subcutaneous administration of octreotide or placebo. Dogs were fed a fat-restricted meal 2 hours after subcutaneous administration. There were no obvious differences in the insulin concentrations observed in response to placebo and octreotide. Dog 1 appears to show increased insulin secretion in response to feeding. Redrawn from Simpson* et al. *(1995) with permission of the* Journal of Small Animal Practice *(BVA Publications). (Conversion factor for insulin μIU/ml to pmol/l is* × *7.18)*

suggests that the activity of insulin-like growth factors (IGFs) may be altered in these individuals, with subsequent manifestations of insulin excess despite low circulating insulin levels (Phillips and Robertson, 1993; Zapf, 1994). Insulin-like growth factors 1 (IGF-1) and 2 (IGF-2) are proteins with structural similarities to insulin and relaxin. In normal individuals, hepatic production of IGF-1 is stimulated by GH, whereas synthesis of IGF-2 is essentially independent of GH levels. Although circulating levels of IGFs are much higher than those of insulin, attachment to specific binding proteins keeps their bioavailability low. Two distinct subclasses of binding proteins (IGFBP) have been identified based on size (40–50 kD or 150–200 kD), with varying affinities for the IGFs. Synthesis of the larger IGFBP complexes is GH dependent; they have a longer half-life and are unable to cross endothelial walls. Serum from patients with extra-pancreatic tumour hypoglycaemia contains elevated levels of big (pro) IGF-2 which disappears after successful removal of the tumour. Oversecretion of big IGF-2 leads to suppression of GH. As a consequence, formation of a GH-dependent 150 kD IGFBP complex, which normally carries 70–80% of total serum IGF-2 and largely restricts its bioavailability, is impaired. Decreased formation of the 150 kD complex leads to a shift of IGF-2 to a 50 kD IGFBP complex, resulting in a 30-fold shorter serum half-life of IGF-2, increased turnover and enhanced bioavailability. Insulin target organs are thus exposed to an enormous insulin-like potential which is continuously provided by oversecreted big IGF-2 and causes increased glucose consumption by skeletal muscle, inhibition of hepatic glucose production, inhibition of lipid mobilisation from adipose tissue and pronounced hypoglycaemia. Increased big IGF-2 has been reported in a dog with non-islet cell tumour-related hypoglycaemia (Boari *et al.*, 1992).

Sepsis is a relatively common cause of hypoglycaemia in dogs and may induce hypoglycaemia via the effects of endotoxin. Endotoxin increases the peripheral uptake of glucose and limits the ability of the liver to keep up with increased demand for glucose (Wolf *et al.*, 1977).

Care must be exercised to detect erroneous causes of hypoglycaemia such as delayed analysis of plasma from non-fluoride-containing sample tubes or samples from patients with relative or absolute polycythaemia. Laboratory error must be kept in mind and should be suspected where hypoglycaemia is documented in the absence of appropriate clinical findings. The analysis of a second appropriately collected and processed sample should be performed to confirm hypoglycaemia.

DIAGNOSTIC APPROACH

When hypoglycaemia (glucose usually <3.5 mmol/l) is confirmed its cause is determined by careful review of the signalment and history, a thorough physical examination, quick laboratory tests and routine clinicopathological testing. Additional tests such as insulin concentration, hepatic function, adrenocorticotropic hormone (ACTH) stimulation, blood culture, radiography, ultrasonography and surgical biopsy are employed on the basis of clinical findings and these initial test results. Where fasting hypoglycaemia is not detected but hypoglycaemia is suspected as the cause of clinical abnormalities, glucose determination should be repeated after an 8-hour fast.

Signalment
The signalment is useful in distinguishing likely causes of hypoglycaemia. Young animals are most likely to develop hypoglycaemia as a result of starvation, congenital liver disease, e.g. portosystemic vascular anomalies (PSVA), sepsis (especially with parvovirus) or glycogen storage disease, whereas middle aged to older animals are more likely to be affected by insulinoma, non-islet cell neoplasia, acquired hepatic disease, hypoadrenocorticism and sepsis.

Clinical signs and physical findings
Weakness, collapse, seizures and altered consciousness (depression, coma) are the most common signs associated with hypoglycaemia. Muscle fasciculations, bizarre

History and examination	Findings
Signalment	Middle aged (mean age 8–10 years) No sex predilection Any breed: Standard Poodle, Boxer, Fox Terrier, German Shepherd Dog, Irish Setter may be predisposed
Major complaints	Intermittent weakness, collapse Ataxia, posterior weakness Seizures
Minor complaints	Muscle fasciculations Polyphagia, weight gain Polyuria, polydipsia
Physical examination	Often unremarkable May be obese Peripheral neuropathy may be evident – proprioceptive deficits, muscle atrophy
Routine laboratory tests: 　Complete blood count	Usually unremarkable May see 'stress leucogram' Lymphocytosis or eosinophilia should increase the suspicion of hypoadrenocorticism
Serum chemistry profile	Hypoglycaemia: blood glucose may be normal on random testing, patient should be re-sampled after 8-hour fast No other specific findings have been described Essential to include electrolytes to rule out hypoadrenocorticism
Urinalysis	Unremarkable

***Table 17.2**: Clinical and clinicopathological findings in dogs with insulinoma.*

behaviour, lethargy and polyphagia may also be present. In addition to these signs, dogs with insulinoma may have persistent ataxia, weakness or recumbency, unrelated to circulating blood glucose concentrations (Table 17.2). Both fore- and hindlimbs may show signs of lower motor neuron dysfunction such as decreased spinal reflexes which are related to the presence of a peripheral neuro-pathy. Possible causes of the neuropathy include permanent neurological damage due to persistent hypoglycaemia, or the release of an unidentified neurotoxin from the tumour.

Clinical signs and physical findings which are not related solely to hypoglycaemia, such as small stature, diarrhoea, vomiting, gastrointestinal blood loss, jaundice, hyperaemia, petechiae, bradycardia, renomegaly, hepatomegaly, abdominal masses and hyperthermia, are helpful in localising the cause of hypoglycaemia. Dogs with insulinoma usually have few physical and biochemical abnormalities whereas sepsis is often associated with fever and the brick-red mucous membranes and tachycardia typical of hyperdynamic shock. Sepsis should be particularly suspected in patients who have received chemotherapy or are splenectomised, those with gastroenteritis, particularly when associated with parvovirus enteritis or gastrointestinal blood loss, and those with abnormal hepatic function or endocarditis. PSVA may be

associated with small stature or poor growth, and renomegaly. Acquired or end-stage liver disease may be associated with jaundice or ascites. Glycogen storage disorders are rare but are most often documented in young dogs with hepatomegaly. Hypoadrenocorticism typically manifests with signs of gastrointestinal disease, dehydration and bradycardia. Non-islet cell tumours causing hypoglycaemia often have localising signs such as abdominal masses or effusions.

Laboratory evaluation

The rapid analysis of haematocrit, total protein, glucose, urea and electrolytes (Na^+, K^+, Ca^{2+}) should be performed while awaiting the results of more comprehensive clinicopathological testing. These tests will enable the confirmation of hypoglycaemia and help to distinguish hypoglycaemia from other causes of weakness, collapse or seizures such as hypo/hypercalcaemia. They also enable the identification of patients with hypoadrenocorticism, electrolyte abnormalities, renal disease and anaemia, and facilitate appropriate initial therapy. An ACTH stimulation test should be performed in animals with suspected hypoadrenocorticism. Where hepatic encephalopathy is present, or is suspected, blood ammonia or total bile acid concentrations should be determined. When hypoglycaemia is documented, particularly in a patient with few clinical abnormalities, blood sampling technique should be reviewed, and the value confirmed on a fresh plasma sample if necessary.

Laboratory findings apart from hypoglycaemia are uncommon in dogs with insulinoma. An increased white cell count with a left shift, or neutropenia, may point towards sepsis. Decreases in mean cell volume, mean corpuscular haemoglobin, creatinine, blood urea nitrogen, total protein and cholesterol, isosthenuria with or without ammonium biurate crystals, and a mild increase in hepatic enzymes are frequent findings in PSVA. Patients with acquired liver disease may have elevated hepatic enzymes, hypoalbuminaemia and hyperbilirubinaemia. Non-islet cell tumours causing hypoglycaemia may show changes related to disruption of the target organ, e.g. increased liver enzymes or hyperbilirubinaemia in hepatocellular carcinoma. Laboratory findings with hypoadrenocorticism include hyperkalaemia, hyponatraemia, hypochloraemia, hypercalcaemia, azotaemia, lymphocytosis, eosinophilia and a variable degree of anaemia. Evaluation of plasma cortisol before and after ACTH stimulation confirms or rules out hypoadrenocorticism. Blood and urine cultures can be used to confirm sepsis. Hepatic function can be evaluated using bile acids, and hepatic pathology and non-islet cell neoplasia are identified by combined imaging and biopsy techniques.

DIAGNOSIS OF INSULINOMA

The tentative diagnosis of insulinoma and non-islet cell tumour is often suspected after examining the patient and reviewing routine clinical pathology results. The diagnosis is confirmed by documentation of insulin secretion in the face of hypoglycaemia, along with evidence of a pancreatic mass. Histological evaluation and immunocytochemical staining for insulin provides the definitive diagnosis.

Insulin measurement

A blood sample for insulin determination should be collected during a period of hypoglycaemia. Many dogs with insulinoma will have serum insulin concentrations within the reference range (often reported as 5–20 µIU/ml, but refer to laboratory); a normal insulin concentration in the face of hypoglycaemia is inappropriate and indicates excessive insulin release.

Sample guidelines for the interpretation of fasting insulin concentration are:

- Insulin >20 µIU/ml (>144 pmol/l) — absolute hyperinsulinaemia consistent with insulinoma
- Insulin 10–20 µIU/ml (72–144 pmol/l) — relative hyperinsulinaemia consistent with insulinoma
- Insulin 5–10 µIU/ml (36–72 pmol/l) — possible insulinoma
- Insulin <5 µIU/ml (<36 pmol/l) — inconsistent with insulinoma.

Several formulae have been recommended for determination of appropriate circulating insulin and glucose

Breed	Age	Sex	Basal insulin (µIU/ml)	Basal glucose (mmol/l)	IGR (IU/mol)
German Shepherd Dog	10	FS	18	3	6
Border Collie	7	F	33	2.7	12.2
Springer Spaniel	7	FS	38	2.6	14.6
Dobermann	7	M	77	3.3	23.3
German Shepherd Dog	7	FS	120	1.2	100
Crossbreed	9	FS	18	3.3	5.5
Crossbreed	8	FS	13.4	1.7	7.9
Golden Retriever	9	M	31	2.3	13.5
German Shepherd Dog	9	M	25	2.6	9.6
Springer Spaniel	11	M	9.7	2.2	4.4
Crossbreed	9	FS	30	2.1	14.3
Rottweiler	6	F	96	3.8	25.3
Jack Russell Terrier	8	FS	36	2.1	17.1
Springer Spaniel	9	M	21.7	1.4	15.5
Springer Spaniel	7	M	69	1.1	62.7
Irish Setter	9	M	39	3	13
Springer Spaniel	11	F	19.6	1.8	10.9
Boxer	10	F	15.7	3.7	4.2
Crossbreed	8	F	28.7	1.6	17.9
Golden Retriever	7	FS	21.7	1.6	13.6
Irish Setter	9	FS	58	2.1	27.6
Golden Retriever	9	M	41	1.9	21.6
Short-haired Pointer	9	M	34	3.2	10.6
Mean ± SD	8.6 ± 1.3		38.8 ± 27.8	2.4 ± 0.8	19.6 ± 21.2
Control (n=7)			8.0 ± 2.3	5.1 ± 0.8	1.6 ± 0.6

Table 17.3: *Insulin and glucose concentrations in 23 dogs with insulinoma that were referred to the teaching hospitals of the Royal Veterinary College, University of London, and Cambridge University. (IGR, insulin:glucose ratio; FS, neutered female.) Data compiled from Dunn* et al. *(1992), Simpson* et al. *(1995) and Lamb et al. (1995). (Conversion factor for insulin µIU/ml to pmol/l is ×7.18)*

concentrations. Note that the formulae for insulin:glucose ratios use common rather than SI units. The conversion factor from μIU/ml to pmol/l is $\times$ 7.18; the conversion factor for pmol/l to μIU/ml is $\times$ 0.139. The ratio of insulin to glucose (IGR) and the amended insulin:glucose ratio (AIGR) have been described. These formulae can be employed when absolute hyperinsulinaemia is not present and results of basal insulin measurements are equivocal. The IGR (IU/mol) compares the concentration of insulin (μUI/l) to that of glucose (mmol/l). An IGR of 4.2 IU/mol or greater is consistent with insulinoma (Dunn et al., 1992). The AIGR is based on the assumption that insulin levels should be zero if blood glucose falls below 30 mg/dl. The AIGR is calculated as follows:

$$AIGR = \frac{\text{plasma insulin (μIU/ml)} \times 100}{\text{plasma glucose (mg/dl)} - 30}$$

The conversion factor for glucose from mmol/l to mg/dl is 18.02. If glucose is ≤30mg/dl, the divisor becomes 1.

An AIGR greater than 30 is consistent with an insulinoma, although abnormal ratios have been reported in dogs with other causes of hypoglycaemia. Some workers consider the AIGR to be more helpful than the IGR, although this is controversial (Kruth et al., 1982; Mehlhaff et al., 1985; Feldman et al., 1986; Leifer et al., 1986; Caywood et al., 1988; Dunn et al., 1992; Nelson, 1995).

The insulin and glucose concentrations of 23 dogs with confirmed insulinoma are summarised in Table 17.3. Absolute hyperinsulinaemia (>20 mIU/l) and hypoglycaemia (<3.5 mmol/l) were present in 16/23 dogs. The IGR was >4.2 IU/mol in all 23 dogs. It was not necessary to employ the AIGR in these cases. The repeated determination of plasma glucose and insulin may be necessary to document equivocal cases.

Stimulation tests

A number of substances that are known to stimulate insulin secretion, such as glucagon, intravenous glucose and adrenaline, have been used in provocative tests designed to identify neoplastic islet tissue (Kruth et al., 1982; Leifer et al., 1986; Dunn et al., 1992). The potential benefits of these tests are not well established and the risk of complications (potentially severe hypoglycaemia) have restricted evaluation and application to date.

Abdominal radiography and ultrasonography

Most insulinomas are small (<4 cm in diameter) and preoperative identification is difficult (Saunders, 1991; Lamb et al., 1995). Abdominal radiographs are usually of little benefit, although hepatomegaly or decreased serosal detail may be present with metastatic disease. As experienced ultrasonographers identified an insulinoma in only 8/30 and 9/13 proven cases (see Figure 17.1) a negative scan does not rule out the presence of a tumour (Lamb et al., 1995; Nelson, 1995). The smallest insulinoma detected in one series was 7 mm in diameter. Ultrasonographic examination of the hepatic parenchyma and regional lymph nodes is worthwhile, as these are the commonest sites for metastases, but it can be insensitive. Endoscopic and intra-operative ultrasonography may enable more accurate detection of primary pancreatic tumours and their metastases in the future (Galiber et al., 1988; Glover et al., 1992; King et al., 1994). Scintigraphic studies with radio-labelled somatostatin analogues have enabled the detection of insulinoma and metastases in 50–60% of humans with insulinoma (Reubi et al., 1994; Krenning et al., 1994). Localisation of the insulinoma with these analogues reflects the presence of somatostatin receptors on the insulinoma. The presence or absence of receptors is variable and is thought to account for differences in detection. The demonstration of somatostatin receptors on insulinomas also has important therapeutic implications as these analogues can reduce insulin secretion.

Exploratory laparotomy

Surgery permits visualisation of the pancreas and identification of some macroscopic metastases and provides the opportunity to remove or to debulk the tumour. Intraoperative ultrasonography may be employed to detect pancreatic tumours and metastases.

INITIAL MANAGEMENT

Restoring blood glucose concentrations should rapidly terminate a seizure in a hypoglycaemic patient. Intravenous dextrose should be administered in small amounts, slowly. Large boluses of intravenous dextrose may trigger a massive release of insulin from insulinomas, resulting in rebound hypoglycaemia and severe seizuring (Nelson, 1995).

- Administer 1 ml/kg 50% dextrose intravenously over 5–10 minutes and repeat if necessary
- Administer B vitamins intravenously (24–100 mg for a dog, 25 mg for a cat; thiamine is a coenzyme for CNS glucose utilisation)
- Maintain on intravenous infusion (2.5–5% glucose or dextrose)
- Rub glucose syrup over the gums if patient is at home or if vascular access is difficult
- Encourage the patient to eat as soon as possible.

In non-seizuring patients, frequent feeding of small amounts of food (3–6 small meals of commercial foods high in protein, fat and complex carbohydrate) may alleviate clinical signs. Where signs of hypoglycaemia persist despite feeding, intravenous glucose can be administered as a 2.5% solution in half strength saline, a 5% solution in water, or added to a balanced electrolyte solution being administered to correct electrolyte abnormalities. Glucose concentrations should be monitored in response to therapy. Most patients with non-tumour-related hypoglycaemia respond rapidly to feeding or intravenous glucose, and plasma glucose concentrations normalise. Patients with insulinoma and non-islet cell tumour-related hypoglycaemia may respond poorly to feeding or glucose. Blood glucose concentrations in dogs with insulinoma often remain subnormal in the face of continuous infusion of solutions containing 5% glucose. Some patients with insulinoma may release excessive insulin in response to food or glucose, which can result in rebound hypoglycaemia and seizuring. In these patients the blood glucose concentration should be maintained at a level that alleviates clinical signs (usually around 2.5 mmol/l).

If hepatic encephalopathy is suspected or confirmed (high ammonia), a lactulose or neomycin enema can be administered. Patients with suspected hepatic encephalopathy can be initially maintained on intravenous 0.9% NaCl with 20–30 mmol KCl/l. Alkalosis and hypokalaemia should be detected and treated in these patients as these can potentiate encephalopathy. Patients with acquired or chronic hepatic disease are usually maintained on 0.45% NaCl to avoid Na^+ retention.

Where clinical findings are consistent with sepsis, blood and urine cultures should be obtained and broad-spectrum antibiotics (e.g. a cephalosporin with enrofloxacin or amikacin) and gastrointestinal mucosal protectants administered, in concert with aggressive fluid therapy and patient monitoring while the site of origin is investigated. Plasma glucose concentration should be maintained between 5.5 and 11 mmol/l.

Patients with suspected hypoadrenocorticism are usually treated with intravenous glucocorticoids and 0.9% NaCl, with glucose if hypoglycaemia is present.

THERAPY FOR INSULINOMA

Patients with insulinoma may be managed medically, surgically, or with a combination of both (Kruth *et al.*, 1982; Mehlhaff *et al.*, 1985; Leifer *et al.*, 1986; Caywood *et al.*, 1988; Meleo, 1990; Dunn *et al.*, 1993; Nelson, 1995; Simpson *et al.*, 1995). Although the chance of a complete surgical cure is low, many patients will benefit from tumour debulking and may enjoy long disease-free intervals. Older dogs, or those with preoperative evidence of extensive metastasis, are poor surgical candidates and are best managed medically from the outset.

Surgery

Tumour resection is the treatment of choice for dogs with solitary pancreatic masses. Approximately 50% of dogs with solitary pancreatic masses were alive 18 months postoperatively, 20% at 24 months (Caywood *et al.*, 1988). Death by 24 months is likely to be due to inadequate pancreatic resection or the presence of undetected metastases. When metastatic disease is detected, the median survival times range from around 6 months for dogs with distant metastases, to 18 months for those with localised disease (pancreas and regional nodes). Improvement of prognosis is therefore determined by the presence or absence of metastases. The mean survival time for medically managed patients is reported as 12 months from onset of signs of hypoglycaemia. Surgical candidates should be referred to hospitals with intensive care facilities as these cases are difficult to manage in a normal practice.

Preoperative management

Management of the seizuring patient is outlined above. In the stable patient, hypoglycaemic episodes can usually be avoided with cage rest and frequent feedings of diets consisting of palatable, complex carbohydrates, every 3–6 hours. Therapy with corticosteroids (0.5 mg/kg prednisolone orally twice daily) can be initiated if seizures persist. Intravenous 5% dextrose added to a balanced electrolyte solution can be started 12 hours before surgery to maintain blood glucose at about 2.5 mmol/l.

Intraoperative management

The goal of surgery is to remove the primary tumour and any visible metastases. The primary tumour may be located anywhere in the pancreas, and can be difficult to recognise. If it is not found despite gentle palpation, one limb of the pancreas can be resected in the hope of removing microscopic neoplasia. The use of intravenous methylene blue to identify tumour tissue has not been very helpful in the authors' experience and is avoided because of potential adverse effects. Intraoperative ultrasonography is potentially useful but requires prospective evaluation. Common sites for metastasis are adjacent lymph nodes and liver; a thorough inspection of the abdomen is necessary to identify and remove any suspicious lesions. Glucose-containing fluids should be administered during surgery at a rate of 5 × maintenance.

Postoperative management

The patient may be hyper-, hypo- or euglycaemic after surgery. Persistence of hypoglycaemia indicates inadequate tumour removal and carries a poorer prognosis. Although normal or high blood glucose levels at this point are encouraging, most of these dogs will eventually succumb to metastatic disease, with recrudescence of their original signs. Pancreatitis is a significant complication of insulinoma surgery, and patients should be managed accordingly:

- All patients: Nothing by mouth for at least 48 hours, with fluid therapy at twice maintenance level. Electrolytes and glucose should be evaluated at least twice daily and analgesia provided if indicated. The patient should be gradually introduced to food after 2–3 days
- Patients with hyperglycaemia: Insulin therapy can be initiated if hyperglycaemia is severe or lasts for more than 3 days. The patient should be re-evaluated frequently (every 7–14 days) for resolution of diabetes mellitus or return of hypoglycaemic episodes
- Patients with persistent hypoglycaemia: Intravenous 5% dextrose can be administered to maintain a blood glucose concentration of about 2.5 mmol/l and then slowly decreased as food is introduced. Medical management can be introduced 3–4 days after surgery
- The pre- and postoperative administration of the somatostatin analogue octreotide may also be indicated in patients undergoing pancreatic resection due to its potential beneficial effects on insulin release and pancreatitis (Konturek *et al.*, 1988; McKay *et al.*, 1993).

Medical therapy

Either because of inoperable tumour or metastases, most dogs with insulinomas will require medical therapy. The aim of medical therapy is not to restore blood glucose levels to normal, but simply to reduce the clinical signs of hypoglycaemia. Most clinicians add drugs in a sequential fashion, and multidrug therapy is common.

Glucocorticoids (prednisolone 0.5–2 mg/kg twice daily): Glucocorticoids are generally the first drugs to be used in patients where dietary modification alone does not reduce the signs of hypoglycaemia. Steroids increase blood glucose concentrations by promoting hepatic glycogenolysis and by inhibiting insulin-mediated peripheral utilisation of glucose. The smallest effective dose should be used, as signs of iatrogenic hyperadrenocorticism are common and may prompt diazoxide administration.

Diazoxide (5–30 mg/kg twice daily): Diazoxide inhibits the release of insulin from pancreatic islet cells by blockade of intracellular Ca^{2+} release. Diazoxide also stimulates the sympathetic nervous system and the adrenal medulla, with subsequent promotion of hepatic glycogenolysis and gluconeogenesis and reduced peripheral glucose uptake.

Although the majority of dogs appear to show clinical improvement with this medication, side effects may be a problem; vomiting, anorexia, diarrhoea, blood dyscrasias and pancreatitis have been reported. Hyperglycaemia may also occur, in which case the dosage should be reduced. Concurrent hepatic disease may result in side effects at low doses.

It is advisable to start at the bottom of the dose range, and gradually increase the dosage if necessary. Diazoxide is a diuretic of the benzothiadiazide class, and its hyperglycaemic effects may be enhanced by concurrent administration of thiazide diuretics (e.g. hydrochlorthiazide).

Propranolol (0.1–0.4 mg/kg three times daily): Propranolol inhibits release of insulin from islet cells through β-adrenergic blockade. Propranolol also has some peripheral insulin-antagonistic effects, by alteration of insulin receptor affinity. Adverse effects are usually due to its negative inotropic and chronotropic effects (e.g. hypotension) or alterations in airway function (bronchospasm). It is not widely used in dogs with insulinoma as its potency appears to be low.

Octreotide (10–40 μg or 2–16 μg/kg subcutaneously three times daily): Octreotide is a long-acting synthetic somatostatin analogue that is rapidly absorbed after subcutaneous administration (see Figure 17.2). Octreotide inhibits the synthesis and secretion of insulin from normal islet cells, and has been effective in alleviating hypoglycaemia in some human patients with insulinoma (Maton *et al.*, 1989; Timmer *et al.*, 1991; Buchanan, 1993; von Yben *et al.*, 1994). While anecdotal reports have suggested that somatostatin reduces the signs of hypoglycaemia in dogs (Lothrop, 1989; Meleo, 1990), a placebo-controlled study did not demonstrate any improvement in clinical signs or blood glucose and insulin levels in three dogs with insulinoma (see Figure 17.2) (Simpson *et al.*, 1995). However, a recent report which describes the response of six dogs with insulinoma to intravenous octreotide, demonstrates the suppression of serum insulin at 10, 20 and 30 minutes after administration (Nelson, 1995). These contradictory results are likely to be due to the variable expression of somatostatin receptors by neoplastic islet cells. The identification of somatostatin receptors on insulinomas either *in vivo* (scintigraphy) or *in vitro* (in biopsy specimens) will hopefully enable selective application in the future. At present, expense, the need for parenteral administration and poor efficacy have limited the application of somatostatin analogues.

PROGNOSIS

The long-term prognosis for dogs with insulinoma is grave, and most patients will die of their disease. Surgery is the recommended approach for patients with solitary masses, 80% of which will probably die within 24 months. Where metastatic disease is detected, the median survival times range from around 6 months for dogs with distant metastases to 18 months for those with localised disease (pancreas and regional nodes). Some individuals remain disease free, or are maintained medically, for prolonged periods after surgical debulking. The mean survival time for medically managed patients is reported as 12 months from onset of signs of hypoglycaemia.

TREATMENT OF NON-ISLET CELL TUMOUR HYPOGLYCAEMIA

Surgical removal of the underlying tumour is the therapy of choice for non-islet cell tumour hypoglycaemia, using the perioperative strategies described for insulinoma patients to control hypoglycaemia. If complete surgical resection is impossible, symptoms of hypoglycaemia may be reduced with frequent feedings and oral glucocorticoids. The prognosis depends on the tumour type. Hepatocellular carcinomas appear to be the commonest cause of non-islet cell tumour-associated hypoglycaemia in dogs, and carry a grave prognosis. However, the long-term outcome may be good in patients with benign tumours.

REFERENCES

Beaudry D, Knapp DW, Montgomery T, Sandusky GS, Morrison WB and Nelson R (1995) Hypoglycaemia in four dogs with smooth muscle tumors. *Journal of Veterinary Internal Medicine* **9**, 415–419

Boari A, Venturili M and Minuto F (1992) Non-islet cell tumor hypoglycaemia in a dog associated with high levels of insulin-like growth factor II. *XVII World Small Animal Veterinary Association Conference Proceedings*, pp. 678–679

Buchanan KD (1993) The effects of Sandostatin on neuroendocrine tumors of the gastrointestinal system. *Recent Results in Cancer Research* **129**, 45–55

Caywood DD, Klausner JS, O'Leary TP, Withrow SJ, Richardson RC, Harvey HJ, Norris AM, Henderson RA and Johnston SD (1988)

Pancreatic insulin-secreting neoplasms: Clinical, diagnostic and prognostic features in 73 dogs. *Journal of the American Animal Hospital Association* **24**, 577–584

Dunn JK, Bostock D, Herrtage ME, Jackson KF and Walker MJ (1993) Insulin-secreting tumors of the canine pancreas: clinical and pathological features of 11 cases. *Journal of Small Animal Practice* **34**, 325–331

Dunn JK, Heath MF, Herrtage ME, Jackson KF and Walker MJ (1992) Diagnosis of insulinoma in the dog: a study of 11 cases. *Journal of Small Animal Practice* **33**, 514–520

Feldman EC, Schall WS and Kruth SA (1986) Amended insulin:glucose ratio (letter). *Journal of the American Veteinary Medical Association* **188**, 1227–1230

Galiber AK, Reading CC, Charboneau JW, Sheedy PF, James EM, Gorman B, Grant CS, van Heerden JA and Telander RL (1988) Localization of pancreatic insulinomas: comparison of pre- and intraoperative US with CT and angiography. *Radiology* **166**, 405–408

Glover JR, Shorvon PJ and Lees WR (1992) Endoscopic ultrasound for localization of islet cell tumours. *Gut* **33**, 108–110

Hawkins KL, Summers BA, Kuhajda FP and Smith CA (1987) Immunocytochemistry of normal pancreatic islets and spontaneous islet cell tumors in dogs. *Veterinary Pathology* **24**, 170–179

Johnson SE (1995) Diseases of the liver. In: *Textbook of Veterinary Internal Medicine*, 4th edn, ed. SJ Ettinger and EC Feldman, pp. 1313–1357. WB Saunders, Philadelphia

King CMP, Reznek RH, Dacie JE and Wass JAH (1994) Imaging islet cell tumours. *Clinical Radiology* **49**, 295–303

Kirby R (1995) Septic shock. In: *Current Veterinary Therapy XI*, ed. JD Bonagura, pp. 139–146. WB Saunders, Philadelphia

Konturek SJ, Bilski J, Jaworek J, Tasler J and Schally AV (1988) Comparison of somatostatin and its highly potent hexa- and octapeptide analogs on exocrine and endocrine pancreatic secretion. *Proceedings of the Society for Experimental Biology and Medicine* **187**, 241–249

Krenning EP, Kwekkeboom DJ, Oei HY, DeJong RJB, Dop FJ, Reubi JC and Lamberts SWJ (1994) Somatostatin-receptor scintigraphy in gastroenteropancreatic tumors. *Annals of the New York Academy of Sciences* **733**, 416–424

Kruth SA, Feldman EC and Kennedy PC (1982) Insulin-secreting islet cell tumors: establishing a diagnosis and the clinical course for 25 dogs. *Journal of the American Veterinary Medical Association* **181**, 54–58

Lamb CR, Simpson KW, Boswood A and Matthewman LA (1995) Ultrasonography of pancreatic neoplasia in the dog: retrospective review of 16 cases. *Veterinary Record* **137**, 65–68

Leifer CE, Peterson ME and Matus RE (1981) Hypoglycemia associated with non-islet cell tumors in 13 dogs. *Journal of the American Veterinary Medical Association* **186**, 53–55

Leifer CE, Peterson ME and Matus RE (1986) Insulin-secreting tumor: diagnosis and medical and surgical management in 55 dogs. *Journal of the American Veterinary Medical Association* **188**, 60–64

Lothrop CD (1989) Medical treatment of neuroendocrine tumors of the gastroenteropancreatic system with somatostatin. In: *Current Veterinary Therapy X*, ed. RW Kirk, pp. 1020–1024. WB Saunders, Philadelphia

Madison JE (1995) Medical management of chronic hepatic encephalopathy. In: *Current Veterinary Therapy, XII*, ed. JD Bonagura, pp. 1153–1157. WB Saunders, Philadelphia

Maton PN, Gardner JD and Jensen RT (1989) Use of long-acting somatostatin analog SMS201-995 in patients with pancreatic islet cell tumors. *Digestive Diseases Science* **34**, 28S–39S

McKay CJ, Imrie CW and Baxter JN (1993) Somatostatin and somatostatin analogues — are they indicated in the management of acute pancreatitis? *Gut* **34**, 1622–1626

Mehlhaff CJ, Peterson ME, Patnaik AK and Carillo JM (1985) Insulin-producing islet cell neoplasms: surgical considerations and general management in 35 dogs. *Journal of the American Animal Hospital Association* **21**, 607–612

Meleo K (1990) Management of insulinoma patients with refractory hypoglycaemia. *Problems in Veterinary Medicine* **2**, 602–609

Nelson RW (1995) Insulin-secreting islet cell neoplasia. In: *Textbook of Veterinary Internal Medicine*, 4th edn, ed. SJ Ettinger and EC Feldman, pp. 1501–1509. WB Saunders, Philadelphia

Phillips LS and Robertson DG (1993) Insulin-like growth factors and non-islet cell hypoglycaemia. *Metabolism* **42**, 1093–1101

Reubi JC, Laissue J, Waser B, Horisberger U and Schaer JC (1994) Expression of somatostatin receptors in normal, inflamed, and neoplastic human gastrointestinal tissues. *Annals of the New York Academy of Sciences* **733**, 122–137

Saunders HM (1991) Ultrasonography of the pancreas. *Problems in Veterinary Medicine*, **3**, 583–603

Simpson KW, Stepien RL, Elwood CM, Boswood A and Vaillant C (1995) Evaluation of the long acting somatostatin analogue octreotide in the management of insulinoma in three dogs. *Journal of Small Animal Practice* **36**, 161–165

Timmer R, Koniingsberger JC, Erkelens DW, Thijssen JHH, Lips CJM and Koppeschaar HPF (1991) No effects of the long-acting somatostatin analogue octreotide in patients with insulinoma. *Netherlands Journal of Medicine* **38**, 199–203

von Yben FE, Grodum E, Gjessing HJ, Hagen C and Neilsen H (1994) Metabolic remission with octreotide in patients with insulinoma. *Journal of Internal Medicine* **235**, 245–248

Wolf RR, Dariush E and Spitzer J (1977) Glucose and lactate kinetics after endotoxin administration in dogs. *American Journal of Physiology* **232(2)**, E180–E185

Zapf J (1994) Role of insulin-like growth factor II and IGF binding proteins in extrapancreatic tumour hypoglycaemia. *Hormone Research* **42**, 20–26

CHAPTER EIGHTEEN

Disorders of Water and Sodium Balance

John K. Dunn

INTRODUCTION

Body water is distributed between the extracellular and intracellular fluid (ICF) compartments. The extracellular fluid (ECF) compartment is made up of fluid in the vascular and interstitial spaces. The distribution of fluid between the vascular and interstitial spaces is controlled by the intracapillary hydrostatic and plasma oncotic pressures. The movement of water between the extracellular and intracellular compartments is regulated primarily by changes in ECF osmolality. If ECF osmolality is high, water is drawn out of the cells and the cells 'shrink'; conversely low ECF osmolality leads to swelling and ultimate lysis of cells.

NORMAL WATER BALANCE

The intake of water must compensate for daily losses that occur via the skin, gastrointestinal and respiratory tracts, and kidneys. The balance between water intake (50–60 ml/kg/day) and loss is normally so precise that daily fluctuations in body weight are less than 1%. The amount of water lost in faeces in the normal animal is unimportant (approximately 5 ml/kg/day) compared with the volumes lost in urine (approximately 20–40 ml/kg/day) and evaporation via the respiratory tract and skin (approximately 15 ml/kg/day). An obligatory loss of urine is required for the excretion of the end products of dietary protein metabolism (urea, sulphate and phosphate ions). Variations in the rate of release of vasopressin (antidiuretic hormone, ADH) from the neurohypophysis ensure that a minimal volume of maximally concentrated urine is produced.

Cats derive a higher percentage of their daily water requirements from their food. The volume of water drunk depends on the type of diet (cats on dry rations drink more water; Seefeldt and Chapman, 1979) and the frequency of feeding (cats fed periodically drink less than those fed continuously; Finco *et al.*, 1986).

Water balance is closely related to the osmolality of the ECF, and since ECF osmolality is almost entirely determined by the concentration of sodium ions, it is also inextricably linked to sodium regulation. The two main mechanisms for balancing water loss with water intake are the thirst mechanism, and renal control of salt and water excretion. Disturbances in water balance may arise as a result of a defective thirst mechanism and/or defective renal concentration mechanisms. Most disorders of water balance are the result of impaired ability of the kidney to conserve water. Under normal circumstances renal concentration defects which result in polyuria initiate compensatory changes in the thirst mechanism and the animal becomes polydipsic. Hence polydipsia, in most cases, can be regarded as a compensatory mechanism to maintain total body fluids within normal limits.

VOLUME CONTRACTION

Contraction of ECF volume may involve simultaneous loss of both sodium ions and water (in which case ICF volume may be spared), or pure water loss where fluid depletion is distributed throughout total body water. Volume contraction may be caused by reduced fluid intake or by renal and non-renal loss of water and solute.

The hydration status of an animal is usually expressed as a percentage of body weight and is assessed by checking skin elasticity. Skin elasticity only provides a crude estimation of hydration status; in thin animals the degree of dehydration may be overestimated and, conversely, in obese animals with large subcutaneous fat deposits the degree of dehydration may be underestimated. Packed cell volume (PCV) and total plasma protein concentration can also be used to estimate hydration status; a 20% reduction in ECF volume results in a 20% increase in PCV and total plasma protein concentration. Other clinical and laboratory parameters used to assess an animal's hydration status are listed in Table 18.1.

The earliest clinical signs of dehydration become evident when body weight is reduced by 5–8%. These signs become more pronounced until there is a 15% reduction in body weight, at which stage the animal will be showing

Skin 'tents' when lifted as it loses its normal elasticity
Mucous membranes appear dry and congested
Eyes retract in their sockets
Increased packed cell volume and total plasma protein concentration
Increased plasma sodium and chloride concentrations
Increased plasma urea and creatinine concentrations with concentrated urine (if renal function normal)
Increased plasma and urine osmolalities (if renal function normal)

Table 18.1: Clinical and laboratory parameters used to assess hydration status.

Weak rapid pulse

Dry, pale mucous membranes

Prolonged capillary refill time

Sunken eyes

Poor skin elasticity

Cool distal extremities

Decreased urine output

Evidence of microcardia (thoracic radiographs)

Table 18.2: Clinical signs of volume depletion (hypovolaemic shock).

signs characteristic of hypovolaemic shock (Table 18.2). The severity of clinical signs observed depends on the type of fluid lost (e.g. blood, solute or pure water), the rate of fluid loss, and the fluid compartment from which it is lost (e.g. ECF only or ECF and ICF).

Fluid therapy must take account of the fluid deficit and daily maintenance requirements to compensate for urinary and insensible losses described above. Additional ongoing losses which may be occurring through vomiting and diarrhoea, burns or body cavity effusions should be estimated and added to the total daily fluid requirements. Measurement of urine output is essential in cases where continued rapid administration of fluids is likely to result in overhydration and pulmonary oedema, e.g. animals with oliguric renal failure or congestive heart failure (CHF).

VOLUME EXPANSION

Expansion of the ECF compartment occurs when sodium and water intake exceeds renal excretion. Causes include overzealous administration of fluids that contain sodium, especially to animals with oliguric renal failure or CHF, and hypoproteinaemia (severe chronic liver disease, nephrotic syndrome, and protein-losing enteropathy). Extracellular fluid is redistributed from the plasma space to the interstitium; this results in a reduction in effective arterial blood volume and reduced tissue perfusion. Reduced tissue perfusion leads to activation of the renin–angiotensin system (RAS), sodium retention, and expansion of interstitial volume which is manifested clinically as oedema. Other clinical signs associated with hypervolaemic states are listed in Table 18.3.

Increased respiratory rate/coughing

Vomiting

Subcutaneous oedema/ascites

Chemosis/exophthalmos

Increased urine output

Table 18.3: Clinical signs of fluid volume overload (hypervolaemia).

CONTROL OF WATER AND SODIUM BALANCE

Thirst mechanism
An intact thirst mechanism is necessary to replace physiological renal and non-renal water loss. Neurons of the thirst centre respond to an increase in ECF osmolality and a decrease in effective blood volume. Thirst can be stimulated by a 2% increase in plasma osmolality, via hypothalamic osmoreceptors, or by an 8–10% reduction in blood volume via input from peripheral volume receptors located in major vessels.

Renal control of water and sodium balance
The primary mechanism for preventing excessive fluid loss is the renal conservation of water, which is dependent on the synthesis and release of ADH from the posterior pituitary. The ability of the kidney to concentrate urine depends on three factors: the amount of circulating ADH; the responsiveness of the distal tubules and collecting ducts to ADH; and the degree of hypertonicity of the renal medulla. In response to ADH, water is reabsorbed along the concentration gradients established in the renal medulla by the countercurrent multiplier system involving the loop of Henle and vasa recta. High concentrations of sodium chloride and urea within the medullary interstitium preserve this concentration gradient thereby maximising the antidiuretic effect of the hormone

Secretion of ADH
ADH is synthesised by the supraoptic and paraventricular nuclei of the hypothalamus which are located near the neurons of the thirst centre. The hormone is stored and released from the nerve endings of the neurohypophysis (posterior pituitary), acts on the cells of the distal tubules and alters water permeability of the collecting ducts by a specific receptor mechanism. The production and release of ADH is controlled by osmoreceptors in the hypothalamus, which sense changes in plasma osmolality, and by volume receptors located in the left atrium, carotid sinus, and aortic arch which respond to alterations in vascular pressure and volume. The osmoreceptors which control thirst are considered to be separate from those that control the secretion of ADH.

The normal physiological response to a decrease in plasma osmolality is a decrease in ADH secretion so that the urine becomes more dilute. Water reabsorption by the collecting ducts decreases and water is lost in excess of solute until osmolality returns to normal. With severe volume contraction, the ECF osmolality receptors are reset at a lower threshold so that the ADH response is enhanced until ECF volume is restored, i.e. plasma volume is maintained at the expense of osmolality and hypotonic hyponatraemia may develop (Senior, 1995). Delivery of solute to the distal renal tubule may also be compromised during hypovolaemic states which may further limit the loss of water.

Renal tubular function
Glomerular filtrate is isosthenuric, i.e. has a specific

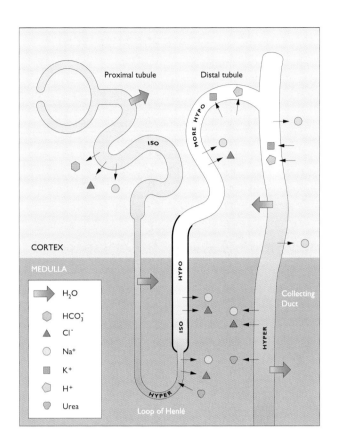

Figure 18.1: Changes in urine osmolality and movement of ions and other solutes in various parts of the nephron. The thickened wall of the ascending limb of the loop of Henlé indicates relative impermeability of the tubular epithelium to water. In the presence of ADH, the fluid in the collecting ducts becomes hypertonic, whereas in the absence of this hormone, fluid in the distal tube and collecting duct remains hypotonic. Aldosterone promotes resorption of Na^+ and secretion of H^+ and K^+ in the distal convoluted tubule. In addition to Na^+ and Cl^-, urea contributes to the high solute concentration in the interstitial medulla of the kidney. Urea diffuses from the inner medullary collecting duct (under the influence of ADH) into the interstitium before diffusing into the thin segment of the ascending loop of Henlé. This recirculation mechanism for urea is important for maintaining medullary hypertonicity. Loss of these medullary concentration gradients (medullary washout) results in submaximal concentration of urine. (Redrawn after Cannon, 1977.)

gravity equal to that of plasma (1.008–1.012). Approximately 70% of the filtered load of sodium is actively reabsorbed in the proximal tubule by a process that is dependent on the activity of a sodium/potassium ATPase pump in the renal tubular epithelial cells. The reabsorption of sodium and other solutes, such as glucose, amino acids, potassium, chloride and bicarbonate, sets up osmotic gradients for the passive reabsorption of water.

Up to 25% of the filtered sodium is absorbed with chloride from the thick ascending limb of the loop of Henle, which contributes significantly to maintenance of renal medullary hypertonicity. This part of the nephron is impermeable to water which means that the glomerular filtrate is actively diluted so that on entering the distal tubule it is hypotonic to plasma.

In the distal tubule less than 10% of filtered sodium and water are reabsorbed while potassium is actively secreted into the tubular lumen under the action of aldosterone (see below). In the presence of ADH, water is absorbed with urea from the collecting ducts and some distal tubule segments which results in the production of concentrated urine. The changes in urine osmolality that occur in different parts of the nephron are shown in Figure 18.1.

Aldosterone

Aldosterone is produced by the zona glomerulosa of the adrenal cortex, and acts on the distal tubular epithelial cells where it promotes the reabsorption of sodium and the excretion of potassium and hydrogen ions. Aldosterone is secreted in response to an increase in plasma potassium concentration via a direct effect of potassium on the adrenal cortex.

Alterations in plasma sodium concentration influence aldosterone release via the RAS (Figure 18.2). Sodium

depletion causes a reduction in circulating blood volume which results in decreased renal perfusion. The decrease in renal perfusion is detected by specialised myoepithelial cells of the juxtaglomerular apparatus which secrete renin. Any condition therefore which decreases ECF volume and/or results in a fall in arterial blood pressure, e.g. severe dehydration, shock, haemorrhage or CHF, will also result in the release of renin into the systemic circulation.

Renin cleaves angiotensin I from angiotensinogen, a plasma α-2 globulin produced in the liver. Angiotensin converting enzyme (ACE) converts angiotensin I to angiotensin II. Angiotensin II is a powerful vasoconstrictor which increases peripheral vascular resistance. It has a direct negative feedback effect on the secretion of renin and stimulates the release of aldosterone from the adrenal cortex thereby replacing the ECF volume deficit and increasing arterial blood pressure.

Natriuretic factors

Natriuretic factors or hormones may influence sodium balance in the short term. One such hormone, known as atrial natriuretic factor (ANF), is released by atrial and ventricular myocardial cells in response to chronic volume overload in animals with decompensated CHF. ANF acts directly on the kidney to increase sodium excretion and also has hypotensive effects by inhibiting the renin–angiotensin–aldosterone system (RAAS).

DISORDERS OF ADH SECRETION AND RELEASE

ADH plays a pivotal role in the regulation of water

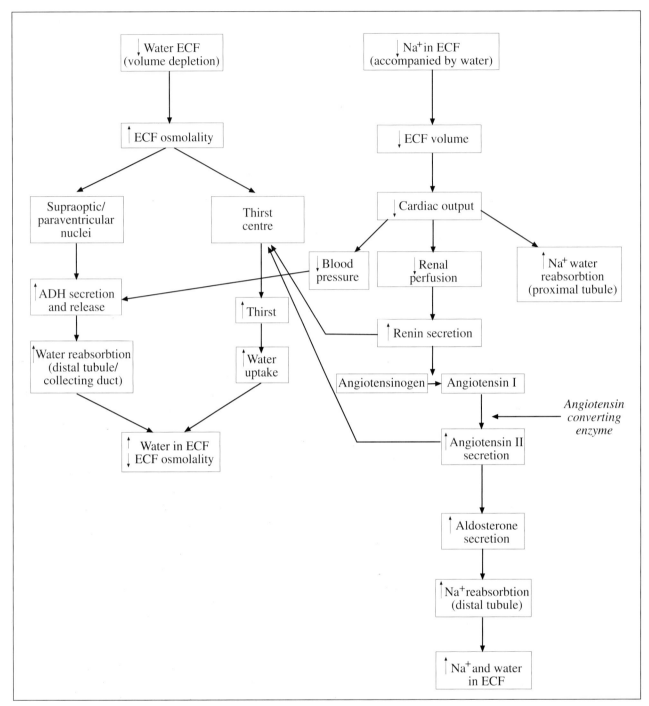

Figure 18.2: *Water and sodium balance. ECF = extracellular fluid; ADH = antidiuretic hormone.*

balance. ADH is released primarily in response to an increase in plasma osmolality and decreases in blood volume and blood pressure. Nausea, hypoglycaemia, activation of the RAAS, pain, emotion, and physical exercise may also result in release of ADH.

Diabetes insipidus

Diabetes insipidus is characterised by polydipsia and the production of large volumes of hyposthenuric urine. Diabetes insipidus exists in two forms. The central form (CDI) is caused by the defective synthesis or release of ADH from the posterior pituitary, while nephrogenic diabetes insipidus (NDI) represents an inability of the distal renal tubules and collecting ducts to respond to ADH.

Central diabetes insipidus

Central diabetes insidipus is caused by either an absolute or relative deficiency of ADH. In the dog, CDI is usually classified as idiopathic although it may occur secondary to head trauma or large pituitary or hypothalamic tumours. Congenital CDI in the dog is a rare disease. Acquired (idiopathic) and congenital forms of CDI, involving a partial or absolute deficiency of ADH, occur infrequently in the cat.

History and clinical signs: Animals with CDI present with a history of severe polydipsia and polyuria. There is no breed, age or sex predisposition for this disorder. The polydipsia may be so marked that affected animals constantly seek water, and may drink any liquid available including their own urine. As a result they may become restless and inappetant, and lose weight. Animals with diabetes insipidus frequently present with a history of nocturia and urinary incontinence. Clinical examination is often unremarkable. Central nervous system (CNS) signs (visual deficits, incoordination, aimless wandering, and seizures) may become apparent if the diabetes insipidus is associated with a large expanding pituitary or hypothalamic tumour.

Laboratory abnormalities: Routine haematological and biochemical results from animals with CDI are often within normal limits. If the animal has been deprived of water or is marginally dehydrated the PCV, total plasma protein concentration, and plasma urea, creatinine, sodium and chloride levels may be increased. Urine specific gravity is typically <1.005; a partial deficiency of ADH may result in the production of urine in the isosthenuric range.

Nephrogenic diabetes insipidus

Stimulation of specific V2 receptors on renal tubular epithelial cells by ADH results in the generation of intracellular cAMP which increases the number of aqueous channels on the luminal membrane of the tubular epithelial cells. This results in the absorption of free water and formation of concentrated urine. Nephrogenic diabetes insipidus is the result of a defect in the V2 receptor that leads to blunting of the renal tubular response to ADH. Congenital (primary) NDI is rare; most cases are acquired and occur secondary to a number of renal, metabolic and electrolyte disorders (see Chapter 1). Non-responsiveness of V2 receptors to ADH may be partial or complete.

Diagnosis of diabetes insipidus

The aims of the diag-nostic investigations for diabetes insipidus are two-fold. First, it is necessary to rule out other causes of polyuria and polydipsia (see Chapter 1). In most cases, this is easily achieved on the basis of routine haematological and biochemical analyses, but additional diagnostic tests for covert hepatic disease or hyperadrenocorticism may be indicated.

Having excluded most of the systemic and metabolic causes of polyuria and polydipsia, diagnostic tests should be directed at differentiating central and nephrogenic forms of diabetes insipidus from primary (psychogenic) polydipsia associated with renal medullary washout. Measurement of plasma osmolality may be helpful in this respect. Dogs with primary polydipsia tend to have lower plasma osmolality values than animals with diabetes insipidus because of chronic volume overload. Plasma ADH measurements have been found to be helpful in humans for distinguishing CDI and NDI and primary polydipsia. ADH assays are as yet not a practical proposition for animals because of their limited availability and prohibitive cost.

Water deprivation test: The aim of a water deprivation test is to establish whether ADH is released in response to dehydration. Plasma urea, creatinine and calcium concentrations should be determined beforehand. Water deprivation is contraindicated in animals that are

1. Fast for 12 hours
2. Catheterise and empty bladder
3. Check urine specific gravity
4. Record body weight
5. Record urine and plasma osmolalities, packed cell volume, total plasma protein and blood urea concentrations
6. Withold all water
7. Catheterise bladder every 1 or 2 hours, and repeat parameters listed above

Table 18.4: Protocol for performing a standard water deprivation test.

azotaemic or hypercalcaemic, or showing clinical evidence of dehydration. The standard protocol for performing a water deprivation test is described in Table 18.4. The test is discontinued when the animal has lost 5% of its body weight or the urine specific gravity exceeds 1.030. Failure to concentrate urine above 1.010 is highly suggestive of CDI or NDI. Values between 1.020 and 1.030 indicate submaximal concentration of urine and should be regarded as equivocal. Equivocal results may be obtained in animals with only a partial deficiency of ADH or when prolonged polydipsia results in loss of renal medullary concentration gradients (medullary washout).

Cats with diabetes insipidus may become severely dehydrated and lose more than 5% of their body weight in less than 10 hours following abrupt water deprivation, and therefore require particularly close monitoring. A urine specific gravity of 1.025 represents an adequate response to water deprivation in the cat.

A modified or partial water deprivation test is indicated when medullary washout is suspected, for example when equivocal results are obtained using the protocol described above or following the administration of ADH. The modified test involves a gradual reduction in daily water intake (10–15% per day) over a 3-day period. On day 1 no more than twice the normal daily maintenance requirements should be given i.e. water intake should not exceed 100 ml/kg body weight; this volume should be offered in 6–8 drinks over 24 hours. Hydration status and urine specific gravity should be monitored on a daily basis. The test is useful for differentiating CDI or NDI from primary polydipsia associated with medullary washout. Failure to adequately concentrate urine at the end of the 3-day period suggests that medullary washout is not the cause of the polyuria.

ADH (vasopressin) response test: An ADH response test is indicated in animals that fail to concentrate urine adequately in response to water deprivation. ADH can be administered following a standard or modified water deprivation test. The bladder should be catheterised and emptied. Urine specific gravity, and if possible urine and plasma osmolalities, should be determined before the ADH is given. Desmopressin (1-desamino-8-D arginine vasopressin, DDAVP), a synthetic ADH analogue, can be injected subcutaneously, intramuscularly or intravenously (2 µg for dogs <15 kg, and cats; 4 µg for dogs >15 kg); alternatively 20 µg DDAVP intranasal drops (approximately four drops of the 100 mg/ml preparation) can be instilled into the conjunctival sac. Thereafter the bladder should be catheterised and urine specific gravity and urine and plasma osmolalities measured every 30–60 minutes for 2–4 hours. An increase in urine specific gravity to >1.025 (or in most cases 1.030) or a greater than 10% increase in urine osmolality is consistent with a diagnosis of CDI or partial NDI. A positive response to ADH is not significant unless it has been demonstrated that the animal cannot concentrate its urine in response to water deprivation. Failure to concentrate urine in response to DDAVP (i.e. a <10% increase in urine osmolality) suggests NDI or primary polydipsia with medullary washout.

Following completion of the test, small amounts of water (e.g. 5 ml/kg) can be offered at regular (e.g. 30–60 minute) intervals. Large amounts of water given either during or after the test may result in water intoxication and a variety of CNS signs due to cerebral oedema.

ADH trial: Animals that respond equivocally to ADH may show a positive response if ADH is administered over a longer period. Intranasal drops can be administered via the conjunctival sac (1–4 drops twice daily for 5–7 days). A decrease in water consumption by more than 50% during the first day is highly suggestive of CDI or partial NDI (Nichols and Thompson, 1995). Renal medullary washout can blunt the response to ADH in some dogs which are severely polydipsic. Continued ADH administration in such cases may result in a gradual improvement in concentrating ability as the polyuria diminishes and renal medullary concentration gradients are re-established.

The Hickey–Hare test: In the author's experience there are few indications for performing the Hickey–Hare test since most polyuric states, even those complicated by renal medullary washout, can be readily differentiated on the basis of a modified water deprivation test when used in combination with an ADH response test. The Hickey–Hare test assesses the ability of the hypothalamic–pituitary–renal axis to decrease urine volume in response to increasing plasma osmolality. Its main use therefore is to distinguish polyuric states where medullary washout is a suspected complication. The test involves the administration of hypertonic saline to a water-loaded animal. The protocol is given in Table 18.5.

In normal dogs, and dogs with primary polydipsia, urine volume gradually decreases as urine specific gravity

1.	Give 20 ml/kg of water by stomach tube
2.	Catheterise and empty the bladder
3.	Administer 2.5% sodium chloride intravenously at a rate of 2.5 ml/kg/min over 45 minutes
4.	Measure urine volume, specific gravity and osmolality every 15 minutes after the start of the infusion

Table 18.5: *Protocol for the Hickey–Hare test.*

and osmolality increase. Failure to do so is suggestive of CDI or NDI. A potential hazard of this test, which has prevented its extensive use, is sodium overload which may lead to the development of CNS signs.

Treatment of diabetes insipidus

CDI or partial NDI: The synthetic analogue of ADH (DDAVP) is available as an injectable preparation (4 µg/ml) for intravenous and subcutaneous administration, and also as an intranasal solution (100 µg/ml; 2.5 ml). The dose of DDAVP varies considerably from animal to animal and is also dependent on the preparation used and route of administration. Intranasal administration is poorly tolerated in most dogs and cats. For long-term management, DDAVP can be injected subcutaneously (0.5–2 µg once or twice daily) or the intranasal drops can be instilled into the conjunctival sac (1–4 drops once or twice daily). Duration of action following subcutaneous or conjunctival administration is extremely variable (8–24 hours); in most cases ADH has its maximal effect between 6 and 10 hours. DDAVP has recently become available in tablet form (0.1 or 0.2 mg). The oral administration of DDAVP for the treatment of canine and feline diabetes insipidus has yet to be evaluated. A dose of 10 µg/kg given before food twice daily has been used successfully to treat one dog with CDI (IK Ramsey, personal communication).

Side effects of DDAVP therapy are uncommon. Water intoxication and hyponatraemia occasionally occur if large volumes of water are ingested during the initial stages of treatment.

Thiazide diuretics have been used to treat both the central and nephrogenic forms of diabetes insipidus and may help to reduce water intake by as much as 50% (see NDI below).

Chlorpropamide is an oral sulphonylurea hypoglycaemic agent which has been used with variable success at a dose of 10–40 mg/kg/day to treat canine CDI caused by a partial ADH deficiency (Feldman and Nelson, 1996). The drug potentiates the renal tubular effects of ADH and therefore some endogenous ADH is required. A regular feeding schedule is essential to avoid problems associated with hypoglycaemia.

Nephrogenic diabetes insipidus: Thiazide diuretics such as chlorothiazide and hydrochlorothiazide are the mainstay of treatment for NDI. Water intake in some cases may be reduced by 30–50%. Thiazide diuretics act by reducing total body sodium by inhibiting sodium reabsorption in the ascending loop of Henle. The decrease in plasma sodium and osmolality inhibits the thirst centre thereby reducing water consumption. This in turn leads to ECF volume contraction, a decrease in glomerular filtration rate, and increased proximal tubular reabsorption of sodium and water with resultant decreased delivery of sodium to the distal tubule. The net result is a reduction in urine volume. The suggested doses of hydrochlorothiazide and chlorothiazide are 2.5–5 mg/kg twice daily and 10–20 mg/kg twice daily, respectively. Salt intake should be restricted to potentiate the action of these drugs. Side effects are rare.

DISORDERS OF SODIUM BALANCE

Hyponatraemia

Normal plasma sodium concentrations vary from approximately 142 to 155 mmol/l. Hyponatraemia, which in most cases is a reflection of plasma hypo-osmolality, is a relatively rare abnormality in small animal medicine. It may result from abnormalities in either the thirst mechanism or the hypothalamic–pituitary–renal axis, and may be classified as hypotonic (hypo-osmolar), hypertonic (hyperosmolar), or isotonic (euosmolar). Causes of hyponatraemia are listed in Table 18.6.

Hypotonic hyponatraemia
Hypoadrenocorticism
Syndrome of inappropriate antidiuretic hormone secretion
Primary polydipsia
Postobstructive diuresis
Congestive heart failure
Severe liver disease
Nephrotic syndrome
Oliguric renal failure
Gastrointestinal haemorrhage
Postoperative pain, stress
Diuretic therapy
Hypertonic hyponatraemia
Diabetes mellitus
Mannitol administration
Isotonic hyponatraemia (pseudohyponatraemia)
Hyperlipaemia
Hyperglobulinaemia

Table 18.6: Causes of hyponatraemia.

Hypotonic (hypo-osmolar) hyponatraemia

The pathophysiological mechanisms for hypotonic hyponatraemia include plasma volume depletion, inappropriate secretion of ADH, and primary polydipsia.

Decreased circulating plasma volume: A decrease in effective circulating plasma volume may be caused by true volume depletion (resulting from either loss of blood or solute and water) or hypervolaemic states, such as CHF and the nephrotic syndrome, where there is redistribution of fluid from the vascular to the interstitial space resulting in reduced tissue perfusion. True volume depletion may be caused by haemorrhage, vomiting and diarrhoea, and severe burns. Water and solute may also be lost in excessive amounts via the kidneys. In most cases the loss of solute occurs in fluid which is either isotonic or hypotonic so that the plasma sodium concentration usually does not decrease, for example most animals with non-oliguric renal disease maintain a normal plasma sodium concentration as long as water is not retained and solute is not lost by other routes such as vomiting and diarrhoea. Hyponatraemia may develop if the renal losses that occur, for example during postobstructive diuresis in cats, are replaced using hypotonic (e.g. sodium-free) fluids and/or if the ability of the kidneys to excrete free water is

impaired. Excessive renal loss of solute and water may also occur postoperatively (pain and stress are thought to enhance ADH production independent of ECF osmolality) and as a result of overzealous diuretic therapy.

Hyponatraemia is a common feature of hypoadrenocorticism. The deficiency of aldosterone results in excessive renal sodium loss which leads to volume depletion, release of ADH, and stimulation of the thirst centre. In most cases the hyponatraemia is associated with hyperkalaemia. Hypovolaemia stimulates ADH release at a lower ECF osmolality, and the continued secretion of ADH is enhanced by the lack of glucocorticoids.

With hypervolaemic states such as CHF, water may be retained in excess of sodium resulting in hyponatraemia despite a normal or increased total body sodium content.

Syndrome of inappropriate ADH secretion: The syndrome of inappropriate ADH secretion (SIADH) is a relatively rare disorder where ADH secretion occurs in the absence of the osmotic and volume stimuli normally required for ADH release. Retention of ingested water leads to inhibition of aldosterone secretion, loss of sodium in the urine, and hyponatraemia. Affected animals do not appear hypovolaemic or clinically dehydrated (they are usually normovolaemic). Despite the hyponatraemia, a significant amount of sodium is excreted in urine. Renal, adrenal and thyroid function are normal. Fluid restriction corrects both the hypotonic hyponatraemia and natriuresis. SIADH has been reported in dogs with dirofilariasis and hypothalamic tumours (Scott-Moncrieff, 1995); in humans SIADH has been associated with malignant tumours, some of which are thought to secrete an ADH-like substance. Certain drugs, including cyclophosphamide, vincristine, barbiturates and non-steroidal anti-inflammatory drugs, are known to impair water excretion in humans by either stimulating ADH release or potentiating its action at the receptor level.

Primary polydipsia: Primary polydipsia, sometimes referred to as psychogenic polydipsia, commonly occurs in young dogs. Water intake is often markedly increased although affected animals retain the ability to concentrate urine. Plasma sodium concentration and osmolality may be low if water intake overwhelms the ability of the kidney to excrete free water. The aetiology of the condition is uncertain. It may represent a behavioural abnormality triggered by an environmental or emotional stimulus. The differentiation of primary polydipsia from the central and nephrogenic forms of diabetes insipidus has been discussed above.

Hypertonic (hyperosmolar) hyponatraemia

When a solute such as glucose accumulates in large amounts in the ECF, as occurs in uncontrolled diabetes mellitus, fluid is drawn from cells and this decreases the sodium concentration in the ECF. The reduction in ECF sodium concentration is therefore the result of altered distribution of water between the ICF and ECF and does not represent an alteration in total body water, i.e. it is a dilutional hyponatraemia. A similar situation may arise following the administration of hypertonic solutions such as mannitol. The hyponatraemia may be expected to resolve spontaneously if the concentration of solute in the ECF is reduced.

Isotonic (euosmolar) hyponatraemia

Under normal circumstances the concentration of dissolved substances in the small non-aqueous fraction of plasma does not significantly interfere with measurement of solutes such as sodium which are contained in the aqueous fraction. If, however, the concentration of dissolved solutes in the non-aqueous phase of plasma (or serum) significantly increases, the concentration of solutes in the aqueous phase is artefactually reduced. Hence severe hyperlipidaemia or hypergammaglobulinaemia results in displacement of the aqueous phase and an erroneously low

plasma sodium concentration (pseudohyponatraemia) although the concentration of sodium in the aqueous phase and plasma osmolality are essentially unaltered. Such errors can be avoided by using ion-specific electrodes which measure plasma sodium concentration only in the aqueous phase.

Investigation of hyponatraemia

History and clinical signs: Hyponatraemia causes weakness, depression, vomiting, muscle fasciculations, seizures and coma. Expansion of ICF results in CNS signs due to cerebral swelling; these signs become more pronounced if hyponatraemia develops rapidly. Clinical signs reflecting the underlying condition causing the hyponatraemia may also be present.

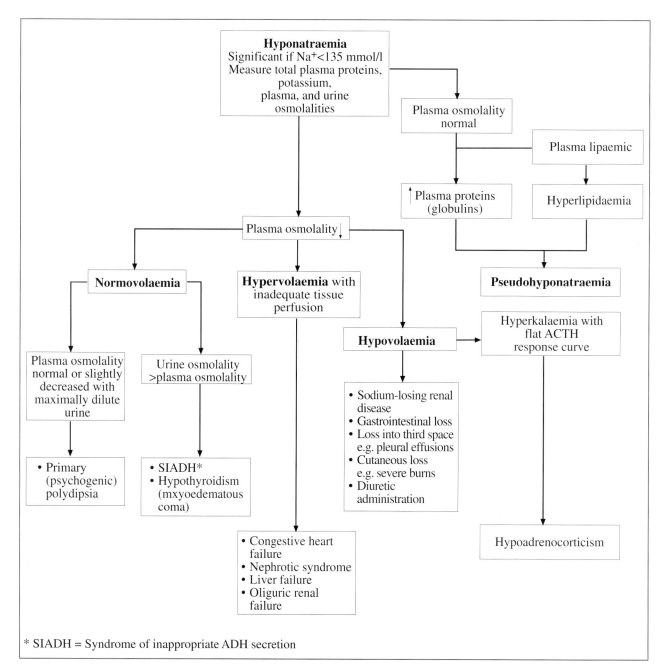

Figure 18.3: Diagnostic approach to hyponatraemia.

Laboratory investigation of hyponatraemia: In addition to the history and clinical signs, the investigation of hyponatraemia should include visual examination of plasma (serum) for evidence of lipaemia, measurement of total plasma protein concentration, and full routine haematological and biochemical examinations. In many cases the cause of hyponatraemia is immediately obvious. An ACTH stimulation test should be performed to rule out hypoadrenocorticism. Plasma and urine osmolalities should be determined immediately if plasma sodium is <135 mmol/l. In cases of SIADH, plasma osmolality will be low and urine osmolality will be unexpectedly high. The diagnostic approach to hyponatraemia is outlined in Figure 18.3.

Management of hyponatraemia

Isotonic saline should be administered if volume depletion is evident and, or, plasma sodium is >120 mmol/l. If hyponatraemia is particularly severe (plasma sodium <120 mmol/l) and CNS signs are present, a hypertonic saline solution (e.g. 2.5% sodium chloride) and frusemide (2–4 mg/kg twice daily) should be given. Plasma osmolality should be corrected over a 24–48 hour period; rapid correction may cause shrinkage of brain cells. Long-term restriction of water may be required to manage cases of SIADH and primary polydipsia. Dietary sodium restriction and diuretics are indicated if hyponatraemia is associated with oedema or ascites (e.g. CHF).

Hypernatraemia

Hypernatraemia may be caused by three mechanisms: loss of hypotonic fluid (e.g. diarrhoea), loss of pure water (e.g. diabetes insipidus), and salt gain (e.g. increased salt intake). As such, hypernatraemia can be classified as hypovolaemic, normovolaemic or hypervolaemic (Table 18.7). It is important to note that an increase in plasma sodium concentration does not indicate increased total body sodium reserves; the amount of total body sodium may be decreased, normal, or increased depending on the underlying pathogenesis.

Hypernatraemia due to loss of hypotonic fluid (hypovolaemic hypernatraemia)
Vomiting/diarrhoea
Osmotic diuresis (e.g. diabetes mellitus, mannitol)
Postobstructive diuresis

Hypernatraemia due to pure water loss (normovolaemic hypernatraemia)
Diabetes insipidus (especially if deprived of water)
Hypodipsia associated with central nervous system lesions, e.g. large hypothalamic tumours
Hypodipsia in young female Miniature Schnauzers

Hypernatraemia due to sodium gain/overload (hypervolaemic hypernatraemia)
Excessive administration of intravenous sodium chloride, e.g. in dogs with oliguric renal failure
Essential hypernatraemia
Primary hyperaldosteronism

Table 18.7: Causes of hypernatraemia.

Loss of hypotonic fluid (hypovolaemic hypernatraemia)

Loss of hypotonic fluid due to diarrhoea, often with a concurrent disturbance in water intake, is the most common cause of hypernatraemia in dogs and cats. Water is lost in excess of sodium, resulting in decreased ECF volume and a decrease in total body sodium. The animal appears clinically dehydrated but the kidneys retain the ability to conserve water and sodium resulting in production of concentrated urine. The osmotic diuresis that occurs with diabetes mellitus, mannitol administration, or following relief of urethral obstruction in a cat may also result in hypotonic fluid loss.

Pure water loss (normovolaemic hypernatraemia)

Diabetes insipidus results in pure water loss without the loss of electrolytes such as sodium. Contraction of plasma volume only occurs if water intake is restricted. Under such circumstances water moves from cells to the ECF. Initially, skin elasticity is normal but continued water deprivation results in clinical evidence of dehydration. Continued diuresis results in severe hypernatraemia, plasma volume contraction, azotaemia due to renal ischaemia, and eventually renal shutdown. Plasma osmolality is increased while urine osmolality is markedly decreased.

Animals with CNS lesions, for example large tumours impinging on the hypothalamus, may become hypodipsic. Hypodipsia due to an abnormal thirst mechanism has been reported in Miniature Schnauzers (Crawford *et al.*, 1984)

Sodium gain (hypervolaemic hypernatraemia)

Hypernatraemia due to excessive sodium intake is usually iatrogenic, e.g. an excessive volume of intravenous sodium chloride solution administered to a dog with acute oliguric renal failure. Total body sodium and ECF volume increase and the urine has a high sodium content.

Essential hypernatraemia is a rare condition of dogs and cats caused by failure of osmoreceptors to respond to an increase in serum osmolality (ADH response to volume contraction is normal). The condition is characterised by the gradual onset of hypernatraemia. Affected animals are usually adipsic but have normal skin turgor. Plasma osmolality is increased and urine concentrating ability is maintained. CNS signs usually do not appear until plasma sodium exceeds 175 mmol/l. Primary hyperaldosteronism is a rare cause of hypernatraemia in dogs and cats (see Chapter 24).

Investigation of hypernatraemia

History and clinical signs: Clinical signs of hypernatraemia usually do not become apparent until plasma sodium exceeds 175 mmol/kg and plasma osmolality is >350 mOsm/kg. Clinical signs of hypernatraemia include depression, weakness, anorexia, vomiting, increased thirst (variable and depends on the cause), disorientation, and a variety of other CNS signs. Plasma hyperosmolality causes contraction of ICF volume; movement of water from the intracellular to the

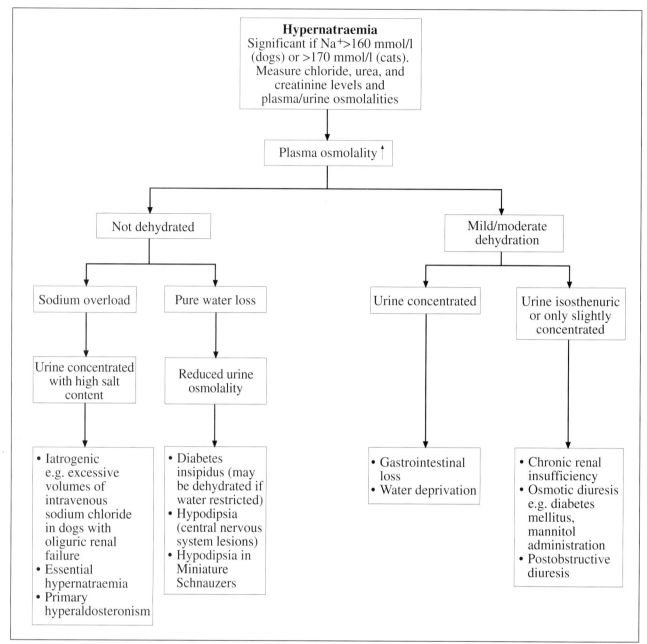

Figure 18.4: *Diagnostic approach to hypernatraemia.*

extracellular compartment results in cellular dehydration. When plasma osmolality increases gradually, brain cells accumulate substances known as 'idiogenic osmoles' in an attempt to maintain cell volume. CNS signs are more likely to develop if plasma osmolality increases rapidly because these 'idiogenic osmoles' have insufficient time to form and prevent shrinkage of brain cells. Shrinkage of brain cells causes tearing of fine meningeal vessels, and subarachnoid and subcortical haemorrhages. CNS signs include irritability, muscle twitching, spasticity and seizures. Coma and death occur when plasma osmolality exceeds 400 mOsm/kg.

When hypernatraemia is associated with hypotonic fluid loss and low total body sodium, signs of hypovolaemia may become evident. If sufficiently severe, hypovolaemia can result in renal ischaemia, acute tubular necrosis and ultimately renal failure.

Laboratory investigation of hypernatraemia: In most cases the increase in plasma sodium is accompanied by an increase in chloride concentration. Plasma and urine osmolalities should be determined (normal plasma osmolality varies from 290 to 310 mOsm/kg) and may be helpful in establishing the cause of the hypernatraemia. The diagnostic approach to hypernatraemia is outlined in Figure 18.4.

Management of hypernatraemia

Treatment of hypernatraemia should be directed at the primary underlying cause. Animals that are hypernatraemic but which are showing signs of hypovolaemia (i.e. have low total body sodium) should be given isotonic saline until the ECF volume deficit is restored.

Thereafter half-strength saline can be given followed by a 5% dextrose solution. Hypernatraemia due to pure water loss should be treated by oral water replacement or the administration of sodium-free fluids, e.g. 5% dextrose solution. Hypernatraemia caused by excessive sodium intake should be treated with a 5% dextrose solution and frusemide to promote urinary sodium excretion. Treatment of essential hypernatraemia involves adding the daily water requirements to food to compensate for the adipsia. Meals should be split into three or four portions.

In animals with chronic hypernatraemia, plasma osmolality should be reduced slowly over a 48-hour period since the idiogenic osmoles that accumulate in brain cells to prevent cellular dehydration do not rapidly dissipate. If fluids are administered too quickly, cerebral oedema may develop which may lead to seizures, muscle fasciculations and coma.

REFERENCES

Cannon PJ (1977) The kidney and heart failure. *New England Journal of Medicine* **296**, 26

Crawford MA, Kittleson MD and Fink GD (1984) Hypernatraemia and adipsia in a dog. *Journal of the American Veterinary Medical Association* **184**, 818–821

Feldman EC and Nelson RW (1996) Water metabolism and diabetes insipidus. In: *Canine and Feline Endocrinology and Reproduction, 2nd edn*, ed. EC Feldman and RW Nelson, pp.2–37. WB Saunders, Philadelphia

Finco DR, Adams DD, Crowell WA, Stattleman AJ, Brown SA and Barsanti JA (1986) Food and water intake and urine composition in cats: influence of continuous versus periodic feeding. *American Journal of Veterinary Research* **47**, 1638–1642

Nichols R and Thompson L (1995) Pituitary-hypothalamic disease. In: *Textbook of Veterinary Internal Medicine, 4th edn*, ed. SJ Ettinger and EC Feldman, pp. 1422–1436. WB Saunders, Philadelphia

Scott-Moncrieff JCR (1995) Hyponatraemia and hypokalaemia. In: *Textbook of Veterinary Internal Medicine, 4th edn*, ed. SJ Ettinger and EC Feldman, pp. 40–45. WB Saunders, Philadelphia

Seefeldt SL and Chapman TE (1979) Body water content and turnover in cats fed dry and canned rations. *American Journal of Veterinary Research* **40**, 183–185

Senior DF (1995) Fluid therapy, electrolytes and acid-base control. In: *Textbook of Veterinary Internal Medicine, 4th edn*, ed. SJ Ettinger and EC Feldman, pp. 294–312. WB Saunders, Philadelphia

CHAPTER NINETEEN

Endocrine Emergencies

Mark E. Peterson

INTRODUCTION

There are six endocrine disorders in dogs and cats that can be emergencies. These include:

- Acute adrenocortical insufficiency
- Diabetic ketoacidosis
- Non-ketotic hyperosmolar diabetic syndrome
- Hypoglycaemia
- Hypercalcaemia
- Hypocalcaemia.

ACUTE ADRENOCORTICAL INSUFFICIENCY

Adrenocortical insufficiency, or hypoadrenocorticism, results from deficient adrenal production of glucocorticoids and/or mineralocorticoids. Either destruction of the adrenal cortex (i.e. primary adrenocortical insufficiency or Addison's disease) or deficient pituitary adrenocorticotropic hormone (ACTH) production (i.e. secondary adrenocortical insufficiency) may impair adrenocortical function and cause hypoadrenocorticism. However, because serum electrolyte disturbances do not develop in dogs or cats with secondary adrenal insufficiency, the vast majority of animals that develop severe adrenal crisis have the primary form of hypoadrenocorticism, i.e. Addison's disease.

In animals with primary adrenocortical insufficiency, adrenal destruction can result from a variety of causes. Idiopathic atrophy of the adrenal cortex, which accounts for most cases of primary hypoadrenocorticism in dogs and cats, is likely to result from autoimmune destruction of the adrenal cortex. Less common causes of primary adrenocortical insufficiency include destruction of the adrenal cortices by granulomatous disease, metastasis of cancer to the adrenal glands, and iatrogenic destruction of the adrenal cortices by the adrenocorticolytic drug, o,p'-DDD (mitotane).

The main clinical manifestations of primary hypoadrenocorticism are attributable to deficiencies of both aldosterone and cortisol (Schaer and Taboada, 1992). Lack of aldosterone results in an impaired ability to conserve sodium and excrete potassium. Deficiency of total body sodium results in a low circulating blood volume with subsequent hypotension, reduced cardiac output, and reduced perfusion of the kidneys. The most prominent manifestations of hyperkalaemia are in the heart, including depressed myocardial excitability, prolonged refractory period of the myocardium, and slowed conduction. Lack of cortisol results in the commonly observed gastrointestinal signs of anorexia, vomiting, abdominal pain, and weight loss.

Diagnosis

A tentative diagnosis of acute adrenocortical insufficiency can be made on the basis of the history and results of physical examination. Progressive weight loss, periodic vomiting or diarrhoea, and lethargy are generally present for weeks to months before culminating in an acute hypotensive state of collapse. The adrenal crisis, however, can occur more acutely with or without an associated stress to trigger the emergency.

On physical examination, the acutely decompensated dog or cat with Addison's disease is usually either hypo- or normothermic and may be dehydrated (Peterson *et al.*, 1989; Kintzer and Peterson, 1994; Melin and Peterson, 1996). The animal is often very depressed, and muscle weakness is usually profound. The respiratory rate can be normal or rapid, the latter due to shock and compensation for metabolic acidosis. The mucous membranes are usually pink, but the capillary refill time is prolonged. Cardiac auscultation might reveal a normal sinus rhythm or bradyarrhythmia. The pulse quality is weak, and the rate varies from normal to slow.

The electrocardiogram (ECG) is a useful tool for detecting the various electrophysiological abnormalities of the heart associated with hyperkalaemia. The most common abnormalities include flattened P waves, high positive or negative deflection in the T waves, broadened QRS complexes, bradycardia, sinoventricular complexes, and atrial standstill.

The definitive diagnosis of Addison's disease is based on biochemical test results. The hallmark findings include hyperkalaemia and hyponatraemia (Na:K ratio <23:1). Additional associated abnormalities include mild to moderate hypochloraemia, azotaemia, hyperphosphataemia, and metabolic acidosis. About 20% of cases have mild hypercalcaemia but hypoglycaemia is rare.

Although the historical, physical, clinicopathological, and ECG abnormalities described strongly suggest acute hypoadrenocorticism and constitute the basis for a clinical diagnosis and need for immediate treatment, the absolute diagnosis depends on demonstration of absent or minimal adrenocortical response to synthetic ACTH injection. To avoid an unnecessary delay of treatment for the sake of performing a diagnostic test, the following procedure is recommended soon after the dog or cat's admission:

1. Obtain blood for a haemogram, serum biochemical analysis, and basal cortisol determination, and perform a baseline urinalysis.
2. Administer fluids intravenously.
3. Immediately administer synthetic ACTH. A total dosage of 0.25 mg is administered intravenously or intramuscularly to dogs, and 0.125 mg intravenously to cats.
4. Obtain a second blood sample for cortisol determination, one hour later.

With this technique, the patient derives the benefit of prompt treatment while confirmatory diagnostic tests are performed. Dexamethasone is often administered before the ACTH stimulation test because it has little or no influence on measurement of endogenous cortisol concentrations. However, it is important to realise that many glucocorticoid preparations, including hydrocortisone, prednisone, and prednisolone, cross react in most cortisol assays to falsely elevate endogenous cortisol determinations, and should not be administered until the ACTH stimulation test is completed. Alternatively, ACTH stimulation testing could be performed within a few days once the dog or cat is stable. If hydrocortisone, prednisone, or prednisolone are given, dexamethasone should be substituted as glucocorticoid replacement, and testing postponed for 2–3 days to ensure reliable results.

Treatment

Whenever a diagnosis of Addisonian crisis is likely, treatment should be initiated without delay. The therapeutic objectives include:

- Resuscitation of intravascular volume
- Provision of glucocorticoids
- Reversal of the hyponatraemia and hyperkalaemia
- Recognition and reversal of any life-threatening cardiac arrhythmias.

Intravascular volume resuscitation

Since death from acute adrenocortical insufficiency is usually attributed to vascular collapse and shock, rapid correction of hypovolaemia is the first priority in treating the condition. An indwelling intravenous catheter should be placed in the jugular or cephalic vein and 0.9% normal saline infused at the initial rate of 20–40 ml/kg/h during the first 1–2 hours. If the animal is markedly hypotensive, the rate of saline infusion should be increased to 40–80 ml/kg/h during this period. Caution must be used if very high fluid rates (i.e. 90 ml/kg/h) are administered to animals with severe volume contraction and bradycardia, as pulmonary oedema could result. Once volume replacement has occurred, the fluid rate can be decreased to a maintenance rate of approximately 2–3 ml/kg/h (50–70 ml/kg/day). The fluids are discontinued when hydration, urine output, serum electrolytes, and serum creatinine concentrations are restored to normal (usually after 48–72 hours of treatment).

Glucocorticoid supplementation

Glucocorticoid deficiency is best corrected initially by intravenous administration of a rapid-acting glucocorticoid. Mineralocorticoid supplementation is not strictly necessary but some of the drugs do have significant mineralocorticoid activity (e.g. hydrocortisone) which may enhance renal distal tubular sodium resorption and potassium excretion. A wide variety of glucocorticoids is available for use in the crisis situation, including:

- Dexamethasone solution: a single dose of 0.5–2.0 mg/kg given intravenously
- Dexamethasone sodium phosphate: a single dose of 0.5–2.0 mg/kg given intravenously
- Methyprednisolone sodium: a single dose of 1–2 mg/kg given intravenously
- Hydrocortisone sodium phosphate and hydrocortisone sodium succinate: 5–10 mg/kg given intravenously every 6 hours or a continuous intravenous infusion at 0.625 mg/kg/h.

If necessary, the initial doses of dexamethasone or methylprednisolone sodium succinate can be repeated 2–6 hours later. As the animal's condition improves, the daily parenteral glucocorticoid supplementation should be continued but the dose gradually reduced over the next 3–5 days until oral drugs can be tolerated without the risk of vomiting. Usually prednisone or prednisolone is used at an initial dose of 0.2–0.5 mg/kg/day (see Chapter 11).

Treatment of hyponatraemia and hyperkalaemia

The above treatment protocol is a safe and reliable means of quickly lowering serum potassium concentrations. While mineralocorticoid supplementation is not strictly necessary in the acute phase of therapy, it forms the mainstay of long-term treatment of primary hypoadrenocorticism. Therefore, treatment with fludrocortisone acetate at a dose of 0.02 mg/kg/day should be started as soon as the animal is stable. Desoxycorticosterone pivalate, an injectable mineralocorticoid preparation, is unavailable in the UK.

Treatment of life-threatening cardiac arrhythmias

Serum potassium concentrations greater than 7.0 mmol/l cause progressive depression of the excitability and conduction velocity of the myocardium. ECG signs of life-threatening myocardial toxicity include widened QRS complexes, sinoventricular complexes, atrial standstill, and other bradyarrhythmias. Rapid intravenous administration of fluids is sufficient to lower the serum potassium concentration within 1–2 hours in most dogs with hypoadrenocorticism. However, if hyperkalaemic myocardial toxicity is life threatening, treatment with one of the following four protocols may be indicated:

- Administer 10% glucose intravenously (4–10 ml/kg intravenously) over 30–60 minutes
- Administer a 10% calcium gluconate solution (0.5–1.0 ml/kg intravenously) slowly over 10–20 minutes, accompanied by continuous ECG

monitoring. Calcium gluconate directly antagonises the myocardial toxic effect of hyperkalaemia but does not lower the serum potassium concentration

- Administer sodium bicarbonate (1–2 mmol/kg intravenously) over 5–15 minutes to lower the serum potassium concentration
- Administer regular crystalline insulin (0.25 IU/kg intravenously) to lower the serum potassium concentration. To avoid the anticipated hypoglycaemic side effects of insulin, also give a bolus injection of dextrose at the dose of 2–3 g per unit of insulin administered. Half of the dextrose should be administered as an intravenous bolus and the other half added to the intravenous fluids and given over the next 6–8 hours.

These emergency measures for the treatment of myocardial toxicity are usually required only once and need not be repeated.

DIABETIC KETOACIDOSIS

Diabetes mellitus is a disorder characterised by an absolute or relative lack of the pancreatic hormone, insulin. Insulin deficiency, together with the abnormally high secretion of glucagon which frequently develops secondary to diabetes in animals, accounts for the fasting hyperglycaemia of this disorder. In animals with mild insulin deficiency, impaired transfer of ingested nutrients into tissues causes mild to moderate hyperglycaemia. Severe insulin deficiency not only hampers uptake of ingested fuels by tissues, but also results in marked glucose overproduction and excessive mobilisation of the body's protein and fat stores. With marked lack of insulin, increased delivery of fatty acids to the liver results in the production of ketone bodies (e.g. β-hydroxybutyrate, acetoacetate, and acetone), responsible for the clinical state of ketoacidosis (Schaer and Taboada, 1992).

Diagnosis

Diabetic ketoacidosis should be suspected when the history includes polydipsia, polyuria, weight loss, and polyphagia, lasting for several weeks or months, that progresses to include signs of lethargy, anorexia, and vomiting during several days before examination. Some dogs and cats, however, have an acute history of polydipsia, polyuria, vomiting, weakness, and depression. On physical examination, the dog or cat with ketoacidosis is often dehydrated, weak, and depressed. A diagnosis of diabetic ketoacidosis is easily confirmed by demonstrating persistent hyperglycaemia, glucosuria, and ketonuria.

Treatment

The main objectives in the treatment of diabetic ketoacidosis are:

- To correct dehydration and electrolyte deficits
- To correct acidosis
- To provide adequate amounts of insulin to normalise intermediary metabolism (i.e. gradually reduce hyperglycaemia and stop ketogenesis)
- To provide a carbohydrate substrate when required during insulin treatment
- To identify precipitating factors (e.g. infection).

Because osmotic and biochemical deficits can be induced by overly aggressive treatment, metabolic abnormalities associated with diabetic ketoacidosis should not be corrected too quickly, but rather over a period of 36–48 hours.

Fluid therapy

Replacement and maintenance of normal fluid balance are of extreme importance in the treatment of diabetic ketoacidosis. In addition to correcting dehydration, fluid therapy lowers plasma glucose concentration by increasing glomerular filtration and urine flow and thus glucose excretion, even in the absence of insulin administration.

Most dogs and cats with moderate to severe ketoacidosis have varying degrees of dehydration on physical examination. The calculated fluid requirement (ml) includes: the animal's dehydration deficits (calculated as the % dehydration x kg body weight x 1000); the 24-hour maintenance needs (60–65 ml/kg/day); and extra losses that occur secondary to vomiting and diarrhoea. If the dog or cat is severely dehydrated, one half of the estimated dehydration deficit can be administered intravenously over the first 2–4 hours of hospitalisation, with the remaining replacement and maintenance volumes given over the following 20–22 hours. An isotonic fluid (i.e. 0.9% saline or lactated Ringer's solution) should be administered during this initial treatment period (Chastain and Nichols, 1981; Schaer and Taboada, 1992; MacIntire, 1995; Feldman and Nelson, 1996a).

Electrolyte therapy

Serum concentrations of potassium and phosphate may be low, normal, or even high in dogs or cats with untreated ketoacidosis. Nevertheless, when treatment begins with insulin, the resulting influx of glucose into cells causes both potassium and phosphate to translocate from plasma into the cytosol (and therefore lower the serum concentrations of these electrolytes). In addition, correction of acidosis also causes both electrolytes to move into the intracellular compartment. Without supplementation, severe hypokalaemia and hypophosphataemia can develop within 2–4 and 12–24 hours of therapy, respectively.

The most common clinical signs associated with hypokalaemia are generalised muscle weakness in both the dog and cat and cervical ventroflexion in cats. Other signs of hypokalaemia may include gastrointestinal stasis with anorexia, vomiting, and abdominal distension, respiratory failure, cardiac arrhythmias, and cardiac arrest. Hypophosphataemia affects primarily the haematological and neuromuscular systems in dogs and cats. Signs of acute hypophosphataemia include haemolytic anaemia, muscle weakness and rhabdomyolysis, and decreased cerebral function leading to seizures, stupor, and coma. Many animals with severe hypophosphataemia, however, may not manifest any overt clinical signs.

In animals with moderate to severe hypokalaemia,

potassium supplementation is best provided by the addition of a potassium solution (either potassium chloride or potassium phosphate) to the parenteral fluids (Table 19.1). In general, potassium supplementation is best begun after the first 2 hours of fluid therapy when dehydration has been at least partially corrected and urine output is adequate. Ideally, the amount of potassium required should be based on the actual measurement of the serum potassium concentration. If an accurate measurement of serum potassium is not possible, 40 mmol of potassium should initially be added to each litre of intravenous fluids administered at maintenance rates. Potassium supplementation should be infused slowly and never be given at a rate greater than 0.5 mmol/kg/h. It is also important to monitor the serum potassium concentration daily in order to adjust the dosage of potassium supplementation.

Serum potassium (mmol/l)	Amount of potassium to add to a litre of fluids (mmol)
>3.5	20
3.0–3.5	30
2.5–3.0	40
2.0–2.5	60
<2.0	80

Table 19.1: *Supplementation of potassium for intravenous fluid therapy at maintenance rates in animals with diabetes mellitus. The rate of potassium administered should not exceed 0.5 mmol/kg/h.*

Severe hypophosphataemia is an indication for the intravenous administration of phosphate. Administration of 0.01–0.03 mmol of phosphate/kg/h for 6 hours before rechecking the serum phosphate concentration has been recommended as a guideline for initial phosphate supplementation in dogs and cats with diabetes, although higher dosages (0.03–0.06 mmol of phosphate/kg/h for 6–12 hours) may be needed to correct hypophosphataemia in some animals (Nichols and Crenshaw, 1995). An alternative approach is to determine the amount of potassium supplementation required in the animal (Table 19.1) and then supplement with 50% as potassium chloride and 50% as potassium phosphate. The serum phosphate concentration should be monitored frequently (at least once to twice daily) during phosphate administration. Adverse effects from overzealous phosphate administration include iatrogenic hypocalcaemia and metastatic calcification, so care must be exercised to avoid oversupplementation. Supplementation with potassium and phosphate are usually discontinued when normal serum electrolyte concentrations are restored and the animal is able to eat and drink without vomiting.

Bicarbonate therapy

Although excessive production of ketones can lead to severe metabolic acidosis in animals with diabetes mellitus, caution must be taken to avoid the injudicious administration of sodium bicarbonate. Rapidly or excessively administered sodium bicarbonate can cause extracellular fluid hyperosmolarity, cerebrospinal fluid acidosis, intracranial haemorrhage, metabolic alkalosis, hypokalaemia, and impaired oxygen transfer from haemoglobin to tissues. Therefore, use of sodium bicarbonate should be reserved for dogs or cats with a blood pH of less than 7.1, or when the plasma bicarbonate (or total CO_2) concentrations are less than 12 mmol/l.

Bicarbonate requirements are calculated using the formula:

[body weight (kg) $\times$ 0.4 $\times$ 12] – [patient's bicarbonate (or total CO_2) $\times$ 0.5]

The difference between the patient's serum bicarbonate concentrations and the critical value of 12 mmol/l represents the treatable base deficit in ketoacidosis. The factor 0.5 provides one half of the required dose of bicarbonate in the infusion. In this manner, a conservative dose is given over 6 hours. Once the blood pH rises to above 7.2, or when the plasma bicarbonate (or total CO_2) concentrations are greater than 12 mmol/l, supplementation with sodium bicarbonate should be discontinued.

Insulin treatment

Regular insulin is generally used in the initial treatment of dogs and cats with diabetic ketoacidosis, especially if depression, dehydration, anorexia, and vomiting are present. By contrast, a ketoacidotic dog or cat with a good appetite and no signs of debilitation could be treated initially with the intermediate- or long-acting insulins, as are cats with uncomplicated diabetes.

One commonly recommended insulin regimen used to control hyperglycaemia and ketoacidosis (while decreasing the possibility of iatrogenic hypoglycaemia and hypokalaemia) involves the use of low-dose insulin administered intramuscularly. With this treatment protocol, regular insulin is administered intramuscularly at a loading dose of 0.2 IU/kg, followed by hourly doses of 0.1 IU/kg intramuscularly, until the blood glucose concentration falls to less than 15 mmol/l. Once this is achieved (usually within 4–8 hours), regular insulin can be administered intramuscularly or subcutaneously every 6 hours (initial dose, 0.25–0.5 IU/kg). Subsequent regular insulin doses should be adjusted by 0.5–1.0 units as needed to maintain the blood glucose concentration between 5 and 15 mmol/l, and glucose supplementation should be added as needed. Once the dog or cat is eating and does not vomit, treatment is continued with an intermediate- or long-acting insulin with the same protocol used to treat uncomplicated diabetes.

Although this hourly intramuscular regimen works well in most dogs and cats with ketoacidosis, use of low-dose regular insulin administered subcutaneously every 6 hours, is also very effective in most patients. This regimen may work especially well for the veterinarian without intensive care facilities. With this method, 0.5 IU/kg of regular insulin administered subcutaneously is followed by subsequent doses every 6 hours, adjusted to maintain the blood glucose concentration between 5 and 15 nmol/l.

Blood glucose monitoring and supplementation

Frequent monitoring of the initial blood glucose response to insulin (every 1–2 hours) is essential for successful management of diabetic ketoacidosis. When laboratory facilities are unavailable for blood glucose determinations, fairly accurate results can be obtained with reagent test strips, particularly when read on an automated test strip analyser. When the blood glucose concentration reaches 12–15 mmol/l, a 2.5–5.0% dextrose drip should be substituted and fluid therapy maintained until the animal is able to eat without vomiting. This dextrose provides a substrate for exogenous insulin and helps prevent hypoglycaemia in the absence of oral intake of food. Because circulating glucose concentrations fall before ketogenesis resolves, exogenous glucose must be provided to cover the regular insulin needed to correct the ketosis.

The use of urine glucose determinations alone is inferior to serial blood glucose measurements in the management of diabetes mellitus for many reasons. These include individual variations in the renal threshold for glucose and the fact that the measured urine glucose value represents circulating glucose which has 'spilled' into the urine over a period of hours, and therefore has no correlation with the present blood glucose concentration. It must also be remembered that the concentration of ketone bodies in the blood or urine should not be used to monitor the insulin dosage during the initial treatment. As diabetic ketoacidosis improves during initial therapy, there is a shift in ketone body production from β-hydroxybutyrate to acetoacetate. Reagent strips may actually become more positive for ketone bodies than at the onset of therapy or time of initial diagnosis due to their greater sensitivity to detect acetoacetate over β-hydroxybutyrate. This should not be taken as an indication to increase the dosage of insulin; such an action will invariably lead to a hypoglycaemic crisis.

Subsequent treatment

Once the dog or cat is stable, eating, and no longer ketoacidotic, fluid therapy and supplementation with potassium can be discontinued. Administration of insulin should be continued with an intermediate- or long-acting insulin preparation (0.25–0.5 IU/kg once or twice daily).

NON-KETOTIC HYPEROSMOLAR DIABETIC SYNDROME

Non-ketotic hyperosmolar diabetic syndrome is an uncommon but serious complication of diabetes mellitus in dogs and cats. It is characterised by severe hyperglycaemia, hyperosmolality, extreme clinical dehydration, and absence of ketoacidosis (Schaer and Taboada, 1992; MacIntire, 1995; Feldman and Nelson, 1996a). Animals with non-ketotic hyperosmolar diabetes usually have stupor or coma on examination.

Before the development of non-ketotic hyperosmolar diabetic syndrome, classical signs of diabetes (e.g. polydipsia, polyuria, polyphagia, and weight loss) are usually observed. In animals with non-ketotic hyperosmolar diabetes, it is thought that at some point the increasing osmolality begins to impair central nervous system (CNS) function, causing mental confusion, reduced water intake, dehydration, and azotaemia. It is believed that concurrent diseases such as cardiac or renal failure, which impair the body's ability to retain water and excrete sodium, may precipitate non-ketotic hyperosmolar coma. Renal excretion prevents blood glucose from exceeding 25 mmol/l, unless the glomerular filtration rate is altered by renal or prerenal factors.

Diagnosis

The diagnosis of non-ketotic hyperosmolar diabetic syndrome is based on typical clinical signs of diabetes progressing to neurological abnormalities, stupor, or coma. Several clinicopathological abnormalities characterise the syndrome. Most dogs and cats have severe azotaemia, which may be renal as well as prerenal in origin. The blood glucose concentration is extremely high (>35 mmol/l). Serum osmolality is high (>350 mOsmol/kg) and can be determined by the freezing point depression method with an osmometer or can be calculated using the following formula:

$$\text{Osmolality (mOsmol/kg)} = 2(\text{serum Na}^+ + \text{K}^+) + \text{glucose (mmol/l)} + \text{Urea nitrogen (mmol/l)}.$$

Treatment

The main objectives in the treatment of non-ketotic hyperosmolar diabetic syndrome are:

- To correct the extreme degree of volume depletion
- To correct the hyperosmolar state
- To provide adequate amounts of insulin to reduce hyperglycaemia
- To detect and correct any underlying precipitating factors, such as illness or drug administration.

In general, parenteral fluid and electrolyte replacement and regular insulin administration are similar to that described for ketoacidosis. As with animals with ketoacidosis, attempts should be made to correct the hyperosmolarity, hyperglycaemia, and dehydration gradually (rather than precipitously). Fluid therapy is the most important factor in the treatment of non-ketotic hyperosmolar diabetes. If circulatory collapse is present, isotonic saline should be initiated. In all other cases, initial fluid replacement with hypotonic (0.45%) saline may be considered because of the hyperosmolar state and considerable loss of body water (Schaer and Taboada, 1992).

Because dogs and cats with non-ketotic hyperosmolar diabetes tend to be critically ill, the prognosis is usually poor to grave. The most common cause of death is renal failure.

HYPOGLYCAEMIA

Hypoglycaemia is a biochemical abnormality rather than a disease. Numerous disorders cause hypoglycaemia in dogs and cats but, regardless of cause, severe hypoglycaemia is a medical emergency, since neuronal function is dependent on an adequate circulating glucose supply. Irreversible damage to the CNS or death can result from prolonged and profound hypoglycaemia.

The manifestations of hypoglycaemia are usually not apparent until the blood glucose level has dropped below 2.5 mmol/l. Clinical signs are related to the rate of fall of blood glucose, the concentration of glucose attained, and the duration of hypoglycaemia. The signs of hypoglycaemia may be roughly divided into two categories:

- Adrenergic manifestations, e.g. tremors, nervousness, hyperactivity, and tachycardia, which are caused by stimulation of the sympathetic nervous system
- Neuroglucopenic manifestations, e.g. mental dullness, confusion, blindness, seizures, and coma, which are caused by glucose deprivation of the CNS. Signs associated with the adrenergic phase usually, but not consistently, precede those of the neuroglucopenic phase.

Differential diagnosis

Numerous causes of hypoglycaemia have been reported, and long-term treatment must be specific (Leifer and Peterson, 1984; Schaer and Taboada, 1992). Insulin-induced hypoglycaemia in diabetic animals receiving exogenous insulin is the most common cause of hypoglycaemia in veterinary practice (see Chapter 12). Functional pancreatic islet cell tumour, usually islet cell adenocarcinoma, is a relatively common cause of hypoglycaemia in dogs. Insulinoma has also been rarely reported in cats. The diagnosis of an islet cell tumour is strongly suggested by the presence of a high serum insulin concentration together with moderate to severe hypoglycaemia.

Hypoglycaemia has also been associated with extra-pancreatic neoplasia in dogs, particularly with hepatocellular carcinoma and lymphosarcoma. Although the mechanism for tumour-induced hypoglycaemia is unclear, it may result from production of insulin-like factors by the tumour, increased glucose utilisation by the tumour, or decreased glucose production.

Many other rarely reported causes of hypoglycaemia should always be considered in the differential diagnosis. Starvation can produce clinical manifestations of hypoglycaemia in puppies or kittens, especially those that are heavily parasitised. Hypoglycaemia in fasted toy breed dogs has been described and may be the result of limited hepatic glycogen storage or merely an exaggeration of the neonate's inability to tolerate fasting. Rarely, clinically apparent hypoglycaemia develops in animals secondary to adrenal insufficiency (i.e. Addison's disease). Severe diffuse liver disease of any cause may result in hypoglycaemia, since the liver is the major site of glycogenolysis and gluconeogenesis. Finally, hypoglycaemia has been described in animals with both experimentally induced and naturally occurring sepsis. Several mechanisms have been postulated, including high glucose utilisation and low glucose production.

Management

The owner of a dog or cat that has a hypoglycaemic reaction may be instructed (over the telephone) to rub glucose syrup or 50% dextrose gel into the buccal mucosa, or administer a glucose solution orally, if possible. Most dogs respond to this treatment within 30–60 seconds. Owners should never attempt, however, to pour the syrup into the mouth of a convulsing or comatose animal.

Once the animal is in the hospital, the initial step should be to obtain a venous blood sample for blood glucose determination. The blood glucose concentration should be estimated quickly with appropriate reagent test strips, and serum submitted to the laboratory for insulin and glucose determinations, especially if an insulin-secreting tumour is suspected. A bolus of 50% dextrose should then be administered intravenously to effect (usually 1.0 ml/kg), and an infusion of 5–10% dextrose continued to maintain normoglycaemia. The underlying cause and precipitating factors should then be investigated.

HYPERCALCAEMIA

In general, hypercalcaemia is defined as a fasting serum total calcium concentration of >3 mmol/l. The development of clinical signs depends on the magnitude of the calcium elevation, how quickly the hypercalcaemia developed, and the duration of the hypercalcaemia. Serum total calcium concentrations between 3.5 and 4.0 mmol/l may not be associated with systemic signs; however, serum concentrations of >4.5 mmol/l are often associated with severe life-threatening signs (Feldman and Nelson, 1996b). Abnormalities in sodium and potassium may magnify clinical signs of hypercalcaemia because of their effects on cell membrane permeability, particularly in nerve and muscle tissue. Soft tissue mineralisation may occur with prolonged hypercalcaemia.

Signs of hypercalcaemia include:

- Polydipsia and polyuria. These are the most common signs, owing to direct stimulation of the thirst centre and an impaired ability of the kidneys to concentrate the urine
- Anorexia, vomiting, and constipation. These can result from depressed contractility of the muscle walls of the gastrointestinal tract
- Generalised weakness. This may develop from depressed contractility of skeletal muscle secondary to lowered excitability of the nervous system
- Depression, muscle twitching, and seizures. These can occur as neurological manifestations
- Cardiac arrhythmias. These can develop from the direct effects on the myocardium or secondary to cardiac mineralisation.

Differential diagnosis

There are a number of conditions that can cause hypercalcaemia in dogs and cats; these are listed in Table 19.2. Malignancy-associated hypercalcaemia is by far the most common cause of persistent hypercalcaemia in dogs and

| **Non-pathological conditions** |
| Growing dogs |
| Lipaemia |
| Haemoconcentration |
| Hyperproteinaemia |
| Laboratory error or improper handling of sample |
| **Pathological conditions** |
| Malignancy-associated hypercalcaemia |
| Lymphoma |
| Adenocarcinoma of the apocrine glands of the anal sac |
| Multiple myeloma |
| Mammary gland tumours |
| Metastatic bone tumours |
| Primary hyperparathyroidism |
| Hypoadrenocorticism |
| Renal failure (tertiary hyperparathyroidism) |
| Hypervitaminosis D |
| Cholecalciferol (rodenticide) toxicity |
| Iatrogenic – dietary supplementation |
| Houseplants (e.g. *Cestrus diurnum*, day-blooming jessamine) |
| Granulomatous disease |

Table 19.2: *Differential diagnosis of hypercalcaemia.*

cats. Other conditions leading to hypercalcaemia are rare. Differentiation of the causes of hypercalcaemia is discussed fully in Chapter 16.

Treatment
The definitive treatment of hypercalcaemia involves correcting the underlying cause. Unfortunately, the cause may not be apparent and supportive measures must be taken to reduce the serum calcium concentration. Emergency treatment and supportive measures include volume expansion, loop diuretics, sodium bicarbonate, glucocorticoids, calcitonin, plicamycin, and bisphosphonates.

Volume expansion
Volume expansion reduces haemoconcentration and encourages renal calcium loss by improving glomerular filtration rate and sodium excretion, which results in less calcium resorption. Normal 0.9% saline given at 2–3 times the maintenance rate (120–180 ml/kg/day) is usually effective in promoting calciuresis (Feldman and Nelson, 1996b). Potassium supplementation is often necessary to prevent hypokalaemia. The animal must also be monitored carefully for adverse effects such as pulmonary oedema resulting from administration of large quantities of fluids intravenously.

Loop diuretics
Diuretics such as frusemide increase calcium excretion; however, a high dosage may be needed to treat hypercalcaemia (one recommended protocol suggests a 5 mg/kg bolus followed by infusion at 5 mg/kg/h). The use of diuretics in a dehydrated animal is contraindicated because volume con-

traction and further haemoconcentration may worsen the hypercalcaemia. Thiazide diuretics, which reduce calcium excretion by the kidneys, are contraindicated.

Sodium bicarbonate
Sodium bicarbonate given as a slow intravenous bolus (1 mmol/kg) and repeated every 10–15 minutes for four treatments (maximal total dose, 4 mmol/kg) has been shown to reduce serum total calcium concentration (Kruger *et al.*, 1986). Although the magnitude of calcium reduction is mild, alkalosis also favours the shift of ionised calcium to protein-bound calcium. Sodium bicarbonate is more beneficial when combined with other treatments.

Glucocorticoids
Glucocorticoids, such as prednisone (1–2 mg/kg twice daily) or dexamethasone (0.1–0.2 mg/kg twice daily), reduce bone resorption of calcium and intestinal calcium absorption, increase renal calcium excretion, and are cytotoxic to malignant lymphocytes, leading to a substantial reduction in serum calcium concentration in animals with hypercalcaemia secondary to lymphoma, myeloma, hypervitaminosis D, and hypoadrenocorticism. However, use of glucocorticoids may make the definitive diagnosis of the underlying cause of hypercalcaemia difficult.

Calcitonin
Calcitonin (4-6 IU/kg two or three times daily subcutaneously) can be administered as an antidote in animals with cholecalciferol (rodenticide) toxicity. However, the reduction of serum calcium concentration may be short term (hours), and multiple treatments may be required.

Plicamycin (mithramycin)
Plicamycin, previously called mithramycin, is a potent inhibitor of osteoclastic bone resorption. However, plicamycin has been associated with many serious side effects, such as thrombocytopenia, hepatic necrosis, renal necrosis, and hypocalcaemia, thereby limiting its use in animals. The dosage is 25 µg/kg, administered by slow infusion over 4–6 hours, once or twice weekly to control hypercalcaemia (Kruger *et al.*, 1986; Rosol *et al.*, 1994).

Bisphosphonates
See Chapter 16.

HYPOCALCAEMIA

Hypocalcaemia is a serum total calcium concentration of <2 mmol/l. The severity of clinical signs may not always be commensurate with the degree of hypocalcaemia. Concurrent acid–base disorders and other electrolyte imbalances which alter the ionised calcium concentration play a role in the development of clinical signs, which are often episodic. These include:

* Tremors, twitching, tetany, muscle spasms, and gait changes (stiffness and ataxia) resulting from an increase in the excitability of the peripheral nervous

---

Causes of mild asymptomatic hypocalcaemia

Hypoalbuminaemia (most frequent cause of hypocalcaemia)

Primary renal disease

Pancreatitis

Intestinal malabsorption syndromes

Chelating agents that bind calcium (e.g. EDTA, oxalates, and phosphates)

Rhabdomyolysis due to soft tissue trauma

Nutritional secondary hyperparathyroidism

Causes of severe symptomatic hypocalcaemia

Puerperal tetany/eclampsia

Hypoparathyroidism

   Spontaneous (lymphocytic parathyroiditis)

   Iatrogenic, secondary to bilateral thyroidectomy

   Postoperative, secondary to removal of parathyroid tumour

Phosphate enema intoxication (reciprocal decrease in serum calcium)

Too rapid intravenous administration of phosphate supplementation

---

Table 19.3: Differential diagnosis of hypocalcaemia.

system. Occasionally, generalised seizure activity may develop because of increasing excitability of the CNS as well

- Behavioural changes (restlessness, aggression, panting, hypersensitivity to stimuli, and disorientation) are common

- Bradycardia, hyperthermia, polyuria, polydipsia, and vomiting are seen in some animals.

Differential diagnosis

Numerous causes of hypocalcaemia are known, many of which fail to produce clinical signs associated with a low circulating calcium concentration (Table 19.3). Of the conditions associated with severe symptomatic hypocalcaemia, puerperal tetany or eclampsia occurs in lactating bitches and queens as a result of calcium loss into the milk and poor dietary calcium intake. This is the most common cause of severe hypocalcaemia in dogs, but is rare in cats (Feldman and Nelson, 1996c).

Hypoparathyroidism, the other major cause of symptomatic hypocalcaemia, is a metabolic disorder characterised by hypocalcaemia and hyperphosphataemia and either transient or permanent parathyroid hormone (PTH) insufficiency (Peterson, 1986). Iatrogenic injury or removal of the parathyroid glands during thyroid surgery (thyroidectomy) is one cause of hypoparathyroidism; a second is excision of a parathyroid tumour for treatment of primary hyperparathyroidism since the remaining parathyroid glands have atrophied due to hypersecretion of PTH by the tumour. Finally, spontaneous (idiopathic) hypoparathyroidism is a rare disorder reported in both dogs and cats. Most animals with idiopathic hypoparathyroidism have complete parathyroid gland destruction and atrophy, and require lifelong treatment to maintain normocalcaemia.

Differentiation of the causes of hypocalcaemia is discussed in Chapter 16.

Treatment

Treatment of hypoparathyroidism includes calcium supplements and vitamin D (Peterson, 1986). Although many parenteral calcium preparations are available, 10% calcium gluconate is generally preferred. Oral calcium supplements are available as gluconate, lactate, chloride, carbonate, and gluconate salts. The most common mistake in the use of a calcium preparation is thinking in terms of weight of salt rather than the quantity of elemental calcium. There are big differences in calcium content between one salt and another, but little difference in effect when prescribed in equimolar amounts. For instance, the elemental calcium content of calcium carbonate (40%) is much higher than that of calcium chloride (27.2%), calcium lactate (13.0%), calcium gluconate (9.2%), or calcium glubionate (6.4%).

The three major vitamin D preparations available include vitamin D_2 (ergocalciferol), dihydrotachysterol, and 1,25-dihydroxycholecalciferol. All vitamin D preparations raise serum calcium concentrations primarily by increasing the gastrointestinal absorption of calcium; however, important differences exist in the dosage of each needed to achieve normocalcaemia in animals with hypoparathyroidism, as well as in the times of maximal onset of effect and duration of action.

Parenteral calcium

If an animal develops overt hypocalcaemia, immediate treatment is essential. Emergency treatment of hypocalcaemia involves intravenous administration of 10% calcium gluconate at a dosage of 1.0–1.5 ml/kg. The drug should be delivered over 10–20 minutes. Infusion should be stopped if signs of toxicity, such as bradycardia, cardiac arrest, vomiting or shortened Q-T interval, occur.

Once the life-threatening signs of hypocalcaemia have been controlled, calcium can be added to the intravenous fluids and administered as a slow infusion of 60–90 mg/kg/day of elemental calcium (e.g. 2.0–2.5 ml/kg 10% calcium gluconate every 6–8 hours). With this regimen, calcium is added to 0.9% sodium chloride (fluids containing bicarbonate, lactate, or acetate should be avoided due to the potential for calcium salt precipitation). Serum calcium concentration should be determined once or twice daily during this treatment period. The rate of calcium administration should be adjusted as necessary to maintain a normal serum calcium concentration, and the infusion should be continued for as long as necessary to prevent recurrence of hypocalcaemia.

If close monitoring is not possible, 10% calcium gluconate can be administered subcutaneously at a dosage of 0.25–0.5 ml/kg three times daily. The 10% calcium gluconate solution should be diluted at least 1:1 with saline before administration to help minimise pain and tissue damage caused by the hypertonicity of the solution.

Although such parenteral calcium administration is effective, signs of hypocalcaemia will recur within hours of stopping calcium administration unless other treatment is given. Therefore, oral calcium and vitamin D should be initiated as soon as they can be tolerated.

Oral calcium

Maintenance treatment of hypoparathyroidism involves the oral administration of calcium supplements as well as vitamin D preparations. Calcium supplementation is recommended at a dosage of 50–100 mg/kg/day of elemental calcium administered in three or four divided daily doses. This degree of calcium supplementation may only be necessary for the first week or two of treatment, after which a normal dietary calcium content is sometimes sufficient to maintain serum calcium concentrations within the normal range.

Vitamin D

Of the three available vitamin D preparations, dihydrotachysterol, a synthetic form of vitamin D, is generally preferred over ergocalciferol (vitamin D2), because dihydrotachysterol raises serum calcium more rapidly and its effects are dissipated more quickly when the drug is discontinued (if hypercalcaemia develops). Dihydrotachysterol is available as an oral solution containing 0.25 mg/ml of the vitamin D preparation. The initial dosage of dihydrotachysterol is 0.03–0.06 mg/kg/day for 2–3 days, then 0.02–0.03 mg/kg/day for 2–3 days, and finally 0.01 mg/kg/day until further dosage adjustments are indicated. Serum calcium should be determined once to twice daily during this initial treatment period until the concentration stabilises in the low–normal range.

Calcitriol (1,25-dihydroxycholecalciferol), the active form of vitamin D, has advantages over other vitamin D preparations, and may be the ideal vitamin D supplement. The time of onset of action (1–4 days) and half-life (<1 day) are shorter than that for dihydrotachysterol and ergocalciferol. The short half-life of calcitriol is an advantage in the management of animals that are overdosed, because the toxic effects resolve more quickly than with other preparations. Despite these advantages, the drug is expensive and the available capsule sizes (250 ng and 500 ng), designed for use in human patients, are not well formulated for the smaller body size of most dogs and cats. The recommended initial dosage of calcitriol (2.5–6.0 ng/kg/day) should be adjusted on the basis of frequent calcium determinations to maintain concentrations within the low–normal range. Because the capsules of calcitriol cannot be readily divided, a pharmacist may need to reformulate these products to a size that is appropriate for the individual pet.

The major complication associated with treatment of chronic hypoparathyroidism is hypercalcaemia, which develops as a consequence of overtreatment with calcium and vitamin D. If a high serum calcium concentration develops during the course of treatment, calcium and vitamin D administration should be temporarily discontinued. Once normocalcaemia has been restored, vitamin D administration should be reinstituted at a lower maintenance dosage (approximately 20% less than that previously administered). In dogs or cats with hypoparathyroidism that might be transient (e.g. after thyroidectomy or parathyroid tumour excision), however, vitamin D and calcium treatment should be reinstated only if marked hypocalcaemia (<2.0 mmol/l) again develops.

REFERENCES AND FURTHER READING

Chastain CB and Nichols CE (1981) Low-dose intramuscular insulin therapy for diabetic ketoacidosis in dogs. *Journal of the American Veterinary Medical Association* **178**, 561-564

Feldman EC and Nelson RW (1996a) Diabetic ketoacidosis. In: *Canine and Feline Endocrinology and Reproduction*, pp. 392–421. WB Saunders, Philadelphia

Feldman EC and Nelson RW (1996b) Hypercalcemia and primary hyperparathyroidism. In: *Canine and Feline Endocrinology and Reproduction*, pp. 455–496. WB Saunders, Philadelphia

Feldman EC and Nelson RW (1996c) Hypocalcemia and hypoparathyroidism. In: *Canine and Feline Endocrinology and Reproduction*, pp. 497–516. WB Saunders, New York

Kintzer PP and Peterson ME (1994) Diagnosis and management of primary spontaneous hypoadrenocorticism (Addison's disease) in dogs. *Seminars in Veterinary Medicine and Surgery (Small Animal)* **9(3)**, 148–152

Kruger JM, Oxborne CA and Polzin DJ (1986) Treatment of hypercalcemia. In: *Current Veterinary Therapy IX: Small Animal Practice*, ed. RW Kirk, pp. 75–90. WB Saunders, Philadelphia

Leifer CE and Peterson ME (1984) Hypoglycemia. *Veterinary Clinics of North America: Small Animal Practice* **14**, 873–889

MacIntire DK (1995) Emergency therapy of diabetic crises: insulin overdose, diabetic ketoacidosis, and hyperosmolar coma. *Veterinary Clinics of North America Small Animal Practice* **25**, 639–650

Melin C and Peterson ME (1996) Diagnosis and treatment of naturally occurring hypoadrenocorticism in 42 dogs. *Journal of Small Animal Practice* **37**, 268–275

Nichols R and Crenshaw K (1995) Complications and concurrent disease associated with diabetic ketoacidosis and other severe forms of diabetes mellitus. *Veterinary Clinics of North America: Small Animal Practice* **25**, 617–624

Peterson ME (1986) Hypoparathyroidism. In: *Current Veterinary Therapy IX*, ed. RW Kirk, pp. 1039–1045. WB Saunders, Philadelphia

Peterson ME, Greco DS and Orth DN (1989) Primary hypoadrenocorticism in ten cats. *Journal of Veterinary Internal Medicine* **3**, 55–58

Rosol TJ, Chew DJ, Hammer AS, Ward H, Peterson JL, Carothers MA and Couto CG (1994) Effect of mithramycin on hypercalcemia in dogs. *Journal of the American Animal Hospital Association* **30**, 244–250

Schaer M and Taboada J (1992) Metabolic and endocrine emergencies. In: *Veterinary Emergency and Critical Care Medicine*, ed. RJ Murtaugh and PM Kaplan, pp. 251–272. Mosby-Year Book, St Louis

CHAPTER TWENTY

Clinical Endocrinology of the Gastrointestinal Tract

Jörg M. Steiner

INTRODUCTION

The gastrointestinal (GI) tract is recognised as the largest endocrine organ of the body (Holst *et al.*, 1996). However, little is known about it, presumably because of its complexity. No other endocrine organ uses as many regulatory substances, yet in no other endocrine organ is the division between communication pathways as blurred as in the GI tract. Traditionally, mechanisms of cell-to-cell communication are divided into autocrine, paracrine, neurocrine, and endocrine (Walsh and Mayer, 1993), but this division is not entirely clear in the GI tract. Almost all regulatory substances synthesised in the GI tract are peptides, but several function as endocrine as well as neurocrine, paracrine, and even autocrine peptides.

In 1902, secretin, the first gut hormone, was discovered. Since then a plethora of GI regulatory peptides has been identified (Table 20.1). Many of these are considered true hormones, although currently only six meet all the physiological criteria for a hormone: insulin, glucagon, gastrin, secretin, cholecystokinin, and motilin (Walsh and Mayer, 1993). It is beyond the scope of this chapter to discuss all of these regulatory peptides in detail, but the main functions of the more important ones are listed in Table 20.2. For further information, the reader is referred to several excellent reviews on the physiology of GI regulatory peptides (Johnson, 1991; Walsh and Mayer, 1993; Zerbe and Washabau, 1995; Holst *et al.*, 1996).

Endocrine disorders are largely associated with a lack or overproduction of hormone. To date, apart from insulin deficiency associated with diabetes mellitus (see Chapters 12 and 13), a lack of GI regulatory peptides has not been identified as causing specific syndromes in dogs, cats, or humans. However, it is likely to be only a matter of time before such syndromes are discovered. Disorders related to overproduction of GI regulatory peptides are well recognised and are caused by neuroendocrine tumours (NETs) of the GI tract. The prevalence of such NETs in humans is estimated at 3–4 cases per million population (Modlin and Tang, 1997). Approximately 50% of all these NETs are carcinoids, 25% insulinomas, 10% gastrinomas, 2% vasoactive intestinal polypeptidomas (VIPomas), 2% glucagonomas, <1% somatostatinomas, and 5-6% non-functioning tumours or pancreatic polypeptidomas. Similar epidemiological data are not available for small animals. Many of these NETs have not been recognised in dogs or cats, and reports are limited to insulinomas, gastrinomas, carcinoids, glucagonomas, and pancreatic polypeptidomas. With the exception of insulinoma (see Chapter 17), these will be discussed separately in the following text.

GASTRINOMA

A syndrome characterised by acid hypersecretion, fulminant peptic ulceration, and a pancreatic non-β islet cell tumour, was first described in a human patient by Zollinger and Ellison (1955). The syndrome was initially called the Zollinger–Ellison syndrome. The ulcerogenic

Regulatory peptide family	Members of regulatory peptide family
Gastrin–cholecystokinin	Cholecystokinin Gastrin
Secretin/glucagon/ vasoactive intestinal polypeptide (VIP)	Gastric inhibitory peptide Glucagon Glucagon-like peptide 1 Glucagon-like peptide 2 Glicentin Growth hormone releasing factor Oxyntomodulin Peptide HI/HM Secretin VIP
Pancreatic polypeptide	Neuropeptide Y Pancreatic polypeptide Peptide YY
Tachykinin/bombesin	Gastrin-releasing peptide (GRP) GRP decapeptide Neuromedin B Neuromedin K Substance K Substance P
Opioid peptide	Adrenocorticotropic hormone β Endorphin β Neoendorphin Dynorphin Leu-encephalin Leumorphin Melanocyte stimulating hormone Met-encephalin
Insulin	Insulin Insulin-like growth factor I
Epidermal growth factor	Epidermal growth factor Transforming growth factor α
Somatostatin	Somatostatin
Calcitonin	Calcitonin Calcitonin gene-related peptide
Miscellaneous	Endothelin Galanin Motilin Neurotensin Thyrotropin releasing hormone

Table 20.1: Overview of families of gastrointestinal regulatory peptides.

Regulatory peptide	Location of secretion	Cell type	Stimulation/inhibition	Most important functions
Gastrin	Stomach, duodenum	G	S Stomach distension Digested proteins and amino acids Bombesin, gastrin-releasing peptide GRP, Ca^{2+} I Luminal acidification Somatostatin	Stimulation of gastric acid secretion Trophic effect on acid-secreting gastric mucosa Stimulation of pepsinogen secretion
Cholecystokinin	Duodenum, jejunum	I	S Fat, fatty acids, proteins, and amino acids Bombesin, GRP I Somatostatin	Stimulation of pancreatic enzyme secretion Gallbladder contraction Regulation of pancreatic growth
Secretin	Duodenum, jejunum	S	S Duodenal acidification	Stimulation of pancreatic bicarbonate secretion
Glucagon	Pancreas	A	S Hypoglycaemia High concentration of amino acids or low concentration of free fatty acids in plasma I Hyperglycaemia	Stimulation of glyco-genolysis Stimulation of gluco-neogenesis from lactate, amino acids, and glycerol
Gastric inhibitory polypeptide (GIP)	Duodenum, jejunum	GIP	S All major classes of nutrients in the gut Bombesin	Inhibition of gastric acid secretion Stimulation of intestinal fluid secretion Stimulation of insulin release
Oxyntomodulin	Ileum, colon	L	S Intraluminal glucose and lipids	Inhibition of gastric acid secretion Stimulation of intestinal mucosal growth
Vasoactive intestinal polypeptide	Entire gastrointestinal (GI) tract		S Vagal stimulation	Relaxation of smooth muscle Vasodilatation Stimulation of pancreatic and intestinal secretion
Peptide YY	Ileum, colon	L	S Intraluminal lipids Bombesin	Inhibition of pancreatic secretion Inhibition of gastric acid secretion Inhibition of gastric emptying
Pancreatic polypeptide	Pancreas	F	S Intraluminal proteins Vagal stimulation	Inhibition of pancreatic enzyme and fluid secretion
Tachykinins	Entire GI tract		S Luminal distension	Regulation of GI motility Transmission of pain impulses
Opioids	Entire GI tract			Inhibition of intestinal water and electrolyte secretion Modulation of GI motility
Insulin	Pancreas	B	S Hyperglycaemia Glucagon I Hypoglycaemia	Stimulation of peripheral glucose uptake Stimulation of glycogen synthesis Stimulation of lipogenesis Stimulation of DNA, RNA, and protein synthesis
Somatostatin	Entire GI tract	D	S Intraluminal lipid, protein, and bile	Inhibition of gastric and pancreatic secretions Inhibition of intestinal amino acid and glucose absorption Inhibition of intestinal motility
Motilin	Duodenum, jejunum	M	S Cyclic release during the fasting state Intraluminal lipids	Initiates phase III of the migratory motility complex
Neurotensin	Ileum, colon	N	S Intraluminal lipids Bombesin	Inhibition of gastric acid secretion

Table 20.2: *Main functions of important gut regulatory peptides.*

factor secreted by the tumour was later identified as gastrin, and the syndrome is now more appropriately referred to as gastrinoma.

Gastrinoma is a rare tumour, having been reported in only 25 dogs and three cats compared with approximately 250 dogs and three cats with insulinoma (Eng *et al.*, 1992; Zerbe, 1992; Green and Gartrell, 1997; Hayden and Henson, 1997; Simpson and Dykes, 1997). Gastrinomas are most commonly single nodules of small size (<2 cm in diameter). Although usually malignant, they grow slowly, and a history spanning several years is not unusual. When first described in humans, the majority were localised in the pancreas, but currently over 50% are found in the duodenum (Solcia *et al.*, 1995). This is probably related to improved localisation techniques rather than a true increase in the incidence of duodenal gastrinomas. By contrast, gastrinomas have not been identified in the duodenum of dogs or cats, although tumours could not be accurately located in several cases.

Gastrinomas synthesise and release supraphysiological quantities of gastrin into the vascular space, leading to gastric acid hypersecretion, hypertrophy of the gastric mucosa, and eventual ulceration (Zerbe, 1992). The constant hyperchlorhydria also leads to a decreased pH in the duodenum, which in turn leads to direct injury to the intestinal mucosa and inactivation of digestive enzymes.

Clinical features

Gastrinomas usually develop in middle-aged to elderly dogs and elderly cats. Females are supposedly more commonly affected than males, but this may be related to the limited number of cases reported.

The most common clinical sign observed in 25 of the reported cases were vomiting (92%), weight loss (88%), anorexia (72%), lethargy (64%), and diarrhoea (60%). In addition, polydipsia, melaena, and abdominal pain were noted in approximately 25%, and haematemesis, haematochezia, fever and a ravenous appetite in 10% of cases. A palpable abdominal mass, tachycardia, and obstipation were reported in a single case each.

Diagnosis

Routine haematological examination does not reveal any specific changes, but over 50% of affected animals exhibit a regenerative anaemia, indicating haemorrhage. Common findings on biochemical analysis include hypoproteinaemia with hypoalbuminaemia, hypokalaemia, increased hepatic enzyme activities, hypochlor-aemia, and hyperglycaemia. More severe changes may be seen, with complications such as pyloric obstruction due to mucosal hypertrophy, or ulcer perforation and peritonitis.

Survey abdominal radiographs are usually unremarkable. Upper GI tract contrast radiography is rarely indicated, but may reveal plaque-like defects in the stomach or duodenum indicating ulceration. Of the small number of dogs examined, abdominal ultrasonography has been unsuccessful in localising the lesion but may be useful for identifying metastatic disease (Lamb *et al.*, 1995). Upper GI tract endoscopy allows the direct visualisation of oesophageal, gastric, and duodenal lesions, but does not

definitively diagnose their underlying cause.

Although rare, gastrinomas should be ruled out in all patients with a history of chronic vomiting, weight loss, anorexia, or diarrhoea in which an alternative diagnosis has not been made. The most important diagnostic tool is measurement of serum gastrin concentration. A species-specific assay is not available, but several human kits have been validated for use in the dog and also seem useful in the cat (Gabbert *et al.*, 1984). Canine gastrin measurements (reference range; 10–40 ng/l) are carried out at the Animal Health Diagnostic Laboratory at Michigan State University, but require rapid separation, freezing (within 1 hour of collection), and shipment on ice. According to the diagnostic recommendations for humans, a presumptive diagnosis of gastrinoma is made if a 24-hour fasting serum gastrin concentration is 10 times the upper limit of the reference range (Orloff and Debas, 1995). Other causes of hypergastrinaemia in the dog such as renal failure, immunoproliferative enteropathy of Basenjis, and gastric dilatation-volvulus (English *et al.*, 1988) are easily ruled out. In cases where serum gastrin concentration is less markedly elevated, provocative testing using the secretin stimulation test is indicated. After a 24-hour fast, serum gastrin concentrations are measured both before and 2, 5, 10, 15, and 20 minutes after the intravenous injection of pure secretin at a dose of 2 IU/kg. An increase of >200 ng/l or a twofold increase at any time is considered diagnostic (Simpson and Dykes, 1997). Alternatively, calcium can be infused at a dose of 5 mg/kg/h with serial measurements of gastrin at 0, 15, 30, 60, 90, and 120 minutes. A twofold increase at any time is diagnostic (Zerbe, 1992). However, in humans the calcium challenge test is less sensitive and is somewhat uncomfortable to the patient (Modlin *et al.*, 1982).

Treatment

Before initiating treatment, the tumour should be staged by localising the primary lesion and searching for metastatic disease. In humans, abdominal ultrasonography, computerised tomography (CT), magnetic resonance imaging (MRI), or selective angiography are all rather unsuccessful in identifying the primary lesion but are useful in assessing metastatic disease (Orloff and Debas, 1995). Endoscopic ultrasonography and somatostatin receptor scintigraphy (SRS) hold more promise and identify the primary lesion in up to 100% of cases. Endoscopic ultrasonography is not yet available for use in small animals, but the successful use of SRS has recently been reported in a dog (Altschul *et al.*, 1997).

After localisation of the primary tumour and exclusion of widespread metastatic disease, exploratory laparotomy is indicated. The goals are:

* Confirmation of diagnosis and localisation of the primary tumour
* Careful evaluation for metastatic lesions
* Removal of the primary tumour
* Removal of single metastatic lesions.

If the primary tumour is not easily identified, the

abdominal cavity, and particularly the duodenum, should be carefully examined for any suspicious lesions. Intraoperative illumination of the duodenal wall may be helpful. If a primary lesion still cannot be identified, biopsy samples of pancreas, lymph nodes, and liver should be taken before closing the abdominal cavity.

Primary lesions should be removed by partial pancreatectomy while minimising pancreatic trauma (Matthiesen and Mullen, 1990). The tumour should be submitted for histopathological examination and immunohistochemical staining for the regulatory peptides most commonly found in gut NETs. Metastatic lesions, which are present in most cases, should only be removed if this is possible without radical excision. Postoperatively, food should be withheld for 24–48 hours, followed by the gradual introduction of water and a low-fat, highly digestible diet.

Medical therapy is indicated before surgery, and in some cases may be discontinued after successful removal of both primary and metastatic lesions. Proton-pump inhibitors are the mainstay of therapy in humans. Omeprazole at a dose of 0.7 mg/kg orally once daily has also been successfully used in the treatment of dogs with gastrinoma (Simpson and Dykes, 1997). Initially, sucralphate (1g per animal orally three times daily) is added to the protocol. Histamine-2 antagonists such as cimetidine, ranitidine, or famotidine at double the standard dose are alternatives when omeprazole is considered too expensive or is ineffective. Octreotide, a long-acting somatostatin analogue, has shown promise in the treatment of human patients. It acts both by inhibiting gastrin release and directly decreasing gastric acid secretion. Octreotide has been used in two dogs with some success at a dose of 2–20 µg/kg subcutaneously three times daily (Lothrop, 1989; Simpson and Dykes, 1997). These two dogs survived for 10 and 14 months, respectively, which is longer than the reported mean survival time of 5.5 months for other affected animals.

Combination chemotherapy using streptozotocin and 5-fluorouracil has been moderately successful in human patients with metastatic gastrinoma (Bieligk and Jaffe, 1995). However, streptozotocin is highly nephrotoxic, and this protocol cannot be recommended for use in dogs or cats without further investigation.

Prognosis

The long-term prognosis for dogs and cats with gastrinoma is grave. However, with appropriate medical management, the short-term prognosis and quality of life can be good. With increased awareness and improved localisation and staging techniques and advanced treatment options, survival times are likely to increase.

GLUCAGONOMA

In 1974, a series of nine human patients with glucagon-producing pancreatic tumours was reported (Prinz et al., 1981). These patients exhibited typical skin lesions characterised by marked erythema and destruction of the superficial epidermis with subsequent healing and progression to other areas, known as necrolytic migratory erythema (NME). The NME occurred in association with diabetes mellitus and a predisposition to thrombo-embolic disease. Despite increasing awareness and improved diagnostic capabilities, the disease remains rare. To date, glucagonoma has not been conclusively diagnosed in veterinary patients. However, two dogs have been reported with characteristic skin lesions and in which diabetes mellitus later developed, and pancreatic NETs staining positive for glucagon were found (Gross et al., 1990). Similar skin lesions, descriptively termed superficial necrolytic dermatitis (SND) have also been reported in several dogs with hepatic disease and/or diabetes mellitus but without glucagonoma (Walton et al., 1986; Turnwald et al., 1989; Miller et al., 1990; Gross et al., 1993). It is more appropriate to consider glucagonoma as a possible differential diagnosis of SND in patients without hepatic disease presenting with or without diabetes mellitus.

Assessment of plasma glucagon concentration may be helpful in confirming a diagnosis. However, veterinary laboratories do not currently offer such an assay although assays developed for use in humans can be used in dogs and cats. The laboratory should be contacted before sampling to ensure proper collection and handling, and a sample from a healthy dog should be evaluated simultaneously. If a glucagon assay is not available, the diagnosis of SND can be confirmed by dermatohistopathology, and exploratory laparotomy then considered. Similar guidelines for localisation and surgical exploration discussed for gastrinomas apply. Medical management involving insulin therapy, intravenous infusion of fatty and essential amino acids, zinc supplementation, and octreotide treatment is indicated if owners refuse surgical exploration, in cases of metastatic glucagonoma and in recurrent cases (Taboada and Merchant, 1997). More clinical information is required before specific treatment recommendations can be given.

PANCREATIC POLYPEPTIDOMA

Gut NETs secreting pancreatic polypeptide have been described in humans (Bieligk and Jaffe, 1995; Perry and Vinik, 1996). Although not often associated with a distinct clinical syndrome, affected patients may suffer from a watery diarrhoea or from rashes. Only one dog with a presumptive diagnosis of pancreatic polypeptidoma has been reported in the veterinary literature (Zerbe et al., 1989). This dog presented for chronic vomiting, anorexia, weight loss, and lethargy. An insulinoma was diagnosed, based on the presence of hypoglycaemia in the face of an elevated serum insulin concentration. Basal serum gastrin concentration was seven times the upper limit of the reference range, but did not increase after secretin or calcium challenge. Serum pancreatic polypeptide concentration was 3500 times the upper limit of the reference range. Multiple pancreatic tumours removed at exploratory laparotomy showed a strongly positive reaction when stained for pancreatic polypeptide, and a positive reaction for insulin, but no reaction when stained for gastrin and other GI regulatory peptides. Unfortunately, assays for pancreatic polypeptide are not available in commercial veterinary laboratories. In addition, it remains unclear if there was a cause and effect relationship between the extremely high value and the clinical signs observed in this patient.

CARCINOIDS

Gastrointestinal carcinoids are a heterogeneous group of tumours arising from the diffuse neuroendocrine system of the GI tract (Klöppel et al., 1996). In human patients, GI carcinoids have been reported to secrete a variety of regulatory substances such as histamine, serotonin, gastrin, somatostatin, tachykinins, peptide YY, pancreatic polypeptide, calcitonin, CCK, motilin, and bombesin. Human gastric carcinoids often secrete large amounts of histamine and lead to a syndrome characterised by flushing, hypotension, lacrimation, cutaneous oedema, and bronchoconstriction. Small intestinal carcinoids secrete serotonin and lead to flushing, diarrhoea, and bronchoconstriction (Nilsson, 1996).

Gastrointestinal carcinoids have also been reported in dogs and cats (Giles et al., 1974; Carakostas et al., 1979; Patnaik et al., 1980; Sykes and Cooper, 1982; Coughlin, 1992). While some of these patients were presented for chronic vomiting or diarrhoea, none showed signs of flushing, hypotension, or bronchoconstriction. This may reflect a lack of synthesis of regulatory substances by canine and feline GI carcinoids, secretion of different regulatory substances compared with human carcinoids or, less likely, a relative resistance of dogs and cats to elevated plasma histamine and serotonin concentrations. Careful evaluation of future cases, including the measurement of urinary histamine and serotonin metabolite excretion, immunohistochemical behaviour, and ultrastructure of the tumour cells, is needed to reach a better understanding of this disease in dogs and cats.

OTHER NETS OF THE GI TRACT

Several other gut NETs have been identified in humans but not yet in dogs or cats.

VIPoma is a NET secreting large amounts of vasoactive intestinal polypeptide (Bieligk and Jaffe, 1995). The clinical syndrome includes watery diarrhoea, hypokalaemia, hypochlorhydria, and acidosis. Diagnosis is established by a markedly increased plasma VIP concentration. Treatment is directed at surgical excision.

Somatostatinoma is a rare NET causing diabetes mellitus, gallstones, and steatorrhoea (Bieligk and Jaffe, 1995). The diagnosis of somatostatinoma is based on a markedly increased plasma somatostatin concentration, and treatment is aimed at surgical excision.

DIAGNOSTIC USES OF GI REGULATORY PEPTIDES

As mentioned previously, secretin can be used in a challenge test for the diagnosis of canine gastrinomas, and radioactively labelled somatostatin can be used to localise gut NETs, especially gastrinomas.

Other diagnostic uses of GI regulatory peptides have been described in humans (Walsh and Mayer, 1993). Pentagastrin, a synthetic gastrin analogue, can be used to assess gastric acid secretory capacity in patients with suspected hypochlorhydria or achlorhydria. Further, secretin can be used to evaluate the bicarbonate secretory capacity of the exocrine pancreas, or to increase exocrine pancreatic blood flow to enhance pancreatic angiography. Finally, glucagon has been used as a relaxing agent of the GI tract to facilitate diagnostic procedures such as colonoscopy, gastroduodenoscopy, or retrograde cholangiopancreatography.

The diagnostic uses of GI regulatory peptides in veterinary patients will also expand in the future.

THERAPEUTIC USES OF GI REGULATORY PEPTIDES

With the exception of insulin treatment for dogs and cats with diabetes mellitus, the range of therapeutic uses of GI regulatory peptides in veterinary patients is limited. The use of octreotide, a long-acting somatostatin analogue, has shown initial promise in the medical management of patients with canine gastrinoma, and may also prove beneficial in the medical treatment of other GI NETs (Lothrop, 1989; Altschul et al., 1997).

Erythromycin, a macrolide antibiotic, can cause motilin release and has been used in dogs at an antimicrobially ineffective dose (1.0 mg/kg orally three times daily) as a gastric prokinetic agent (Walsh and Mayer, 1993; Zerbe and Washabau, 1995).

Other, more exotic applications, such as the treatment of achlorhydria with gastrin analogues, or the treatment of male impotence with VIP, are constantly being investigated in humans and will hopefully lead to future applications in veterinary patients.

REFERENCES

Altschul M, Simpson KW, Dykes NL, Mauldin EA, Reubi JC and Cummings JF (1997) Evaluation of somatostatin analogues for the detection and treatment of gastrinoma in a dog. *Journal of Small Animal Practice* **38**, 286–291

Bieligk S and Jaffe BM (1995) Islet cell tumors of the pancreas. *Surgical Clinics of North America* **75**, 1025–1040

Carakostas MC, Kennedy GA, Kittleson MD and Cook JE (1979) Malignant foregut carcinoid tumor in a domestic cat. *Veterinary Pathology* **16**, 607–609

Coughlin AS (1992) Carcinoid in canine large intestine. *Veterinary Record* **130**, 499–500

Eng J, Du BH, Johnson GF, Kanakamedala S, Samuel S, Raufman JP and Straus E (1992) Cat gastrinoma and the sequence of cat gastrins. *Regulatory Peptides* **37**, 9–13

English RV, Breitschwerdt EB, Grindem CB, Thrall DE and Gainsburg LA (1988) Zollinger–Ellison syndrome and myelofibrosis in a dog. *Journal of the American Veterinary Medical Association* **192**, 1430–1434

Gabbert NH, Nachreiner RF, Holmes-Wood P and Kivela JH (1984) Serum immunoreactive gastrin concentrations in the dog: basal and postprandial values measured by radioimmunoassay. *American Journal of Veterinary Research* **45**, 2351–2353

Giles RC Jr, Hildebrandt PK and Montgomery CA Jr (1974) Carcinoid tumor in the small intestine of a dog. *Veterinary Pathology* **11**, 340–349

Green RA and Gartrell CL (1997) Gastrinoma: A retrospective study of four cases (1985–1995). *Journal of the American Animal Hospital Association* **33**, 524–527

Gross TL, O'Brien TD, Davies AP and Long RE (1990) Glucagon-producing pancreatic endocrine tumors in two dogs with superficial necrolytic dermatitis. *Journal of the American Veterinary Medical Association* **197**, 1619–1622

Gross TL, Song MD, Havel PJ and Ihrke PJ (1993) Superficial necrolytic dermatitis (necrolytic migratory erythema) in dogs. *Veterinary Pathology* **30**, 75–81

Hayden DW and Henson MS (1997) Gastrin-secreting pancreatic endocrine tumor in a dog (putative Zollinger–Ellison syndrome). *Journal of Veterinary Diagnostic Investigation* **9**, 100–103

Holst JJ, Fahrenkrug J, Stadil F and Rehfeld JF (1996) Gastrointestinal endocrinology. *Scandinavian Journal of Gastroenterology* **216** (Suppl), 27–38

Johnson LR (1991) Regulation: peptides of the gastrointestinal tract. In: *Gastrointestinal Physiology, 4th edn*, ed. LR Johnson, pp. 1–14. Mosby Year Book, St Louis

Klöppel G, Heitz PU, Capella C and Solcia E (1996) Pathology and nomenclature of human gastrointestinal neuroendocrine (carcinoid) tumors and related lesions. *World Journal of Surgery* **20**, 132–141

Lamb CR, Simpson KW, Boswood A and Matthewman LA (1995) Ultrasonography of pancreatic neoplasia in the dog: A retrospective review of 16 cases. *Veterinary Record* **137**, 65–68

Lothrop CD (1989) Medical treatment of neuroendocrine tumors of the gastroenteropancreatic system with somatostatin. In: *Current Veterinary Therapy, 10th edn*, ed. RW Kirk, pp. 1020–1024. WB Saunders, Philadelphia

Matthiesen DT and Mullen HS (1990) Problems and complications associated with endocrine surgery in the dog and cat. *Problems in Veterinary Medicine* **2**, 627–667

Miller WH, Scott DW, Buerger RG, Shanley KJ, Paradis M, McMurdy MA and Angarano DW (1990) Necrolytic migratory erythema in dogs: a hepatocutaneous syndrome. *Journal of the American Animal Hospital Association* **26**, 573–581

Modlin IM, Jaffe BM, Sank A and Albert D (1982) The early diagnosis of gastrinoma. *Annals of Surgery* **196**, 512–517

Modlin IM and Tang LH (1997) Approaches to the diagnosis of gut neuroendocrine tumors: the last word (today). *Gastroenterology* **112**, 583–590

Nilsson O (1996) Gastrointestinal carcinoids—aspects of diagnosis and classification. *APMIS* **104**, 481–492

Orloff SL and Debas HT (1995) Advances in the management of patients with Zollinger-Ellison syndrome. *Surgical Clinics of North America* **75**, 511–524

Patnaik AK, Hurvitz AI and Johnson GF (1980) Canine intestinal adenocarcinoma and carcinoid. *Veterinary Pathology* **17**, 149–163

Perry RR and Vinik AI (1996) Endocrine tumors of the gastrointestinal tract. *Annual Review of Medicine* **47**, 57–68

Prinz RA, Dorsch TR and Lawrence AM (1981) Clinical aspects of glucagon-producing islet cell tumors. *American Journal of Gastroenterology* **76**, 125–131

Simpson KW and Dykes NL (1997) Diagnosis and treatment of gastrinoma. *Seminars in Veterinary Medicine and Surgery* (in press)

Solcia E, Fiocca R, Rindi G, Villani L, Luinetti O, Burrell M, Bosi F and Silini E (1995) Endocrine tumors of the small and large intestine. *Pathology, Research and Practice* **191**, 366–372

Sykes GP and Cooper BJ (1982) Canine intestinal carcinoids. *Veterinary Pathology* **19**, 120–131

Taboada J and Merchant SR (1997) Superficial necrolytic dermatitis and the liver. *Conference Proceedings of the 15th Forum of the American College of Veterinary Internal Medicine, Orlando*, pp. 534–537

Turnwald G H, Foil CS, Wolfsheimer KJ, Williams MD and Rougeou BL (1989) Failure to document hyperglucagonemia in a dog with diabetic dermatopathy resembling necrolytic migratory erythema. *Journal of the American Animal Hospital Association* **25**, 363–369

Walsh JH and Mayer EA (1993) Gastrointestinal hormones. In: *Gastrointestinal Disease: Pathophysiology, Diagnosis, Management, 5th edn*, pp. 18–44. WB Saunders, Philadelphia

Walton DK, Center SA, Scott DW and Collins K (1986) Ulcerative dermatosis associated with diabetes mellitus in the dog: a report of four cases. *Journal of the American Animal Hospital Association* **22**, 79–88

Zerbe CA (1992) Islet cell tumors secreting insulin, pancreatic polypeptide, gastrin, or glucagon. In: *Current Veterinary Therapy XI, 11th edn*, eds. RW Kirk and JD Bonagura, pp. 368–375. WB Saunders, Philadelphia

Zerbe CA, Boosinger TR, Grabau JH, Pletcher JM and O'Dorisio TM (1989) Pancreatic polypeptide and insulin-secreting tumor in a dog with duodenal ulcers and hypertrophic gastritis. *Journal of Veterinary Internal Medicine* **3**, 178–182

Zerbe CA and Washabau RJ (1995) Gastrointestinal endocrine disease. In: *Textbook of Veterinary Internal Medicine, 4th edn*, eds. SJ Ettinger and EC Feldman, pp. 1593–1602. WB Saunders, Philadelphia

CHAPTER TWENTY ONE

Clinical Endocrinology of the Kidney

Scott A. Brown

INTRODUCTION

The kidney serves as an end organ for a variety of circulating hormones (Table 21.1), including aldosterone, angiotensin II, atrial natriuretic peptide, glucocorticoids, parathyroid hormone, thyroid hormone, and vasopressin. In addition, the kidney is affected by other cytokines which are generally classified as paracrine or autocrine factors because they are produced and act locally without being carried in the bloodstream. This latter group includes eicosanoids, endothelin, endothelium derived relaxing factor, and the peptide growth factors. Furthermore, the kidney is an endocrine organ, producing components of the renin–angiotensin system (RAS), erythropoietin, and 1,25-dihydroxycholecalciferol. These hormones play a critical role in the control of systemic arterial blood pressure, extracellular fluid volume, haematocrit, and calcium homeostasis.

This chapter will focus on the functions of the kidney as an endocrine organ, with detailed descriptions of the RAS and of erythropoietin. A brief discussion of endothelium derived relaxing factors and growth factors will follow. For in depth discussion of the role of 1,25-dihydroxycholecalciferol in calcium homeostasis and of vasopressin refer to Chapters 16 and 18, respectively.

RENIN-ANGIOTENSIN SYSTEM

Physiology

The systemic or classic RAS (Figure 21.1) plays an important role in maintenance of blood volume and pressure. The rate limiting component of the system, renin, is an enzyme released by specialised smooth muscle cells within the wall of the terminal afferent arteriole of the kidney. Its release is increased by sympathetic stimulation, reduced renal perfusion pressure (systemic hypotension), and reduced solute load to the macula densa portion of the distal tubule. The substrate molecule, referred to as angiotensinogen, or renin substrate, is a circulating peptide of hepatic origin. The terminal 10 amino acid fragment, cleaved from angiotensinogen by renin, is referred to as angiotensin I; this molecule has very limited biological activity. The terminal two amino acids of angiotensin I are removed by angiotensin converting enzyme (ACE). This enzymatic activity is ubiquitous in nature, being present in plasma and endothelium of most vascular beds. The remaining eight amino acid fragment is the active component of this system, angiotensin II. This molecule raises systemic arterial pressure by increasing vascular resistance (direct constriction of vascular smooth muscle) and expansion of extracellular volume (stimulation of renal sodium and water conservation). An effect of angiotensin II receiving increased attention recently is its ability to act as a growth factor by enhancing the proliferation rate of a variety of cells, including glomerular mesangial cells (Wolf *et al.*, 1992).

The sensitivity of the efferent arteriole to angiotensin II-induced vasoconstriction appears to be greater than that of the afferent arteriole. This observation is somewhat controversial but potentially of great importance in the regulation of renal function. The consequence of preferential postglomerular vasoconstriction is that it would allow angiotensin II to raise glomerular capillary pressure and glomerular filtration rate (GFR). Accordingly, therapeutic agents that reduce the rate of generation of angiotensin II would tend to lower glomerular capillary pressure and, possibly, GFR.

In recent years, it has become apparent that several organs, such as brain and kidney, contain all of the components necessary for the local generation of angiotensin II. These local RASs are separate from the classic or systemic system described above. The local RASs may be

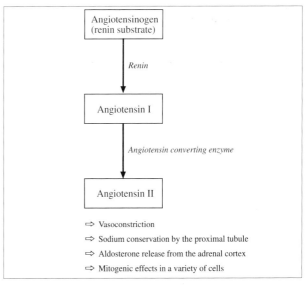

Figure 21.1: The renin–angiotensin system (RAS). The enzyme renin, of renal origin, cleaves the terminal 10 amino acid fragment (angiotensin I) from the plasma peptide molecule angiotensinogen. Converting enzyme activity, which is ubiquitous in location, removes two amino acids, thereby producing the active hormone, angiotensin II. Angiotensin II leads to vasoconstriction, renal retention of sodium (and water), aldosterone release, and proliferation of a variety of cells. The RAS plays an important role in the pathophysiology of congestive heart failure, systemic hypertension, and progressive renal failure.

Circulating factor	Source	Renal effects
Aldosterone	Adrenal cortex	Sodium conservation Kaliuresis and aciduria
Angiotensin II	Plasma (indirectly from kidney via renin generation)	Vasoconstriction Sodium conservation
Atrial natriuretic peptide	Heart (primarily atria)	Natriuresis Vasodilatation
Glucocorticoids	Adrenal cortex	Mild increase in glomerular filtration rate Interference with concentrating mechanism
Eicosanoids	Many sites	Vasodilation and/or vasoconstriction Alteration of tubular sodium/potassium handling
Endothelin	Many sites	Prolonged vasoconstriction
Endothelium derived relaxing factors	Many sites	Intrarenal (and systemic) vasodilation Natriuresis
Erythropoietin	Tubular cells	None, except through secondary effects of increased haematocrit
Growth factors	Many sites	Tubular cells: proliferation (e.g. epidermal growth factor) Mesangial cells: proliferation (e.g. epidermal growth factor) and extracellular matrix formation (e.g. transforming growth factor, type β)
Parathyroid hormone	Parathyroid gland	Phosphaturia
Renin	Afferent arteriole	Enhanced generation of angiotensin II
Thyroid hormone	Thyroid gland	Renal growth Intrarenal (?) and systemic hypertension
Vasopressin	Posterior pituitary and hypothalamus	Permeability of distal nephron segments to water
1,25 dihydroxycholecalciferol	Renal tubular cells	Enhances renal resorption of calcium and phosphorus (other primary effects are enhanced gut absorption of calcium, enhanced bone release of calcium and phosphorus, and reduced secretion of parathyroid hormone by parathyroid gland)

Table 21.1: *Overview of renal endocrinology.*

more important than the systemic system in determining the net effect of angiotensin II on these organs — for example, studies indicate that intrarenal levels of angiotensin II can exceed plasma concentrations by 1000-fold, presumably due to local generation of angiotensin II (Braam *et al.*, 1993). In addition, there is evidence that tissue converting enzyme activity within the kidney is regulated by different mechanisms than plasma activity (Michel *et al.*, 1994) and is less susceptible to inhibition by pharmacological agents than is the plasma enzymatic activity (Allan *et al.*, 1994). This could be critical, since long-term regulation of blood pressure by the kidney appears to be more dependent upon renal, than extrarenal, effects of this hormone (Hall *et al.*, 1977, 1990).

Pathophysiology and therapeutics

The RAS is integral to the pathogenesis of a variety of

diseases. In particular, overactivity of the system plays an important role in the pathogenesis of heart failure, systemic hypertension, and progressive renal failure. Consequently, efforts to reduce the generation of angiotensin II are commonly employed in the treatment of these abnormalities. Renin antagonists, angiotensin converting enzyme inhibitors (ACEI), and angiotensin II antagonists are theoretically useful to achieve this purpose. Clinically, inhibition of converting enzyme activity has been the most commonly used approach, principally because of the widespread availability of ACEI.

Role of the RAS in disorders

Cardiac failure

In dogs with heart failure, ACEI administration (0.5 mg

enalapril/kg body weight orally every 12–24 hours) is of proved benefit (COVE Group, 1995; IMPROVE Group, 1995), presumably by reducing angiotensin II-mediated volume expansion and vasoconstriction. These effects of ACEI will reduce left ventricular afterload and preload, thereby enhancing cardiac performance. The use of ACEI in dogs with congestive heart failure should therefore be associated with an improvement in the quality of life and, or, prolongation of survival time. Although less is known about the use of ACEI in cats, a similar dose has been recommended by others.

In heart failure patients receiving ACEI, plasma concentrations of electrolytes and creatinine should be evaluated before and 10–14 days after the institution of therapy. In dogs with heart failure, the co-administration of high doses of diuretics (e.g. frusemide) and ACEI may lead to a reduction of GFR, clinically manifested as worsening azotaemia. This condition may resolve following a reduction in the dose of the diuretic.

Systemic hypertension

In systemic hypertension, ACEI will reduce angiotensin II-mediated volume expansion and vasoconstriction. If a dog or cat has renal failure, or if systemic hypertension is suspected, baseline values for systemic arterial blood pressure should be obtained before the administration of any antihypertensive agent. Indirect methods for the measurement of blood pressure (e.g. oscillometry or Doppler ultrasonic flowmetry) may provide an adequate estimate of systemic arterial blood pressure.

Although complications related to hypertension can be anticipated with severe elevations of blood pressure, little is known about the actual risk associated with mild to moderate hypertension in dogs and cats. Accordingly, only those animals consistently exhibiting a marked increase in blood pressure (e.g. systolic, mean, diastolic pressures exceeding 200, 140, and 110 mm Hg, respectively) or indications of complications of systemic hypertension (e.g. hypertensive retinopathy, unexplained epistaxis or seizures, left ventricular hypertrophy), should receive antihypertensive therapy.

Because retinal and renal injury appear to be the most likely consequences of systemic hypertension in dogs and cats, a retinal examination and measurement of plasma concentrations of electrolytes and creatinine should be performed before and 10–14 days after the institution of therapy. It seems reasonable to initiate antihypertensive therapy with a low sodium diet, which may lower blood pressure through contraction of extracellular fluid volume and should enhance the efficacy of ACEI. Since animals with renal dysfunction may adapt slowly to changes in sodium intake, any dietary adjustments should be accomplished gradually, by adding increasing amounts of the low sodium diet to the current diet over 10–14 days. An ACEI (e.g. 0.5 mg enalapril/kg body weight twice daily) can be used as first choice pharmacotherapy in hypertensive dogs and cats. Dosage adjustment, based upon precise arterial pressure measurements, will frequently be required. Appropriate doses of antihypertensive therapy must be individualised and should be adjusted to effect,

that is, until hypertension is eliminated. Unless emergency therapy is required, as for retinal detachment or cerebrovascular accident, approximately 14 days should be allowed before assessment of any changes in therapy.

For an ACEI to be effective antihypertensive therapy, blood pressure must be dependent upon circulating or tissue levels of angiotensin II. Human patients with systemic hypertension are often classified on the basis of plasma renin activity. Although little investigative work has been done, hypertensive dogs and cats with high plasma renin activity would be expected to be more responsive to ACEI than those with low plasma renin activity but, because of the possible role of the local RASs in the genesis of hypertension (Hall et al., 1977, 1990; Braam et al., 1993; Allan et al., 1994; Michel et al., 1994), animals with low plasma renin activity may respond to ACEI with a decrement in blood pressure.

The use of combination therapy for systemic hypertension may be more effective in lowering blood pressure than single agent therapy. ACEI may be co-administered with other antihypertensives, such as calcium channel antagonists (e.g. amlodipine 0.625 mg/cat or 1 mg/kg body weight in dogs; every 12–24 hours in both species) or prazosin at a dosage of 0.5–4 mg every 12–24 hours (Cowgill and Kallet, 1983; Ross and Labato, 1989; Snyder and Henik, 1994; Littman and Drobatz, 1995). Prazosin is a vasodilator which may produce systemic hypotension upon initial administration and it may be prudent to hospitalise the animal for observation during the initial 1–2 days of antihypertensive therapy with this agent.

Progressive renal failure

The rationale for the use of ACEI as therapy for progressive renal failure, is based upon the presumed ability of these agents to lower pressure in systemic arteries and, or, glomerular capillaries, and to prevent structural changes within the kidney due to angiotensin II-mediated overproliferation of resident renal cells.

Renal failure can cause alterations in body fluid and electrolyte balance, leading to systemic hypertension (Hall et al., 1990). Elevations of systemic arterial pressure are frequently present in dogs and cats with chronic renal failure (CRF) (Cowgill and Kallet, 1983; Ross and Labato, 1989). Systemic hypertension can also lead to renal injury. This effect has been documented experimentally in rats (Bidani et al., 1990) but studies have not as yet been reported in dogs and cats. The mechanism of renal injury in systemic hypertension appears to involve direct effects of systemic arterial pressure elevation (Bidani et al., 1990), an indirect effect due to transmission of high pressures to the glomerular capillary bed (Anderson et al., 1988), and a mitogenic effect of angiotensin II on glomerular mesangial cells (Wolf et al., 1992). The use of ACEI (0.5 mg enalapril/kg body weight orally every 12–24 hours) to preserve renal structure and function in dogs with progressive renal failure has been advocated on the basis of experimental observations in dogs and rats, and clinical observations in humans. Though less is known about the use of ACEI in cats, a similar dose is generally recommended. The mechanism of the effect is presumably due to lowering of systemic arterial pressure, lowering of intraglomerular pressure due to preferential dilatation of the renal efferent arteriole, and, or, anti-proliferative effects of ACEI. The justification for the use of these agents in animals with renal failure is not dependent upon the presence of systemic hypertension, because the beneficial effects may be independent of the blood pressure lowering effect of ACEI. However, measurement of blood pressure is preferred as it may prove useful in monitoring therapy. In dogs with renal failure, the administration of an ACEI may lead to a reduction of GFR, clinically evidenced as worsening azotaemia. Fortunately, this side effect appears to be less frequent than originally proposed, though plasma concentrations of electrolytes and creatinine should be evaluated before and 10–14 days after the institution of therapy.

Limitations to use of ACEI
Some effects of ACEI may be undesirable. In some animals with azotaemia and systemic hypertension, the ACEI may lower intraglomerular pressure, thus producing a precipitous fall in GFR and worsening of azotaemia. Similar effects may be seen in dogs with heart failure that receive ACEI and diuretic therapy. In people and animals with renal failure but no evidence of cardiac dysfunction, the use of ACEI does not generally exacerbate azotaemia. Additionally, captopril has been associated with an idiosyncratic glomerular disease in some dogs (Knowlen and Kittleson, 1986). The prevalence of this reaction in dogs treated with other agents in this class seems to be infrequent. In people, the ACEI with sulphhydryl groups (e.g. captopril) are associated with a greater prevalence of side effects than other agents (e.g. enalapril, benazepril). Another consideration in the choice of ACEI is the route of clearance of the agent from the body. Some agents in this class, such as benazepril, have substantial hepatic clearance, and dose adjustment may be less important in patients with renal failure.

ERYTHROPOIETIN

Physiology
Erythropoietin is a glycoprotein which regulates erythropoiesis through stimulation of erythrocyte stem cell proliferation and differentiation. Erythropoietin is produced by the liver of fetal and neonatal animals and primarily by the kidney in adults. The production and release of this molecule from the kidney is regulated by arterial oxygen content in a manner that is poorly understood. Some studies have indicated that the proximal tubular cells are a primary source of erythropoietin, though nucleic acid message coding for erythropoietin production has been identified in other cells within the kidney.

Diseases associated with erythropoietin excess
An increase in red blood cell concentration is referred to as polycythaemia. Relative polycythaemia occurs when there is a transient, preferential increase in the ratio of red blood cell mass to plasma volume. Relative polycythaemia occurs with splenic contraction or, more commonly, dehydration. Absolute polycythaemia occurs when there is overproduction of red blood cells, and may be primary or secondary. Primary absolute polycythaemia, referred to as polycythaemia vera, is characterised by the presence of a normal arterial oxygen tension and a normal to low serum erythropoietin concentration. Secondary absolute polycythaemia may be due to: the overproduction of endogenous erythropoietin in response to arterial hypoxia; overzealous administration of exogenous erythropoietin; renal parenchymal disease; or overproduction of other erythrogenic hormones, such as androgens or corticosteroids. The last two causes of secondary absolute polycythaemia (and polycythaemia vera) are generally associated with normal arterial oxygen tension.

Endogenous overproduction of erythropoietin in response to arterial hypoxia may be caused by right-to-left cardiovascular shunting, parenchymal pulmonary disease, alveolar hypoventilation, and chronic hypoxia (e.g. high altitude disease). The cause of endogenous overproduction of erythropoietin associated with renal parenchymal disease, most commonly renal tumours, is often unknown. In animals with renal tumours, neoplastic cells may be producing erythropoietin in an unregulated fashion. In contrast, renal neoplasia or other renal parenchymal diseases, may result in localised intrarenal hypoxia causing erythropoietin overproduction.

Animals with polycythaemia frequently exhibit clinical signs compatible with excessive blood viscosity, including weakness, seizures, dilated retinal vessels, cutaneous and mucous membrane hyperaemia, and seizures. Clinical signs related to dysfunction of the gastrointestinal system (vomiting and, or, diarrhoea) or kidney (polyuria and polydipsia) are often observed. Additional signs referable to the primary cause of the erythropoietin excess may be apparent.

The diagnosis of polycythaemia is based on identification of increased red blood cell numbers. Appropriate ancillary diagnostic tests include measurement of arterial blood gas tensions, urinalysis and serum biochemical tests, thoracic and abdominal radiography and, or, ultrasonography, and measurement of serum erythropoietin concentration.

Diseases associated with erythropoietin deficiency
Dogs and cats with CRF frequently exhibit a non-regenerative, normocytic, normochromic anaemia. While the uraemic environment lowers red blood cell production and lifespan, a relative or absolute lack of erythropoietin is the most important causative factor in the anaemia of renal failure in dogs (King et al., 1992). In cats (Cook and Lothrop, 1994) with renal failure and anaemia, plasma erythropoietin concentration is inappropriately low. In both species, the response to therapy with exogenous erythropoietin is generally dramatic. Thus, erythropoietin deficiency plays the central role in the genesis of the anaemia of CRF in dogs and cats.

The use of exogenous erythropoietin in other causes of anaemia, such as bone marrow suppression associated with feline leukaemia virus infection, is controversial. Some studies have suggested a beneficial effect, despite the fact that deficiency of erythropoietin plays little, if any, role in the genesis of the anaemia.

Use in CRF

Recently, the application of molecular biology techniques has made it possible to administer recombinant erythropoietin to restore a normal haematocrit in many animals with CRF. Some of the clinical signs commonly associated with renal failure in dogs and cats, such as lethargy and inappetance, will improve in response to this therapy (Cowgill, 1992; King *et al.*, 1992).

Before the institution of erythropoietin therapy, ongoing blood loss, infection with feline leukaemia virus, iron deficiency, and other nutritional imbalances should be considered. These abnormalities should be corrected, where possible. Approximately half of dogs and cats with anaemia of CRF exhibit laboratory evidence of iron deficiency, including reduced serum iron concentration and reduced transferrin saturation (Cowgill, 1992). These animals should receive oral iron supplementation at standard doses (i.e. oral iron sulphate, total daily dose of 50–100 mg/day for cats and 100–300 mg/day for dogs, divided and given as multiple subdoses to avoid gastrointestinal upset). Serum iron and transferrin saturation should be monitored to allow dosage adjustment.

In those animals in which the haematocrit is low (generally taken as those with a haematocrit <20%), the use of human recombinant erythropoietin at an initial dosage of 50–100 IU/kg/day subcutaneously three times weekly, should be expected to produce a noticeable increase in haematocrit within 5–10 days. Initially, the haematocrit should be checked twice weekly and the dose adjusted on the basis of these measurements. If a dosage regimen is followed without careful monitoring, some animals will develop life-threatening polycythaemia.

The goal of therapy should be to obtain an haematocrit just below the lower limit of normal range for the species being treated. It is important to avoid overzealous therapy leading to life-threatening polycythaemia, and to evaluate any refractory patient carefully. Dosage adjustments will be required in individual patients. Since individual animals will respond differently, the appropriate times for reassessment of response and determination of future dosage will vary.

Some anaemic animals with CRF are refractory to human recombinant erythropoietin because of iron deficiency, and this problem can be avoided if iron supplementation, as outlined above, is employed. However, because the human recombinant erythropoietin currently available is a product of human genes, some animals will produce antibodies against it. These animals will initially respond but later become refractory due to the production of anti-human recombinant erythropoietin antibodies. Antibody production occurs in about half of all treated animals. These dogs and cats may become refractory to further therapy with human recombinant erythropoietin and generally exhibit a myeloid:erythroid ratio that exceeds 10 (Cowgill, 1992). In these animals, the use of

human recombinant erythropoietin should be discontinued (Cowgill, 1992). Because of the anamnestic response, the further use of human recombinant erythropoietin will not be possible in animals that produce antibodies.

Because nearly half of all treated animals eventually develop antibodies and become refractory to human recombinant erythropoietin therapy, it is unwise to initiate therapy too early in an individual animal. Thus, human recombinant erythropoietin therapy should be reserved for animals with moderate to severe anaemia, generally exhibiting a haematocrit <20%, and for those patients in which it is suspected that the clinical signs of lethargy or inappetance will respond to an increase in haematocrit.

Although apparently uncommon, other potential adverse effects of human recombinant erythropoietin therapy include vomiting, skin reactions, seizures, systemic hypertension, arthralgia, mucocutaneous reactions, and fever (Cowgill, 1992).

PARATHYROID HORMONE

Parathyroid hormone (PTH) has a variety of effects on the kidney, including suppression of renal phosphate resorption, enhanced calcium resorption, and increased renal generation of 1,25 dihydroxycholecalciferol. For a discussion of the control of secretion, and the effects of PTH, see Chapter 16.

ENDOTHELIUM DERIVED RELAXING FACTORS

Endothelium derived relaxing factors (EDRFs) are cytokines produced by the vascular endothelium which cause relaxation of vascular smooth muscle. Nitric oxide is sometimes referred to as an EDRF, however it is apparent that there are a variety of cytokines with a similar effect, such as prostacyclin. Basal production of endothelium derived nitric oxide lowers blood pressure and renal vascular resistance in dogs and cats (Brown, 1992, 1993). Nitric oxide is derived from the amino acid, arginine, and excessive dietary restriction of arginine could produce renal and systemic vasoconstriction, resulting in systemic hypertension and azotaemia. While dietary supplementation with arginine could theoretically reduce systemic blood pressure and enhance GFR in dogs and cats, this has not been carefully studied.

GROWTH FACTORS

Renal disease is often associated with intraglomerular structural abnormalities, including excess deposition of mesangial matrix, which is referred to as glomerulosclerosis. While studies of canine mesangial cells *in vitro* demonstrate the importance of a variety of growth factors in this species (Ennulat and Brown, 1995), the relative importance of growth factors in renal physiology and pathophysiology in dogs and cats remains largely unknown. Growth factors of interest include angiotensin II, epidermal growth factor, insulin-like growth factor-I and II, platelet derived growth factor, and transforming growth factor type-β (Doi *et al.*, 1989; Floege *et al.*, 1990; Barnes and Abboud, 1993; Marti *et al.*, 1994).

OTHER HORMONES

Because many hormones affect the kidney (see Table 21.1), a variety of endocrinopathies can result in abnormalities in renal structure or function. These include interference with the concentrating mechanism by the absence of vasopressin (diabetes insipidus), excess glucocorticoids (hyperadrenocorticism), hypercalcaemia (primary hyperparathyroidism), and hyperglycaemia (diabetes mellitus); increase in the glomerular filtration rate by glucocorticoids (hyperadrenocorticism), thyroid hormone (hyperthyroidism), and hyperglycaemia (diabetes mellitus); development of glomerulosclerosis (hyperadrenocorticism and diabetes mellitus); and interference with renal electrolyte handling by excess or inadequate aldosterone (hypoadrenocorticism or hyperaldosteronism). The reader is referred to corresponding chapters for a discussion of the role of the kidney in these endocrinopathies.

REFERENCES AND FURTHER READING

Allan DR, McKnight JA, Kifor I, Coletti CM and Hollenberg NK (1994) Converting enzyme inhibition and renal tissue angiotensin II in the rat. *Hypertension* **24**, 516–522

Anderson S, Diamond J, Karnovsky MJ and Brenner BM (1988) Mechanisms underlying transition from acute glomerular injury to late glomerular sclerosis in a rat model of nephrotic syndrome. *Journal of Clinical Investigations* **82**, 1757–1768

Barnes JL and Abboud HE (1993) Temporal expression of autocrine growth factors corresponds to morphological features of mesangial proliferation in Habu snake venom-induced glomerulonephritis. *American Journal of Pathology* **143**, 1366–1376

Bidani A, Mitchell K, Schwartz MM, Navar LG and Lewis EJ (1990) Absence of glomerular injury or nephron loss in a normotensive rat remnant kidney model. *Kidney International* **38**, 28–38

Braam B, Mitchell KD, Fox J and Navar LG (1993) Proximal tubular secretion of angiotensin II in rats. *American Journal of Physiology* **264**, F891–F898

Brown SA (1992) Effects of endothelium-derived nitric oxide blockade on renal and glomerular hemodynamics in normal and partially nephrectomized dogs. *Journal of the American Society of Nephrology* **3**, 541(Abstract)

Brown SA (1993) Effects of inhibition of nitric oxide synthase on systemic arterial pressure and renal vascular resistance in cats. *Research in Veterinary Science* **55**, 398–400

Cook SM and Lothrop CD (1994) Serum erythropoietin concentrations measured by radioimmunoassay in normal, polycythemic, and anemic dogs and cats. *Journal of Veterinary Internal Medicine* **8**, 18–25

COVE Group (1995) Controlled clinical evaluation of enalapril in dogs with heart failure: results of the cooperative veterinary enalapril study group. *Journal of Veterinary Internal Medicine* **9**, 243–255

Cowgill LD (1992) Pathophysiology and management of anemia in chronic renal progressive renal failure. *Seminars in Veterinary Medicine and Surgery* **7**, 175–182

Cowgill LD and Kallet AJ (1983) Recognition and management of hypertension in the dog. In: *Current Veterinary Therapy VIII*, ed. RW Kirk, pp. 1025–1028. WB Saunders, Philadelphia

Doi T, Striker LJ, Elliot SJ, Conti FG and Striker GE (1989) Insulin-like growth factor-I is a progression factor for human mesangial cells. *American Journal of Pathology* **134**, 395–404

Ennulat D and Brown S (1995) Canine and equine mesangial cells in vitro. *In Vitro* **31**, 574–578

Floege J, Topley N, Wessel K, Kaever V, Radeke H, Hoppe J, Kishimoto T and Resch K (1990) Monokines and platelet-derived growth factor modulate prostanoid production in growth arrested, human mesangial cells. *Kidney International* **37**, 859–869

Hall JE, Guyton AC, Jackson TE, Coleman TG, Lohmeier TE and Trippodo NC (1977) Control of glomerular filtration rate by renin-angiotensin system. *American Journal of Physiology* **233**, F366–F372

Hall JE, Mizelle HL, Hildebrandt DA and Brands MW (1990) Abnormal pressure natriuresis: a cause or consequence of hypertension. *Hypertension* **15**, 547–559

IMPROVE Group (1995) Acute and short-term hemodynamic, echocardiographic, and clinical effects of enalapril maleate in dogs with naturally acquired heart failure: Results of the invasive multicenter prospective veterinary evaluation of enalapril study. *Journal of Veterinary Internal Medicine* **9**, 234–242

King LG, Giger U, Diserens D and Nagode LA (1992) Anemia of chronic renal failure in dogs. *Journal of Veterinary Internal Medicine* **6**, 264–270

Knowlen G and Kittleson M (1986) Captopril therapy in dogs with heart failure. In: *Current Veterinary Therapy IX*, ed. RW Kirk, pp. 334–339. WB Saunders, Philadelphia

Littman M P and Drobatz K J (1995) Hypertensive and hypotensive disorders. In: *Textbook of Veterinary Internal Medicine*, ed. SJ Ettinger, pp. 93–100. WB Saunders, Philadelphia

Marti HP, Lee L, Kashgarian M and Lovett DH (1994) Transforming growth factor-beta1 stimulates glomerular mesangial cell synthesis of the 72-kd type IV collagenase. *American Journal of Pathology* **144**, 82–94

Michel B, Grima M, Stephan D, Coquard C, Wlesch C, Barthelmebs M and Imbs JL (1994) Plasma renin activity and changes in tissue angiotensin converting enzyme. *Journal of Hypertension* **12**, 577–584

Ross LA and Labato MA (1989) Use of drugs to control hypertension in renal failure. In: *Current Veterinary Therapy X*, eds RW Kirk and JD Bonagura, pp. 1201–1204. WB Saunders, Philadelphia

Snyder PS and Henik RA (1994) Feline systemic hypertension. *Proceedings of the 12th Annual Meeting of the American College of Veterinary Internal Medicine*, p. 126.

Wolf G, Thaiss F, Schoeppe W and Stahl RAK (1992) Angiotensin II-induced proliferation of cultured murine mesangial cells: inhibitory role of atrial natriuretic peptide. *Journal of the American Society of Nephrology* **2**, 1270–1278

PART FOUR

Uncommon Endocrine Disorders

CHAPTER TWENTY TWO

Lipid Disorders

Joan Duncan

INTRODUCTION

Hyperlipidaemia is defined as an increase in plasma cholesterol and/or triglyceride concentrations. The condition may arise as the result of a primary defect in lipoprotein metabolism or as a consequence of an underlying systemic disease.

LIPID METABOLISM

Lipids are essential for normal physiological function and are transported through the plasma to their sites of utilisation in lipid–protein complexes called lipoproteins. There are four discrete populations of lipoproteins recognised in the dog and cat (Table 22.1). Each lipoprotein species has a specific function, and the interactions between lipoprotein populations and tissues ensure the efficient transport of lipid in response to physiological demand (Watson and Barrie, 1993).

CLASSIFICATION OF HYPERLIPIDAEMIA

Physiological hyperlipidaemia

The absorption of dietary fat from the intestines is accompanied by the formation of chylomicrons. The accumulation of these triglyceride-rich lipoproteins lends a turbidity (postprandial lipaemia) to the serum or plasma of normal individuals which clears 4–6 hours after eating. The postprandial rise in triglyceride concentration in healthy dogs is rarely greater than 3 mmol/l and depends upon both the dietary fat intake and the rate of lipoprotein metabolism in that individual. A marginal postprandial rise in cholesterol may also be noted, but this often does not exceed the reference range for the species.

Secondary hyperlipidaemia

Postprandial hyperlipidaemia is the most common cause of hypertriglyceridaemia, but plasma lipid abnormalities are a frequent consequence of systemic disease, particularly endocrine disease. Hypothyroidism, diabetes mellitus, hyperadrenocorticism, cholestatic liver disease, and glomerulonephritis have been associated with hyperlipidaemia (Rogers *et al.*, 1975b; Ford, 1977; Barrie *et al.*, 1993b). In the dog it is proposed that marked hypertriglyceridaemia may predispose the individual to pancreatitis (Whitney *et al.*, 1987).

The mechanism of the lipid abnormalities in each systemic disease is determined by interactions between hormone and plasma protein concentrations and lipoprotein metabolism. Hypercholesterolaemia (mild to marked) is noted in two thirds of dogs with hypothyroidism (Larsson, 1988). It is the author's experience that marked hypercholesterolaemia (>11 mmol/l), is most commonly associated with canine hypothyroidism. The mean (± SD) cholesterol concentration associated with hyperadrenocorticism (8.86 ± 2.32 mmol/l, *n*=14) and diabetes mellitus (9.31 ± 3.76 mmol/l, *n*=11) in the dog are lower than that for hypothyroidism (16.17 ± 9.93 mmol/l, *n*=10) (Barrie *et al.*, 1993b).

Inherited and idiopathic hyperlipidaemia

Primary defects of lipoprotein metabolism in the dog are rare. Idiopathic hyperchylomicronaemia in the Miniature Schnauzer is thought to be the result of an inherited defect, the exact nature of which has not been elucidated (Rogers *et al.*, 1975a; Ford, 1993). The clinical entity is characterised by hypertriglyceridaemia and hyperchylomicronaemia. The degree of hypertriglyceridaemia is variable but clinical signs are usually not noted in dogs until concentrations exceed 5.5 mmol/l (Ford, 1993).

An inherited defect of lipoprotein lipase activity is recognised as the cause of familial hyperchylomicro-

Lipoprotein	Function
Chylomicrons	Transport of dietary lipid (predominantly triglyceride) from the intestines to the peripheral tissues and liver
Very low density lipoproteins	Export of hepatic triglyceride and cholesterol and delivery of triglyceride to peripheral tissues. Modified by the action of the enzymes lipoprotein lipase and hepatic lipase to form low density lipoproteins
Low density lipoproteins	Delivery of cholesterol to peripheral tissues
High density lipoproteins	Transport of cholesterol from peripheral tissues to the liver

Table 22.1: Functions of the lipoprotein classes of the dog and cat.

Physiological hyperlipidaemia
Postprandial hypertriglyceridaemia
Secondary hyperlipidaemia
Diabetes mellitus
Hypothyroidism
Hyperadrenocorticism
Cholestatic liver disease
Glomerulonephritis
Inherited hyperlipidaemia
Idiopathic hyperchylomicronaemia in the Miniature Schnauzer
Inherited hyperchylomicronaemia in the cat
Idiopathic hyperlipidaemia

Table 22.2: Classification of hyperlipidaemia.

Hypertriglyceridaemia
Anorexia
Abdominal pain
Vomiting
Diarrhoea
Abdominal distension
Lipaemia retinalis
Lipid-laden aqueous humor
Seizures
Peripheral neuropathies
Hypercholesterolaemia
Arcus lipoides corneae
Atherosclerosis

Table 22.3: Clinical manifestations of hyperlipidaemia.

naemia in cats (Peritz *et al.*, 1990; Watson *et al.*, 1992). The defect, which has been recognised in kittens and young adult cats, results in the accumulation of chylomicrons and very low density lipoproteins (VLDL) in the plasma of fasted cats (Jones *et al.*, 1986; Peritz *et al.*, 1990).

Where no underlying disease or inherited basis is proven, the hyperlipidaemia is classified as idiopathic (Table 22.2).

CLINICAL MANIFESTATIONS OF HYPERLIPIDAEMIA

The pathological consequences of hyperlipidaemia may be classified according to the role of hypertriglycerid-aemia or hypercholesterolaemia in the induction of certain lesions (Table 22.3).

Hypertriglyceridaemia

Dogs with hypertriglyceridaemia may present with recurrent, but often self-limiting, episodes of abdominal pain, anorexia, vomiting, and diarrhoea (Rogers *et al.*, 1975a). The abdominal pain is frequently difficult to localise (Ford, 1993) and there is rarely demonstrable radiographic or clinical pathological evidence of pancreatitis. In the author's experience, dogs may be at risk of developing such clinical signs when the fasting plasma triglyceride concentration exceeds 5.5 mmol/l.

Lipaemia retinalis (pale pink appearance of the retinal vessels in the non-tapetal fundus) and lipid-laden aqueous humor, are ocular manifestations of marked hypertri-glyceridaemia (Kern and Riis, 1980; Crispin, 1993). Generalised seizures have been noted in Miniature Schnauzers with variable triglyceride concentrations (Rogers *et al.*, 1975a; Bodkin, 1992).

In the cat, hypertriglyceridaemia has been associated with lipaemia retinalis, lethargy and inappetance in kittens and young adult cats (Jones *et al.*, 1983; Watson *et al.*, 1992). Some cases presented at 8–9 months of age with peripheral neuropathies related to the development of xan-thomata (lipid granulomata) over bony prominences (Jones *et al.*, 1983).

Hypercholesterolaemia

In the dog, hypercholesterolaemia has been associated with the development of arcus lipoides corneae, an annular lipid infiltration of the peripheral cornea and perilimbal zone of the sclera. The condition has been recognised in German Shepherd Dogs with hypothyroidism and hyperlipidaemia (Crispin and Barnett, 1978).

Spontaneous atherosclerosis is a rare complication of marked hypercholesterolaemia in the dog but has been noted in dogs with thyroid dysfunction (Patterson *et al.*, 1985; Liu *et al.*, 1986).

INVESTIGATION OF HYPERLIPIDAEMIA

Hyperlipidaemia is often noted during routine laboratory investigations. The lipaemia associated with hypertrigly-ceridaemia may interfere with the production of accurate laboratory results. Pathological hyperlipidaemia should initially be confirmed in a fasting sample (12–16 hours) followed by exclusion of underlying metabolic or endocrine disease. If such a disease is recognised then further lipid investigation is usually unnecessary. In dogs with primary or idiopathic hyperlipidaemia, it may be necessary to categorise the lipid disturbances further (Figure 22.1).

The presence of chylomicrons and VLDL is confirmed in plasma samples stored overnight at 4°C. The chylomicrons float to the top of the sample forming a 'cream layer', while an increase in the VLDL concentration is characterised by an overall opalescence of the plasma infranatant (Figure 22.2). Laboratory confirmation of the presence of these, and the other classes of lipoproteins, is achieved by lipoprotein electrophoresis and combined ultracentrifuga-tion/precipitation techniques (Barrie *et al.*, 1993a).

MANAGEMENT

The plasma lipid concentrations in dogs and cats with secondary hyperlipidaemia return to normal, or near normal, after successful stabilisation or treatment of the underlying disease process. The following guidelines may be

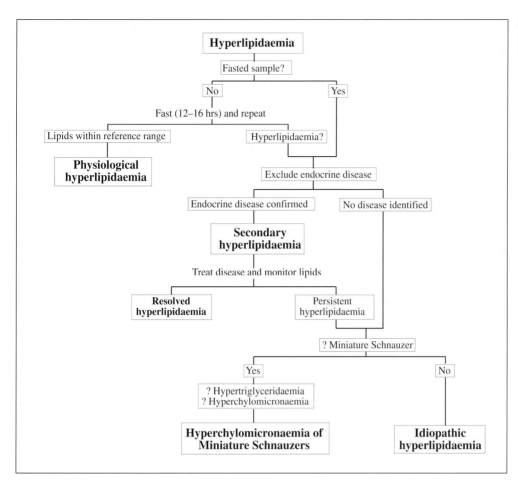

Figure 22.1: The investigation of hyperlipidaemia in the dog.

used for the management of persistent, inherited, or idiopathic hyperlipidaemias.

Dogs with a fasting plasma triglyceride concentration greater than 5.5 mmol/l are considered at risk of developing pancreatitis and lipid-lowering intervention should be instituted. Hypertriglyceridaemic dogs presenting with signs typical of acute pancreatitis should be treated symptomatically, including the maintenance of fluid and electrolyte balance and the withdrawal of food where necessary. The primary approach in the management of hypertriglyceridaemia is the reduction of dietary fat intake. A number of proprietary low fat, high fibre diets are available in canned and dry preparations. The diets should be fed according to the manufacturer's guidelines for maintenance, except in the case of obese animals where a weight reduction programme should be instituted. In many dogs it may be difficult to achieve plasma concentrations within laboratory reference ranges, and therefore the goal of therapy is to maintain a triglyceride concentration less than 5.5 mmol/l.

Kittens with familial hyperchylomicronaemia should be weaned and maintained on a low fat diet. Additional methods for lowering plasma lipid concentrations in the cat have rarely proved necessary.

In some dogs medical therapy may be required in addition to dietary fat restriction. A number of lipid-lowering therapies, including marine oils and gemfibrizol are used in human medicine, where their selection is determined by the nature of the underlying abnormality. These products are not licensed for use in the dog and cat. Until controlled therapeutic trials have been conducted in these species,

lipid-lowering drugs should be used with caution and the animals monitored at frequent intervals. The author has, however, had success with the use of an omega-3 polyunsaturated fatty acid supplement in the treatment of idiopathic hypertriglyceridaemia in the dog. In only one case of idiopathic hypertriglyceridaemia has the author found it necessary to try gemfibrizol therapy, and in this individual the drug was not effective.

SUMMARY

The successful management of the clinical manifestations of hyperlipidaemia in the dog and cat depends upon the reduction of the plasma lipid concentrations followed by regular clinical and laboratory evaluation.

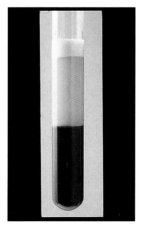

Figure 22.2: Canine serum sample stored overnight exhibiting 'cream layer' indicative of increased chylomicron concentrations, and opalescence of the infranatant indicative of increased very low density lipoprotein concentrations. The affected animal was suffering from concurrent hypothyroidism and diabetes mellitus.

REFERENCES

Barrie J, Nash ASN and Watson TDG (1993a) A method for the quantification of the canine plasma lipoproteins. *Journal of Small Animal Practice* **34**, 226–231

Barrie J, Watson TDG, Stear MJ and Nash ASN (1993b) Plasma cholesterol and lipoprotein concentrations in the dog: The effects of age, breed, gender and endocrine disease. *Journal of Small Animal Practice* **34**, 507–512

Bodkin K (1992) Seizures associated with hyperlipoproteinemia in a Miniature Schnauzer. *Canine Practice* **17**, 11–15

Crispin SM (1993) Ocular manifestations of hyperlipoproteinaemia. *Journal of Small Animal Practice* **34**, 500–506

Crispin SM and Barnett KC (1978) Arcus lipoides corneae secondary to hypothyroidism in the Alsation. *Journal of Small Animal Practice* **19**, 127–142

Ford RB (1977) Clinical applications of serum lipid profiles in the dog. *Gaines Veterinary Symposium* **27**, 12–16

Ford RB (1993) Idiopathic hyperchylomicronaemia in miniature schnauzers. *Journal of Small Animal Practice* **34**, 488–492

Jones BR, Johnstone AC, Hancock WS and Wallace A (1986) Inherited hyperchylomicronemia in the cat. *Feline Practice* **16**, 7–12

Jones BR, Wallace A, Harding DRK, Hancock WS and Campbell CH (1983) Occurrence of idiopathic, familial hyperchylomicronaemia in a cat. *Veterinary Record* **112**, 543–547

Kern TJ and Riis RC (1980) Ocular manifestations of secondary hyperlipidemia associated with hypothyroidism and uveitis in a dog. *Journal of the American Animal Hospital Association* **16**, 907–914

Larsson MG (1988) Determinations of free thyroxine and cholesterol as a screening test for canine hypothyroidism. *Journal of the American Animal Hospital Association* **24**, 209–217

Liu S, Tilley LP, Tappe JP and Fox PR (1986) Clinical and pathologic findings in dogs with atherosclerosis: 21 cases (1970–1983). *Journal of the American Veterinary Medical Association* **189**, 227–232

Patterson JS, Rusley MS and Zachary JF (1985) Neurological manifestations of cerebrovascular atherosclerosis associated with primary hypothyroidism in a dog. *Journal of the American Veterinary Medical Association* **5**, 499–503

Peritz LN, Brunzell JD, Harvey-Clarke C, Pritchard PH, Jones BR and Hayden MR (1990) Characterization of a lipoprotein lipase class III type defect in hypertriglyceridemic cats. *Clinical and Investigative Medicine* **13**, 259–263

Rogers WA, Donovan EF and Kociba GJ (1975a) Idiopathic hyperlipoproteinemia in dogs. *Journal of the American Veterinary Medical Association* **166**, 1087–1091

Rogers WA, Donovan EF and Kociba GJ (1975b) Lipids and lipoproteins in normal dogs and in dogs with secondary hyperlipoproteinemia. *Journal of the American Veterinary Medical Association* **166**, 1092–1100

Watson TDG and Barrie J (1993) Lipoprotein metabolism and hyperlipidaemia in the dog and cat: A review. *Journal of Small Animal Practice* **34**, 479–487

Watson TDG, Gaffney D, Mooney CT, Thompson H, Packard CJ and Shepherd J (1992) Inherited chylomicronaemia in the cat: Lipoprotein lipase function and gene structure. *Journal of Small Animal Practice* **33**, 207–212

Whitney MS, Boon GD, Rebar AH and Ford RB (1987) Effects of acute pancreatitis on circulating lipids in dogs. *American Journal of Veterinary Research* **48**, 1492–1497

CHAPTER TWENTY THREE

Phaeochromocytoma

Elizabeth McNiel and David C. Twedt

INTRODUCTION

Phaeochromocytomas are catecholamine secreting tumours arising from the adrenal medulla. Occasionally, this term is also applied to similar tumours of extra-adrenal origin, or paragangliomas (Feldman and Nelson, 1987; Norton *et al.*, 1993).

The cells comprising phaeochromocytomas are characterised by amine precursor uptake and decarboxylation (APUD). This describes the common biochemical feature of the cells, which involves the synthesis and secretion of biologically active amines (Morrison, 1984; Twedt and Wheeler, 1984; Feldman and Nelson, 1987). Tumours derived from such cells are often called APUDomas and include phaeochromocytomas, insulinomas, gastrinomas, and chemodectomas. APUDomas of various types share morphological features that suggest a common origin from neuroectoderm (Feldman and Nelson, 1987).

Phaeochromocytomas are reported in most domesticated animals including dogs (Bouayad *et al.*, 1987; Gilson *et al.*, 1994a) and cats (Patnaik *et al.*, 1990). These tumours are most commonly unilateral, but are occasionally present in both adrenal glands. Multiple endocrine neoplasia syndromes (MEN), defined as the excessive secretion by more than one endocrine gland, are well documented in people and may involve phaeochromocytoma (MEN type II). Specifically, MEN type IIa is defined by the presence of phaeochromocytoma, medullary thyroid carcinoma, and parathyroid hyperplasia or adenoma. MEN type IIb is defined by the presence of phaeochromocytoma, medullary thyroid carcinoma, and mucosal neuromas. Dogs with MEN have been reported (Peterson *et al.*, 1982). Phaeochromocytomas appear to be rare, especially in the cat, but are important because of the life-threatening sequelae.

Diagnosis of a phaeochromocytoma is a challenge, requiring familiarity with the syndrome. A large proportion of phaeochromocytomas (38–48%) are diagnosed at post-mortem examination (Bouayad *et al.*, 1987; Gilson *et al.*, 1994b). The purpose of this review is to describe the clinical features, diagnosis, and management of phaeochromocytoma in small animals.

PATHOPHYSIOLOGY AND CLINICAL FEATURES

In humans, the catecholamine most frequently secreted by phaeochromocytomas is noradrenaline, although adrenaline or a combination of the two have been reported. Secretion of other biologically active amines or peptide hormones may also occur (Norton *et al.*, 1993). It is not known whether the same is true for the dog.

Catecholamines stimulate receptors of α and β adrenergic classes, resulting in various biological effects. The different effects of adrenaline and noradrenaline are related to differences in potency for various adrenergic receptors. Adrenaline and noradrenaline both stimulate α_1, α_2, and β_1 receptors with equal potency. Adrenaline has greater stimulatory effect on β_2 than noradrenaline.

α and β adrenergic receptors are widely distributed in tissues and their stimulation has wide ranging effects:

- Stimulation of α_1 receptors by circulating catecholamines is responsible for generalised vasoconstriction, decreased gastrointestinal motility, and mydriasis
- Stimulation of β_1 receptors has positive inotropic and chronotropic effects in the heart
- Stimulation of β_2 receptors dilates visceral and skeletal capillary beds, relaxes bronchial smooth muscle, and decreases gastrointestinal motility.

Much of the clinical syndrome associated with secretory phaeochromocytomas may be explained based on these physiological affects.

Clinical signs associated with phaeochromocytomas are related to the secretion of catecholamine or invasive/metastatic characteristics of the tumour. Clinical consequences are diverse, ranging from no apparent clinical signs to cardiovascular collapse. Signs may either develop acutely or be episodic or chronic and progressive. Inconsistency in presentation is probably related to characteristics of the tumour including intermittent or continuous secretion of catecholamines, the amount and type of catecholamine secreted, and whether the tumour invades or thromboses the caudal vena cava (Twedt and Wheeler, 1984; Feldman and Nelson, 1987; Maher, 1994).

Clinical signs associated with phaeochromocytomas are commonly associated with the cardiopulmonary and nervous systems, but may be non-specific. General signs of weight loss, anorexia and depression are frequently reported. Respiratory signs including dyspnoea, panting, or cough are common (Bouayad *et al.*, 1987; Gilson *et al.*, 1994b). A complete list of reported clinical signs is shown in Table 23.1. Most of the clinical signs can be explained by hypertension (α_1 effects) and arrhythmias (β_1 effects)

Non-specific
Weight loss
Anorexia
Depression
Weakness
Collapse
Restlessness
Cardiopulmonary
Dyspnoea
Panting
Cough
Exercise intolerance
Cyanosis
Epistaxis
Neurological
Seizures
Paraparesis
Ataxia
Dilated pupils
Miscellaneous
Polyuria/polydipsia
Abdominal distension
Diarrhoea

Table 23.1: Clinical signs associated with phaeochromocytoma.

resulting from the secretion of catecholamines. Some of the clinical signs are attributable to local invasion by the tumour resulting in thrombosis of the caudal vena cava and haemorrhage into the abdomen.

The average age at presentation of phaeochromocytoma is 10.5 years although some very young (1 year) and old dogs (15 years) are reported. No sex or breed predisposition is apparent in dogs, although in humans the tumour may be familial.

Physical examination findings are usually non-specific. Tachycardia and arrhythmias are often evident. Thoracic auscultation may reveal abnormal lung sounds. Mucous membranes may be hyperaemic as a result of flushing from intermittent catecholamine release. Conversely, the membranes may be pale due to either vasoconstriction or anaemia from haemorrhage.

Thrombosis of the caudal vena cava and other vessels may account for some of the physical findings. Abdominal distension occurs due to vascular obstruction with ascites, but may also result from haemorrhage. Distension of the caudal superficial epigastric veins may rarely be seen. A few dogs have palpable abdominal masses.

Ophthalmic examination may reveal retinal haemorrhages as a result of hypertension. Neurological findings are often non-specific, but may indicate focal central nervous system lesions secondary to haemorrhage or metastasis. Hind limb paraparesis may occur secondary to vascular compromise as well as primary neurological abnormalities.

DIAGNOSIS

Diagnosis of phaeochromocytoma is difficult due to the lack of specific clinical findings and low index of suspicion of the disease. Results of routine laboratory work,

including complete blood count, biochemical profile, and urinalysis, are non-specific (Gilson *et al.*, 1994b; Maher, 1994b). Thrombocytosis may occur with tumours that are chronically bleeding. Liver enzyme elevations may be present but do not appear to correlate with the presence of hepatic metastases. Proteinuria is often found, presumably resulting from hypertensive glomerulopathy. A small number of dogs with pituitary dependent hyperadrenocorticism may have phaeochromocytomas (von Dehn *et al.*, 1995). Signs and laboratory work consistent with hyperadrenocorticism may lead to the impression that an adrenal mass is of adrenal cortical origin. Glucose intolerance occurs in some people with this disease. Dogs with diabetes and concurrent phaeochromocytoma have been recognised.

Radiographs of the abdomen reveal a mass in the perirenal area in 30–56% of cases (Bouayad *et al.*, 1984; Gilson *et al.*, 1994b). Abdominal detail is occasionally decreased due to the presence of fluid. Thoracic radiographs may reveal changes secondary to hypertension, including cardiac enlargement and pulmonary congestion or oedema. Metastases have been recognised in the lungs radiographically in approximately 11% of dogs (Gilson *et al.*, 1994b).

Indirect blood pressure measurements are helpful in identifying dogs with phaeochromocytomas. In one report, six out of seven dogs had hypertension at the time of measurement (systolic >160 mmHg, diastolic >100 mmHg) (Gilson *et al.*, 1994a). Most humans have hypertension in association with this syndrome but in many this is only episodic (Norton *et al.*, 1993). Repeated blood pressure evaluations may be necessary to document hypertension in patients.

Ultrasonography can be helpful in identifying an adrenal mass in cases of suspected phaeochromocytoma, but is limited in determining the extent of disease (Gilson *et al.*, 1994a,b). Echocardiography may reveal left ventricular hypertrophy consistent with systemic hypertension.

Other imaging studies including excretory urography, caudal venography, CT scans, and magnetic resonance imaging (MRI) may be helpful in determining the extent of disease (Norton *et al.*, 1993; Gilson *et al.*, 1994a). Nuclear imaging with [^{123}I]-metaiodobenzylguanidine (I-MIBG) has been performed for diagnosis of phaeochromocytoma in a dog (Berry *et al.*, 1993). MIBG is similar in structure to adrenaline and is taken up by APUD type cells. This method is commonly employed in clinical staging of people and may be used therapeutically in patients with metastatic disease.

Specific diagnostic techniques for phaeochromocytoma are aimed at identifying elevated circulating catecholamines or urinary metabolites of catecholamines. These techniques have been infrequently employed in dogs because of limited availability, poorly established reference ranges, and the problems of 24-hour urine collection. They may be useful in patients in which a phaeochromocytoma is strongly suspected based on clinical signs or the presence of hypertension, but a tumour is not identified with the imaging techniques mentioned. It is imperative that the clinician obtain specific sample handling instructions from the laboratory performing these assays.

Identification of urine catecholamines and metabolites

Circulating catecholamines are metabolised by the hep-atic enzymes, catechol-O-methyl transferase and monoamine oxidase. Unchanged catecholamines and metabolites (metanephrine, vanillylmandelic acid (VMA), and normetanephrine) are excreted primarily in the urine. Therefore, increases in circulating catecholamines which may occur with phaeochromocytoma result in elevations of urine catecholamines and metabolites. To measure urinary excretion of catecholamines, 24-hour urine collection is performed with the patient at rest. Urine must be immediately acidified with hydrochloric acid (pH <3) and refrigerated (Keiser, 1995). Random urine samples may also be used if the catecholamine values are expressed in mg/ml creatinine.

No reference ranges exist for dogs, and these assays have been infrequently performed. In humans, normal total urinary catecholamines are less than 150 µg/day. In patients with phaeochromocytoma values exceed 250 µg/day (Keiser, 1995). Normal human VMA and metanephrine values are <7.0 µg/day and <1.3 µg/day, respectively (Keiser, 1995). Test results may be influenced by exercise, excitement, foods containing vanilla, radiographic contrast agents, and various medications (Keiser, 1995). Improper sample handling and intermittent secretion of catecholamines by the tumour may result in false negative results. Additionally, the specific catecholamine secreted by a tumour and the metabolites produced in an individual patient may vary. Therefore, sensitivity of these tests is increased when multiple catecholamines or metabolites are measured. Finally, impaired renal function may decrease catecholamine excretion resulting in lower values.

Identification of serum catecholamines

Serum catecholamine (noradrenaline, adrenaline, dopamine) levels may be continuously or intermittently elevated in patients with phaeochromocytoma. Chromogranin A, which is secreted simultaneously with catecholamines, may also be elevated when a phaeochromocytoma is present. The function of chromogranin A is unknown. Catecholamine and chromogranin A measurements are performed on samples of heparinised plasma (Keiser, 1995). If the assay can not be performed immediately, the sample should be frozen.

Assays of resting catecholamines are not recommended for diagnostic purposes due to the wide variability of serum concentrations of catecholamines. Normal concentrations of catecholamines do not rule out the diagnosis of phaeochromocytoma, and currently no reference ranges exist for dogs.

Provocative tests

Clonidine suppression test

Clonidine is an α_2 agonist. Administration of clonidine should decrease neurologically mediated release of catecholamines. Phaeochromocytomas secrete catecholamines independent of neurological input. Therefore, concentrations of catecholamines in the bloodstream are not decreased with clonidine administration in patients with phaeochromocytoma. In humans, blood pressure and serum catecholamine concentrations are measured before and 3 hours after administration of 0.3 mg per 70 kg of body weight of clonidine orally (Keiser, 1995).

Catecholamine levels decrease by 50% in normal patients and do not fall in patients with phaeochromocytoma (Keiser, 1995). Blood pressure usually falls in both groups of patients. Results of this test are influenced by the magnitude of the serum catecholamine concentration. It is generally best in patients with high catecholamine concentrations (Keiser, 1995). Fluctuation in catecholamine concentrations with intermittent secretion by the tumour may influence results.

Phentolamine suppression test

When hypertension results from a phaeochromocytoma, α adrenolytic agents will result in a reduction of blood pressure. Phentolamine is an α adrenergic antagonist which can be administered intravenously. In order to perform this test, a hypertensive patient is monitored to obtain a stable baseline arterial blood pressure. Phentolamine is administered at 0.5–1.5 mg as an intravenous bolus (Keiser, 1995). Blood pressure is monitored every 30 seconds for 3 minutes then every minute for 7 minutes. Severe hypotension may result in shock; consequently patients must be monitored very closely.

A positive result is defined as a fall in blood pressure of >35 mm Hg (systolic) and >25 mm Hg (diastolic) for at least 5 minutes (Keiser, 1995). False positive results are common in human patients who are hypertensive for reasons other than a phaeochromocytoma.

Histamine, tyramine, glucagon and metoclopramide provocation tests

Histamine, tyramine, glucagon, and metoclopramide cause increased secretion of catecholamines by the phaeochromocytoma. Tests using these agents are not recommended due to the possibility of inducing a life-threatening hypertensive crisis.

SURGICAL AND MEDICAL MANAGEMENT

Surgery is the treatment of choice for phaeochromocytomas in dogs as in humans. Resection of these tumours tends to be problematic because many of these animals have a high anaesthetic risk as a result of hypertension and arrhythmias, which may worsen with surgical manipulation (Gilson et al., 1994b). Additionally, tumours may invade surrounding structures. Resection of the adjacent kidney and portions of the caudal vena cava are frequently required. Clearly, intensive anaesthetic monitoring and an experienced surgeon are necessary. At the time of surgical resection a thorough exploratory laparotomy is indicated to determine if metastases are present and to rule out the presence of other tumours.

Preoperatively, it may be of value to attempt to normalise blood pressure with α antagonist drugs. Phenoxybenzamine (0.2–1.5 mg/kg orally twice daily) may be the drug of choice due to its long duration of action (Norton *et al.*, 1993; Maher, 1994). Prazosin (0.5–2.0 mg/kg orally twice or three times daily) is an alternative choice. β-blocking agents may be used to control arrhythmias, but should never be used without α-blockade to avoid increasing hypertension (Feldman and Nelson, 1987; Maher, 1994).

When surgical resection is incomplete or animals have metastatic disease, continued management with adrenergic antagonist drugs may be necessary. Chemotherapy has been used in humans, but has not been described in the dog. [^{131}I]-MIBG has also been used in humans with disseminated tumour (Norton *et al.*, 1993). The value of this therapy in the dog is unknown.

PROGNOSIS

The prognosis is difficult to define precisely, as phaeochromocytoma is rare and a limited number of cases have been treated. As in humans, malignant and benign tumours cannot be distinguished solely by histopathology. Clinical evidence of invasion and metastasis defines malignancy (Bouayad *et al.*, 1987; Norton *et al.*, 1993; Gilson *et al.*, 1994a). Fifty per cent of phaeochromocytomas reported in dogs were considered malignant based on invasion and metastatic characteristics. Many dogs with non-invasive tumours may live normal lifespans. Extended survivals of 18 months to 2 years have been reported in dogs with successful surgical resection (Twedt and Wheeler, 1984; Gilson *et al.*, 1994b). Surgery has been effective in dogs with invasive tumours and has allowed for extended survival in dogs with metastases.

REFERENCES AND FURTHER READING

Berry CR, Wright KN, Breitschwerdt EB and Feldman JM (1993) Use of 123Iodine Metaiodobenzylguanidine scintigraphy for the diagnosis of a pheochromocytoma in a dog. *Veterinary Radiology and Ultrasound* **34**, 52–55

Bouayad H, Feeney DA, Caywood DD, Hayden DW (1987) Pheochromocytoma in dogs: 13 cases (1980–1985). *Journal of the American Veterinary Medical Association* **191**, 1610–1615

Feldman EC and Nelson RW (1987) Gastrointestinal endocrinology: The APUDomas. In: *Canine and Feline Endocrinology and Reproduction*, ed. EC Feldman and RW Nelson, pp. 387–395. WB Saunders, Philadelphia

Gilson SD, Withrow SJ and Orton EC (1994a) Surgical treatment of pheochromocytoma: technique, complications and results in six dogs. *Veterinary Surgery* **23**, 195–200

Gilson SD, Withrow SJ, Wheeler SL and Twedt DC (1994b) Pheochromocytoma in 50 dogs. *Journal of Veterinary Internal Medicine* **8**, 228–232

Keiser HR (1995) Pheochromocytoma and related tumors. In: *Endocrinology, 3rd edn*, ed. LJ Degroot, pp. 1853-1877. WB Saunders, Philadelphia

Maher ER (1994) Pheochromocytoma in the dog and cat: Diagnosis and management. *Seminars in Veterinary Surgery (Small Animal)* **9**, 158–166

Morrison WB (1984) The clinical relevance of APUD cells. *Compendium of Continuing Education for the Practising Veterinarian* **6**, 884–889

Norton JA, Levin B and Jensen RT (1993) Cancer of the endocrine system: the adrenal gland. In: *Cancer: Principles and Practice of Oncology, 4th edn*, ed. VT Devita *et al.*, pp. 1365–1371. Lippincott, Philadelphia

Patnaik AK, Erlandson RA, Lieberman PH, Welches CD and Marretta SM (1990) Extra-adrenal pheochromocytoma (paraganglioma) in a cat. *Journal of the American Veterinary Medical Association* **19**, 104–106

Peterson ME, Randolph JF, Zaki FA and Hunter H III (1982) Multiple endocrine neoplasia in a dog. *Journal of the American Veterinary Medical Association* **180**, 1476–1479

Twedt DC and Wheeler SC (1984) Pheochromocytoma in the dog. *Veterinary Clinics of North America: Small Animal Practice* **14**, 767–782

von Dehn BJ, Nelson RW, Feldman EC and Griffey SM (1995) Pheochromocytoma and hyperadrenocorticism in dogs: Six cases (1982–1992). *Journal of the American Veterinary Medical Association* **207**, 322–324

CHAPTER TWENTY FOUR

Hyperaldosteronism

Michael E. Herrtage

INTRODUCTION

Aldosterone is the major mineralocorticoid and is produced by the zona glomerulosa of the adrenal cortex. The release of aldosterone is influenced primarily by the renin–angiotensin system and by plasma potassium concentration (see Chapter 11). The excessive release of aldosterone from the zona glomerulosa is associated with profound electrolyte, fluid and metabolic disturbances.

CAUSES OF HYPERALDOSTERONISM

Hyperaldosteronism can be primary or secondary. Primary hyperaldosteronism, or Conn's syndrome, is defined as an increased production of aldosterone by an abnormal zona glomerulosa in the presence of low plasma renin concentrations. Aldosterone excess leads to increased sodium and water retention, potassium depletion, and suppression of the renin–angiotensin system (RAS). Secondary hyperaldosteronism is more common and is associated with continued stimulation of the RAS. It should be considered in any patient with cardiac failure, renal disease, and severe hepatocellular dysfunction where there is generalised oedema or activation of the juxtaglomerular apparatus. In secondary hyperaldosteronism, plasma renin activity is increased as a result of hypovolaemia or decreased effective circulating fluid volume and this in turn leads to increased secretion of aldosterone from the zona glomerulosa.

Primary hyperaldosteronism seems to be very rare in dogs and cats and there are few well documented cases. In humans, primary hyperaldosteronism is associated with marked muscle weakness, sometimes progressing to flaccid paralysis, polyuria, polydipsia, headache, paraesthesia, and hypertension. The source of the abnormally high concentration of circulating aldosterone is usually a small, solitary, aldosterone-producing adenoma of the adrenal cortex. Adrenocortical carcinomas associated with excessive aldosterone secretion are rare in human patients. About one third of human cases are caused by idiopathic, bilateral adrenocortical hyperplasia involving only the zona glomerulosa. This form of primary hyperaldosteronism has not been recognised in dogs or cats.

Two cases of primary hyperaldosteronism have been reported in the veterinary literature, one in a cat with a large adrenocortical carcinoma (Eger *et al.*, 1983) and one case in a dog which was more vague and less conclusive (Breitschwerdt *et al.*, 1985). Ahn (1994) mentioned several other cats with primary hyperaldosteronism due to adrenocortical carcinomas or adrenocortical adenomas, but few other details were given.

CLINICAL SIGNS

Aldosterone excess leads to sodium and water retention and potassium depletion with a loss of total body potassium and a reduction in plasma potassium concentration. The shift of potassium from its intracellular location to the extracellular fluid compartment results in intracellular movement of hydrogen ions, increased renal excretion of hydrogen ions and the development of metabolic alkalosis. Most of the clinical signs seen in hyperaldosteronism relate to hypokalaemia, which increases the cellular resting membrane potential, resulting in a larger difference between the resting and threshold potential necessary for an action potential and muscle contraction. This results in difficulty in stimulating muscles to contract, producing clinical signs of weakness and disturbed cardiac conduction.

The clinical signs of hyperaldosteronism tend to be vague and non-specific. Signs include weakness, lethargy, depression, and polydipsia and polyuria, all of which can be associated with hypokalaemia. The one documented cat with primary hyperaldosteronism was aged and presented with a history of chronic relapsing weakness and depression (Eger *et al.*, 1983). On physical examination, the generalised muscular weakness may be manifest in the cat by characteristic cervical ventroflexion, reluctance to

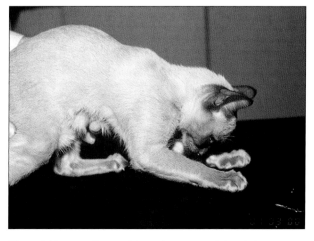

Figure 24.1: *Ventroflexion of the neck in a cat with hypokalaemia.*

move, poor muscle tone, and apparent muscle pain (Figure 24.1). Systemic hypertension due to sodium and fluid retention may be present in some cases of hyper-aldosteronism, and this can be confirmed by blood pressure measurement.

Decreased intake
Anorexia
Low potassium diets
Potassium poor fluid infusion
Increased gastrointestinal losses
Vomiting
Diarrhoea
Enemas
Increased renal loss
Chronic renal failure
Diabetic ketoacidosis
Hyperaldosteronism
Post-obstructive diuresis
Renal tubular acidosis
Hyperadrenocorticism
Diuretic administration
Excess glucocorticoid administration
Transcellular shifts
Metabolic alkalosis
Bicarbonate administration
Insulin administration
Undetermined causes
Hyperthyroidism
Young Burmese cats
Factitious

Table 24.1: Potential causes of hypokalaemia.

LABORATORY FINDINGS

Hypokalaemia with serum potassium concentrations <3.0 mmol/l is a consistent finding in cases of hyperaldosteronism. The differential diagnosis of hypokalaemia is detailed in Table 24.1 and should be considered before a diagnosis of hyperaldosteronism is pursued. Urinary potassium concentrations are increased.

Serum creatine phosphokinase activity is raised but blood urea concentrations are usually normal, and this distinguishes it from the more common causes of hypokalaemia in cats (Dow *et al.*, 1987; Herrtage and McKerrell, 1995).

Profound hypokalaemia detected in association with inappropriately increased plasma aldosterone concentrations provides a definitive diagnosis of hyperaldosteronism. Elevated plasma aldosterone concentrations with normal or low fasting plasma renin concentrations are consistent with primary hyperaldosteronism. An increase in both plasma aldosterone and plasma renin concentrations would be consistent with secondary hyper-aldosteronism. Plasma concentrations of aldosterone and renin must be measured by an assay validated for dogs and cats.

DIAGNOSTIC IMAGING

Imaging of the adrenal gland is discussed in detail in Chapter 10.

Radiographic examination of the abdomen may reveal a mass or mineralisation in the region of the adrenal gland, which could indicate the cause of primary hyperaldosteronism. Adrenal mineralisation, however, can be a normal feature of ageing cats. Thoracic radiographs should be examined for pulmonary metastasis.

Abdominal ultrasonography can be used to image each adrenal gland for evidence of pathology. Adrenocortical adenomas and carcinomas can be identified. The caudal vena cava and liver should also be examined ultrasonographically for evidence of metastases.

TREATMENT

The initial treatment of primary hyperaldosteronism should be directed towards the correction of the hypokalaemia. Hypokalaemia may be treated by intravenous or oral supplementation. Intravenous potassium supplementation is detailed in Chapter 19. Oral supplementation with potassium gluconate should be introduced early in the treatment because it is the most effective method for achieving sustained potassium delivery to the body. Potassium gluconate is administered orally at a dose of 2–6 mmol/day with dosage adjustment based on daily serum potassium concentrations.

The potassium-sparing diuretic spironolactone, is a powerful aldosterone receptor antagonist and has been shown to be successful in augmenting potassium supplementation in the treatment of hypokalaemia in cases of primary hyperaldosteronism. Spironolactone is administered at a dose of 2–4 mg/kg/day. Spironolactone acts by binding cytoplasmic receptor proteins in aldosterone-responsive cells located in the distal convoluted tubules and collecting ducts, thereby inhibiting sodium-potassium exchange, conserving potassium for the body, and facilitating natriuresis.

Surgical adrenalectomy for adrenocortical tumours is recommended and can be curative. It is of paramount importance that the patient's electrolyte, fluid, and metabolic disturbances are corrected first so as to minimise the perioperative complications. The technique of adrenalectomy is discussed in Chapter 10. If the adrenal mass cannot be removed or removal is incomplete, then continued medical management is required using oral potassium supplementation and spironolactone.

The long-term prognosis is difficult to assess until more cases have been documented.

REFERENCES

Ahn A (1994) Hyperaldosteronism in cats. *Seminars in Veterinary Medicine and Surgery (Small Animal)* **9**, 153–157

Breitschwerdt EB, Meuten DJ, Greenfield CL, Anson LW, Cook CS and Fulghum RE (1985) Idiopathic hyperaldosteronism in a dog. *Journal of the American Veterinary Medical Association* **187**, 841–846

Dow SW, Fettman MJ, Curtis CR and LeCouteur RA (1987) Hypokalaemia in cats: 186 cases (1984–1987). *Journal of the American Veterinary Medical Association* **194**, 1604–1608

Eger CE, Robinson WF, and Huxtable CRR (1983) Primary aldosteronism (Conn's syndrome) in a cat; a case report and review of comparative aspects. *Journal of Small Animal Practice* **24**, 293–307

Herrtage ME and McKerrell RE (1995) Episodic weakness. In: *Manual of Dog and Cat Neurology, 2nd edn*, ed. SL Wheeler, pp.189–207. BSAVA, Cheltenham

CHAPTER TWENTY FIVE

Feline Hypothyroidism

Boyd R. Jones

INTRODUCTION

Naturally occurring feline hypothyroidism is a rare disease. Congenital hypothyroidism may occur as a result of thyroid gland agenesis (Figure 25.1) or dysgenesis or from dyshormonogenesis (Arnold *et al.*, 1984; Peterson, 1989; Peterson *et al.*, 1994; Stephan and Schütt-Mast, 1995). Defects in thyroid peroxidase activity resulting in impaired organification of iodide have been reported in domestic shorthaired cats (Sjollema *et al.*, 1991) and in the Abyssinian breed (Jones *et al.*, 1992). In addition, hypothyroidism due to the inability of the thyroid gland to respond to thyrotropin (thyroid stimulating hormone (TSH)) has been described in a family of Japanese cats (Tanase *et al.*, 1991). These defects causing congenital hypothyroidism are usually inherited as an autosomal recessive trait.

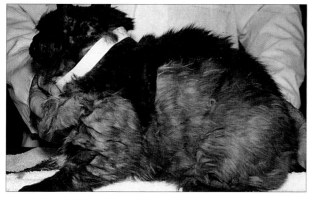

Figure 25.1: *Hypothyroid (thyroid gland agenesis) 16-month-old domestic shorthaired cat with a matted unkempt hair coat.*

Spontaneous acquired primary hypothyroidism due to lymphocytic thyroiditis has been described in an adult cat (Rand *et al.*, 1993) but the most common cause of hypothyroidism in the adult cat is as a sequel to destruction or removal of the thyroid gland after radioiodine or surgical treatment of hyperthyroidism.

CLINICAL FINDINGS

The clinical signs of congenital hypothyroidism may be severe or mild depending on the nature of the metabolic defect which, as in humans, may be partial or complete (Table 25.1). Many affected kittens die before hypothyroidism is suspected or diagnosed; most appear normal at birth, but by 4 weeks their growth rate slows and their small size becomes pronounced compared with their

| Dwarfism |
| Stunted growth |
| Short, broad head |
| Enlarged cranium |
| Shortened limbs |
| Delayed closure of growth plates |
| Retained deciduous teeth |
| Short, rounded body |
| Small ears |
| Apathy |
| Mental dullness |
| Inappetance |
| Lethargy |
| Constipation |
| Thickened skin |
| Soft, fluffy coat |
| Seborrhoea |
| Possible alopecia |
| Possible goitre |

Table 25.1: *Clinical signs expected with feline congenital hypothyroidism (cretinism).*

euthyroid littermates. Affected kittens show signs of disproportionate dwarfism, with an enlarged, broad head, short limbs, and short, rounded bodies. They are lethargic, mentally dull and less active than their healthy littermates. Other signs include bradycardia, hypothermia, constipation and weight loss. Teeth are frequently underdeveloped and replacement of deciduous teeth is often delayed until 18 months of age or older (Figure 25.2). Evidence of delayed closure of ossification centres of long bones is present. Alopecia is not a feature of congenital hypothyroidism, the haircoat being predominantly undercoat with a few guardhairs.

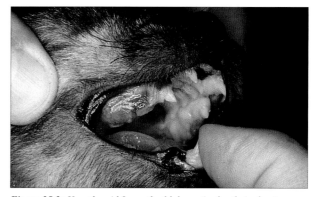

Figure 25.2: *Hypothyroid 9-month-old domestic shorthaired cat showing delayed eruption of permanent dentition.*

Survival of untreated hypothyroid kittens depends on the underlying defect. Kittens with TSH resistance deteriorate rapidly and most die before 16 weeks of age. However, kittens with defective peroxidase activity develop goitre and when they become adults their abnormal appearance and activity is often less noticeable.

In hypothyroid adult cats, skin changes (seborrhoea sicca, matting) are the predominant feature, along with lethargy, depression, hypothermia and bradycardia. Hair may be epilated easily, and regrowth is prolonged where the coat has been clipped. Alopecia is not a feature, but some cats do lose hair from the pinnae. Rand *et al.* (1993) reported puffy facial features associated with myxoedema and obesity in an affected cat.

DIAGNOSIS

Routine haematological and biochemical features

Consistent laboratory findings have not been reported for feline hypothyroidism. Haematological changes may not be present although a mild anaemia is occasionally detected. Serum cholesterol concentrations may be elevated but this finding is not consistent (Jones *et al.*, 1992). Peterson *et al.* (1994) reported that mild to moderate hypercholesterolaemia and anaemia are consistent findings in previously hyperthyroid cats which become hypothyroid after treatment.

Basal serum thyroid hormone concentrations

The total thyroxine (T4) concentration in newborn kittens should be approximately half the serum concentration of their mother. In 2 weeks, total T4 doubles and by 4 weeks of age is within the range 52–72 nmol/l (BR Jones, unpublished data). Basal serum thyroid hormone concentrations are below or at the low end of this range in kittens with the congenital disease and below the adult reference range in adult cats with hypothyroidism (Jones *et al.*, 1992).

Non-thyroidal illness

Many factors affect and diminish basal total T4 concentration, especially illnesses such as diabetes mellitus, renal and hepatic disease, and systemic neoplasia. Peterson and Gamble (1988) showed that the more severe the illness the lower the total T4 concentration. Mooney *et al.* (1996) also identified lower serum total T4 concentrations in sick cats compared with healthy cats. Serum total T4 concentrations were inversely correlated with mortality, supporting the findings of Peterson and Gamble (1988). Most cats with non-thyroidal illness had free T4 concentrations within the reference range or occasionally elevated, even though total T4 values were low. The above systemic diseases and other non-thyroidal diseases must be considered and excluded by thyroid function testing before a diagnosis of primary hypothyroidism is confirmed.

Treatment of hyperthyroidism

After treatment for hyperthyroidism with radioiodine or thyroidectomy, hypothyroidism can be expected. Cats treated with carbimazole or methimazole may have consistently low serum total T4 concentrations in the absence of detectable clinical signs of hypothyroidism. In these cats, the serum triiodothyronine (T3) concentrations are frequently within the reference range, even though the total T4 concentration is below that range (Peterson *et al.*, 1994).

If there is a high index of suspicion of hypothyroidism from the history and clinical findings, then measurement of a low basal T4 concentration supports the diagnosis. However, a definitive diagnosis should be made only after confirmation with a thyrotropin releasing hormone (TRH) stimulation test or a TSH response test.

TRH response test

The TRH response test is the most suitable and reliable provocative test for the diagnosis of hypothyroidism. A blood sample is collected for the measurement of total T4 before and 4 hours after the *slow* intravenous injection of 100 μg of TRH. Some cats may vomit after administration of TRH. In healthy cats and in cats with non-thyroidal disease, a 50–100% rise in serum total T4 concentration is expected. Hypothyroid cats have a low basal value which does not increase after TRH administration.

TSH response test

There are a number of different protocols reported for TSH response testing in cats (Peterson *et al.*, 1994). Most protocols require a blood sample to be collected for serum T4 measurement before and 6 or 7 hours after the intravenous administration of 0.5–1.0 IU/kg of bovine TSH.

Cats with hypothyroidism show little or no rise in T4 concentration above the basal value, whereas healthy cats will show consistent doubling or tripling of basal T4 concentrations (Sparkes *et al.*, 1991).

Additional diagnostic tests

Establishing the nature of the underlying defect in thyroid hormone metabolism may require additional investigations. TSH concentrations were elevated in Japanese cats with suspected TSH resistance (Tanase *et al.*, 1991), although the validity of the TSH assay for cats must be questioned, as a validated radioimmunological assay is not yet available for this species.

[131]I uptake

There may be no uptake of ^{131}I in thyroid agenesis, but in thyroperoxidase deficiency there is an increased uptake and increased discharge after the intravenous administration of sodium perchlorate. [131]I (0.125–1 MBq) is administered intravenously and thyroid uptake measured by a gamma camera. Unorganified ^{131}I is discharged 2 hours after administration by the injection of sodium perchlorate indicating impaired organification. Radioiodine uptake and perchlorate discharge testing are used to establish an organification defect. Thyroid gland biopsy for histopathological examination and biochemical investigations, including measurement of the tissue iodine content, peroxidase activity, and the presence or absence of thyroglobulin, are additional investigations for selected cases. Such studies are best completed at referral centres or at research institutions that have a special research capability for investigation of thyroid diseases.

MANAGEMENT

The recommended dose of L-thyroxine for treating a hypothyroid cat is 10–20 µg/kg daily by mouth. This dose should be increased or decreased depending on the response. In acquired hypothyroidism an excellent response should be expected. However, in the congenital disease the response is more variable and complete resolution of signs may not occur. Some kittens may remain apathetic and lethargic, and their small stature may persist despite treatment.

REFERENCES AND FURTHER READING

Arnold U, Opitz M, Grosser I, Bader R and Eigenmann JE (1984) Goitrous hypothyroidism and dwarfism in a kitten. *Journal of the American Animal Hospital Association* **20**, 753–58.

Jones BR, Gruffydd-Jones TJ, Sparkes AH and Lucke VM (1992) Preliminary studies on congenital hypothyroidism in a family of Abyssinian cats. *Veterinary Record* **131**, 145–48.

Mooney CT, Little CJL and Macrae AW (1996) Effect of illness not associated with the thyroid gland on serum total and free thyroxine concentrations in cats. *Journal of the American Veterinary Medical Association* **208**, 2004–2008

Peterson ME (1989) Feline hypothyroidism In: *Current Veterinary Therapy, 10th edn*, ed. RW Kirk, pp. 1000–1001. WB Saunders, Philadelphia

Peterson ME and Gamble DA (1988) Effect of non-thyroidal illness on serum thyroxine concentration in cats: 494 cases. *Journal of the American Veterinary Medical Association* **197**, 1205–1209

Peterson ME, Randolph JF and Mooney CT (1994) Endocrine diseases. In: *The Cat: Diseases and Clinical Management, 2nd edn*, ed. RG Sherding, pp. 1403–1506. Churchill Livingstone, New York

Rand JS, Levine J, Best SJ and Parker W (1993) Spontaneous adult-onset hypothyroidism in a cat. *Journal of Veterinary Internal Medicine* **7**, 272–276

Sjollema BE, den Hartog MT, de Vijlder JJM, van Dijk JE and Rijnberk A (1991) Congenital hypothyroidism in two cats due to defective organification: data suggesting loosely anchored thyroperoxidase. *Acta Endocrinologica* **125**, 435–441

Sparkes AH, Jones BR, Gruffydd-Jones TJ and Walker MJ (1991) Thyroid function in the cat: assessment by the TRH response test and the thyrotrophin stimulation test. *Journal of Small Animal Practice* **32**, 59–63

Stephan I and Schütt-Mast I (1995) Kongenitale Hypothyreose mit disproportioniertem Zwergwuchs bei einer Katze. *Kleintierpraxis* **40**, 701–706

Tanase H, Kudo K, Horikoshi H, Mizushima H, Okazaki T and Ogata E (1991) Inherited primary hypothyroidism with thyrotrophin resistance in Japanese cats. *Journal of Endocrinology* **129**, 245–251

CHAPTER TWENTY SIX

Autoimmune Polyglandular Syndromes

Richard M. Dixon

INTRODUCTION

Many of the common endocrine diseases in small animals result from immune-mediated destruction of the affected endocrine gland (e.g. primary hypoadrenocorticism or Addison's disease, primary hypothyroidism, insulin-dependent diabetes mellitus (IDDM), primary hypoparathyroidism). Although in most cases the underlying cause remains obscure, a genetic predisposition, together with one or more environmental triggers, is likely. Therefore it is not surprising that more than one endocrinopathy can occur simultaneously within individuals. In addition, these conditions may be found in association with other non-endocrine autoimmune diseases.

While autoimmune polyglandular syndromes (APS) have been recognised in man for many decades, until recently there has been scant information on similar conditions in the dog (Hargis *et al.*, 1981). Although APS remain uncommon in practice, their identification is crucial if the diseases are to be managed optimally.

AETIOLOGY AND PATHOPHYSIOLOGY

The destruction of affected endocrine glands results from both humoral and cell-mediated autoimmune processes, presumably through loss of normal regulatory suppressor T-cell activity (Verghese *et al.*, 1981). This process may progress over months to years but clinical signs only develop once function is below a critical threshold. During the destructive phase, circulating antibodies to the tissues or their products may develop; later in the course of the disease, when little normal tissue remains, these autoantibodies may disappear (Kintzer, 1992). In humans, detection of these autoantibodies can predict an impending endocrinopathy and therefore has prognostic value. The techniques for detecting these antibodies are becoming more widely available in veterinary medicine and may aid in the diagnosis of APS in domestic animals (Haines *et al.*, 1984; Hoenig and Dawe, 1992).

Genetic susceptibility plays a significant role in the development of APS in humans (Thomsen *et al.*, 1975) but similar data are lacking in the dog. There is overwhelming support for a genetic tendency in some common canine

Disease combinations	Reference	Number of dogs
Hypothyroidism and diabetes mellitus	Feldman and Nelson (1996)	13
	Hargis *et al.* (1981)	11
	Graham (1995)	8
	*Haines and Penhale (1985)	6
	Ford *et al.* (1993)	3
	Eigenmann *et al.* (1984	2
Hypothyroidism and hypoadrenocorticism	Melendez *et al.* (1996)	10
	Peterson *et al.* (1996)	9
	Feldman and Nelson (1996)	3
	Bowen *et al.* (1986)	1
	Kooistra *et al.* (1995)	1
Hypothyroidism and diabetes mellitus	Feldman and Nelson (1996)	9
	*Haines and Penhale (1985)	2
	Peterson *et al.* (1996)	1
Hypothyroidism, hypoadrenocorticism, and diabetes mellitus	Feldman and Nelson (1996)	2
Hypothyroidism, hypoadrenocorticism, diabetes mellitus, and hypoparathyroidism	Peterson *et al.* (1996)	1

Table 26.1: Autoimmune polyglandular syndromes recognised in dogs.
* Evidence of subclinical disease based on presence of autoantibodies.

Type I	Type II
Hypoparathyroidism	Hypoadrenocorticism
Mucocutaneous candidiasis	Autoimmune thyroid disease
Hypoadrenocorticism	Insulin-dependent diabetes mellitus
Chronic active hepatitis	Primary hypogonadism
Pernicious anaemia	Myasthenia gravis
Alopecia	Coeliac disease
Malabsorption syndrome	

Table 26.2: Human Type I and Type II autoimmune polyglandular syndromes. All diseases are not present in every case and other conditions may co-exist.

endocrinopathies such as hypothyroidism, Addison's disease, and IDDM (Kramer *et al.*, 1988). In addition, the finding of APS within close families and particular litters of dogs is further evidence of a genetic predisposition (Hargis *et al.*, 1981). The environmental triggers which result in clinical disease in patients who are genetically susceptible to APS are largely unknown, although infectious, chemical, and pharmacological agents have been implicated. Limiting exposure to these factors is not yet feasible but, because of a possible genetic component, breeding from affected animals must be seriously questioned. In addition, the investigation of both clinical and subclinical disease in related individuals may prove useful.

CLINICAL PRESENTATION

The clinical signs of APS relate to the endocrinopathies present (Table 26.1). A subclinical disease may become clinically apparent once another endocrine disease develops or is treated. Complications in an animal with a previously well controlled endocrinopathy, or an inappropriate response to adequate therapy, should also alert the clinician to the possibility of APS.

In dogs, hypothyroidism with diabetes mellitus and hypothyroidism with Addison's disease are most frequently recognised (Table 26.1). Additionally, hypoparathyroidism, hypogonadism, and other immune-mediated diseases such as immune-mediated bone marrow suppression, may also be recognised in varying combinations. In human medicine,

a comprehensive classification scheme exists which identifies different combinations of diseases as particular syndromes (Neufeld *et al.*, 1980; Eisenbarth and Jackson, 1992). Those canine conditions that are commonly recognised are equivalent to human Type II disease (Table 26.2).

The order in which conditions appear in human patients with APS is frequently predictable, e.g. candidiasis followed by hypoparathyroidism and subsequently hypoadrenocorticism in Type I disease, or hypoadrenocorticism and concurrent thyroiditis followed by diabetes mellitus in Type II disease. This allows appropriate sequential monitoring for each additional disease. In dogs, such progression is less well recognised.

DIAGNOSIS

Diagnosis of APS follows the guidelines for each individual endocrine disease, although caution should be exercised when interpreting the results of these tests in the presence of concurrent diseases. If possible, additional endocrine tests should be performed following treatment and stabilisation of the original condition. Clearly an exception to this is when two serious or life-threatening conditions are suspected simultaneously (e.g. addisonian crisis and myxoedema coma), and therapy in this situation may have to be given on the basis of historical and clinical findings before laboratory results are available. Fortunately, most components of APS will develop separately over months or years.

Antibodies against insulin, pancreatic β cells, adrenal cells, thyroid hormones, and thyroglobulin are all markers of immune-mediated endocrine disease. Their presence does not imply failure of the target gland, but should serve as a warning of possible future complications. Appropriate client education and patient monitoring is then possible. Currently, measurement of antibodies to thyroglobulin, thyroxine (T4), triiodothyronine (T3), and insulin is available in some commercial veterinary laboratories in the UK, and others may become available in the future. Given the relatively short lifespan of dogs compared with humans, it is possible that some endocrinopathies may never progress to a state of overt disease. The finding of autoantibodies may remain the only obvious abnormality in these patients.

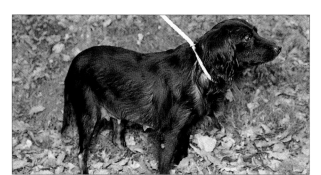

Figure 26.1: A 9 year old female crossbreed dog with bilateral cataracts and symmetrical alopecia, subsequently diagnosed with concurrent insulin-dependent diabetes mellitus and primary hypothyroidism. Courtesy of Carmel T. Mooney.

TREATMENT

Treatment of APS should be aimed at correction of the underlying endocrine disorders. Care should be taken when instituting therapy because the treatment of one condition may result in destabilisation of another, previously well controlled, disease.

There are no reports suggesting that immunosuppression of dogs with APS is indicated, and the use of high doses of glucocorticoids is likely to upset the management of some patients, e.g. diabetic or hypothyroid animals.

SPECIFIC CANINE APS

Hypothyroidism and diabetes mellitus

Hypothyroidism with diabetes mellitus is the most commonly reported of the canine APS. In one study, autoantibodies to pancreatic islet cells were recognised in 6 of 28 (21%) hypothyroid dogs (Haines and Penhale, 1985). In other studies, 13 of 124 (10%) and 11 of 62 (18%) hypothyroid dogs also had concurrent overt diabetes mellitus (Hargis *et al.*, 1981; Feldman and Nelson, 1996). The age of onset of IDDM may be important in determining the likelihood of a dog also becoming hypothyroid. Dogs diagnosed as diabetic under 7 years of age are 15 times more likely to develop hypothyroidism than those diagnosed when older (Graham, 1995). The progression of the two diseases is variable, with clinical signs of thyroid deficiency developing both before and after the diagnosis of diabetes mellitus (Hargis *et al.*, 1981; Graham, 1995). While hypothyroidism has been suggested as a possible cause of increased insulin sensitivity in one diabetic dog (Eigenmann *et al.*, 1984), it generally increases insulin requirement. Therefore hypothyroidism should be considered as a differential diagnosis for unusually high insulin requirements (Ford *et al.*, 1993). Additional clinical findings in affected dogs include those features characteristic of hypothyroidism but not IDDM (e.g. skin thickening, alopecia, lethargy). The diagnosis of hypothyroidism is complicated by the fact that diabetes mellitus often depresses serum total T4 concentrations. Ideally thyroid function testing should be performed after stabilisation of the diabetes. Thyroxine replacement therapy may result in a dramatic reduction in the insulin requirement and thus careful monitoring is required, at least initially, to avoid signs of hypoglycaemia.

Hypothyroidism and Addison's disease

Approximately 50% of all human patients with autoimmune Addison's disease develop at least one additional endocrinopathy, usually hypothyroidism (Greco and Harpold, 1994). This combination of diseases has also been reported, albeit less frequently, in the dog. In one study of 225 addisonian dogs, nine (4%) had concurrent hypothyroidism (Peterson *et al.*, 1996). Hypothyroidism should be suspected in any addisonian dog which exhibits inappropriate hypercholesterolaemia, obesity, dermatological signs, a poor clinical response to mineralocorticoid supplementation or persistent lethargy, heat-seeking behaviour, hyponatraemia, or bradycardia (Melendez *et al.*, 1996). Obvious clinical signs of Addison's disease may only become apparent following the treatment of hypothyroidism, suggesting that the former is precipitated or worsened by treatment of the latter (Bowen *et al.*, 1986). Partial adrenocortical failure (isolated glucocorticoid deficiency) has also been recognised in a dog with hypothyroidism (Kooistra *et al.*, 1995). As with IDDM, thyroid function tests will be adversely affected by Addison's disease and ideally these should be performed after stabilisation of the adrenal disease. When treating affected patients, T4 replacement therapy is likely to increase mineralocorticoid and glucocorticoid requirements. Careful monitoring is therefore required, and steroid dosages increased as necessary.

Addison's disease and diabetes mellitus

Concurrent Addison's disease and diabetes mellitus is less common than hypothyroidism with either Addison's disease or IDDM. Two of 12 (17%) dogs with hypoadrenocorticism were found to have autoantibodies to pancreatic islet cells (Haines and Penhale, 1985). In addition, nine dogs with concurrent Addison's disease and diabetes mellitus were reported by Feldman and Nelson (1996). Of 225 addisonian dogs, only two had concurrent diabetes mellitus (Peterson *et al.*, 1996); of these two dogs, one had concurrent hypothyroidism and hypoparathyroidism. As Addison's disease develops in a diabetic animal, reduced insulin requirements or hypoglycaemic episodes may develop and these should prompt appropriate investigation. Treatment with glucocorticoids in these patients will increase insulin requirements, and restabilisation of the diabetes may then be necessary.

REFERENCES AND FURTHER READING

Bowen D, Schaer M and Riley W (1986) Autoimmune polyglandular syndrome in a dog. *Journal of the American Animal Hospital Association* **22**, 649–654

Eigenmann JE, van deer Haage MH and Rinjberk A (1984) Polyendocrinopathy in two canine littermates: simultaneous occurrence of carbohydrate intolerance and hypothyroidism. *Journal of the American Animal Hospital Association* **20**, 143–148

Eisenbarth GS and Jackson RA (1992) The immunoendocrinopathy syndromes. In: *William's Textbook of Endocrinology, 8th edn*, ed. JD Wilson and DW Foster, pp. 1555–1566. WB Saunders, Philadelphia

Feldman EC and Nelson RW (1996) Hypothyroidism. In: *Canine and Feline Endocrinology and Reproduction*, 2nd edn, pp. 68–117. WB Saunders, Philadelphia

Ford SL, Nelson RW, Feldman EC and Niwa D (1993) Insulin resistance in three dogs with hypothyroidism and diabetes mellitus. *Journal of the American Veterinary Medical Association* **202**, 1478–1480

Graham PA (1995) Diabetes mellitus in association with other syndromes. In: *Clinical and Epidemiological Studies on Canine Diabetes Mellitus*. PhD Thesis, Department of Veterinary Medicine, University of Glasgow, Glasgow

Greco DS and Harpold LM (1994) Immunity and the endocrine syndrome. *Veterinary Clinics of North America* **24**, 765–782

Haines DM, Lording PM and Penhale WJ (1984) Survey of thyroglobulin autoantibodies in dogs. *American Journal of Veterinary Research* **45**, 1493–1497

Haines DM and Penhale WJ (1985) Autoantibodies to pancreatic islet cells in canine diabetes mellitus. *Veterinary Immunology and Immunopathology* **8**, 149–156

Hargis AM, Stephens LC, Benjamin SA, Brewster RD and Brooks RK (1981) Relationship of hypothyroidism to diabetes mellitus, renal amyloidosis, and thrombosis in purebred beagles. *American Journal of Veterinary Research* **42**, 1077–1081

Hoenig M and Dawe DW (1992) A qualitative assay for beta cell antibodies. Preliminary results in dogs with diabetes mellitus. *Veterinary Immunology and Immunopathology* **32**, 195–203

Kintzer PP (1992) Polyendocrine gland failure syndromes. In: *Current Veterinary Therapy XI*, ed. RW Kirk, pp. 383–385. WB Saunders, Philadelphia

Kooistra HS, Rinjberk A and van den Ingh ThSGAM (1995) Polyglandular deficiency syndrome in a boxer dog: thyroid hormone and glucocorticoid deficiency. *Veterinary Quarterly* **17**, 59–63

Kramer JW, Klaassen JK, Baskin DG, Prieur DJ, Rantanen NW, Robinette JD, Graber WR and Rashiti L (1988) Inheritance of diabetes mellitus in Keeshond dogs. *American Journal of Veterinary Research* **49**, 428–431

Melendez LD, Greco DS, Turner JL, Hay DA and VanLiew CH (1996) Concurrent hypoadrenocorticism and hypothyroidism in 10 dogs. *Proceedings of the 14th American College of Veterinary Internal Medicine Forum, San Antonio, Texas* (Abstract)

Neufeld M, MacLaren N and Blizzard R (1980) Autoimmune polyglandular syndromes. *Pediatric Annals* **9**, 154–162

Peterson ME, Kintzer PP and Kass PH (1996) Pretreatment clinical and laboratory findings in dogs with hypoadrenocorticism: 225 cases (1979–1993). *Journal of the American Veterinary Medical Association* **208**, 85–91

Thomsen M, Platz P, Anderson OO, Christy M, Lyngsooe, Nerup J, Rasmussen K, Ryder LP, Nielsen LS and Svejgaard A (1975) MLC typing in juvenile diabetes mellitus and idiopathic Addison's disease. *Transplantation Review* **22**, 125–147

Verghese MW, Ward FE and Eisenbarth GS (1981) Lymphocyte suppressor activity in patients with polyglandular failure. *Human Immunology* **3**, 173–179

CHAPTER TWENTY SEVEN

Pituitary Dwarfism

Elizabeth J. Norman

INTRODUCTION

Somatotropin, or growth hormone (GH), is secreted by somatotroph cells in the anterior lobe of the pituitary gland. Hypothalamic control of GH secretion is mediated by the opposing stimulatory action of somatocrinin, or GH releasing hormone (GHRH), and the inhibitory action of somatostatin. Release of these peptides is controlled by complex neuroregulatory mechanisms, circulating nutrient metabolite concentrations, and by the negative feedback effect of somatomedin C, or insulin-like growth factor-1 (IGF-1), and GH itself (Feldman and Nelson, 1996; Rijnberk, 1996) (Figure 27.1).

GH has both acute catabolic and slow anabolic effects. It acts directly on peripheral cells to restrict glucose uptake by antagonising the actions of insulin, and enhances lipolysis and hepatic gluconeogenesis. It stimulates the hepatic production of IGF-1 which mediates the long-term anabolic actions of GH: protein synthesis, chondrogenesis, and growth (see Figure 27.1). GH may also directly stimulate growth plate cell differentiation and local production of IGF-1 (Rijnberk, 1996).

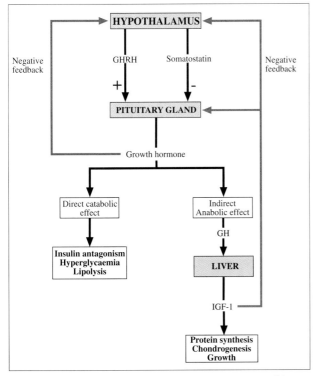

Figure 27.1: *Physiology of growth hormone (GH) secretion and its effects. GHRH, growth hormone releasing hormone; IGF-1, insulin-like growth factor-1; – inhibition; +, stimulation.*

PATHOPHYSIOLOGY

Pituitary dwarfism occurs when there is failure of secretion of GH in the young growing animal. One suggested cause of pituitary dwarfism is pressure atrophy of the adenohypophysis from cystic distension of the embryological craniopharyngeal duct (Rathke's cleft). However, this theory is questionable because such cysts are common, particularly in brachycephalic breeds, and only occasionally enlarge enough to cause pituitary dwarfism. Results of immunohistochemical studies offer an alternative explanation for the development of pituitary dwarfism, as they suggest that embryological oropharyngeal cells fail to differentiate into functional adenohypophyseal cells, and that their inactive secretions form abnormal cystic structures which compress adjacent tissue, resulting in further dysfunction (Capen, 1993). Whatever the underlying developmental abnormality responsible for pituitary dwarfism, there is a failure of secretion of GH alone, or of multiple pituitary hormones including follicle stimulating hormone, luteinising hormone, thyrotropin (thyroid stimulating hormone, TSH), and adrenocorticotropic hormone (ACTH), and their associated end-organ hormones. Panhypopituitarism describes a deficiency of all pituitary hormones. Insensitivity to GH at the cellular level produces secondary pituitary dwarfism in humans but is unproved in the dog or cat (Feldman and Nelson, 1996).

Pituitary dwarfism is rare but has been reported in various breeds of dog, and in the cat (Feldman and Nelson, 1996). The German Shepherd Dog is the most commonly

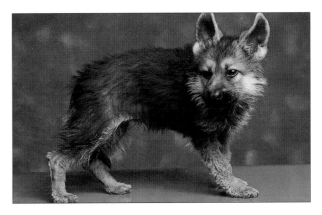

Figure 27.2: *A 7 month old German Shepherd Dog with pituitary dwarfism showing short stature, diffuse caudal truncal alopecia, and retention of the puppy coat. The dog weighed 4.7 kg. Courtesy of Dr C. T. Mooney.*

affected breed, in which pituitary dwarfism has been found to have a simple autosomal recessive mode of inheritance. There is no sex predisposition (Nicholas, 1978).

CLINICAL SIGNS

Growth and dermatological abnormalities

Pituitary dwarfism is characterised by growth and dermatological abnormalities (Figure 27.2), although the clinical picture may be complicated by other secondary hormone deficiencies. Failure to grow is usually easily appreciated by the time an animal is 2–3 months of age but the animal retains its proportional shape. The soft woolly coat of secondary (lanugo) hairs remains, and primary or guard hairs do not develop. The hair is easily epilated and there is gradual development of truncal alopecia, beginning at points of wear and sparing the head and extremities. With time the skin becomes thin and hyperpigmented, and may be scurfy and wrinkled. In many cases, there is delay in tooth eruption and closure of growth plates (Campbell, 1988; Feldman and Nelson, 1996).

Other abnormalities

Pituitary dwarfs are usually bright and alert initially. Aggressive behaviour has been noted in some dogs (Allan *et al.*, 1978). Although normal reproductive function may be maintained, typically there is absence of oestrous activity in females, and testicular atrophy and azoospermia in males (Feldman and Nelson, 1996). Mental retardation, disproportionate dwarfism, and epiphyseal dysgenesis suggest concurrent secondary hypothyroidism, and this may also explain the dullness and decreased activity which usually occurs with time. Other signs of hypothyroidism or hypoadrenocorticism may develop (see Chapters 11 and 14).

Skin and respiratory infections are common long-term complications of pituitary dwarfism (Feldman and Nelson, 1996). Maldevelopment of glomeruli due to lack of GH may impair renal function and, together with low filtration pressure due to glucocorticoid and thyroxine (T4) deficiency, may lead to azotaemia (Rijnberk, 1996). Neurological signs due to enlargement of the cyst are also possible.

The clinical signs of pituitary dwarfism are highly suggestive of the diagnosis but other causes of short stature (Table 27.1) should be excluded. Distinguishing congenital hypothyroidism from pituitary dwarfism can be particularly difficult because the clinical signs are similar and the two diseases may occur concurrently.

LABORATORY INVESTIGATION

In pituitary dwarfism, routine urinalysis and biochemical and haematological examinations are unremarkable but may be useful in differentiating the disorder from other causes of growth failure (see Table 27.1). Hypophosphataemia may be present due to decreased renal tubular phosphate resorption as a result of GH deficiency

Nutritional Underfeeding Poor quality diet
Physiological Accidental mismating between breeds Size variation within breeds
Endocrine Hypothyroidism Diabetes mellitus Hypoadrenocorticism Pituitary dwarfism
Gastrointestinal Parasitism Megaoesophagus Vascular ring anomaly Exocrine pancreatic insufficiency Chronic gastrointestinal obstruction
Cardiac Congenital cardiac disease Endocarditis
Hepatic Portosystemic shunt Hepatitis
Renal Renal dysplasia Polycystic kidney disease Tubular defects Glomerulonephropathies Pyelonephritis
Infectious/inflammatory Chronic inflammatory disease Feline infectious peritonitis
Iatrogenic Inappropriate glucocorticoid administration
Other Lysosomal storage disease Skeletal dysplasia/chondrodystrophy Mucopolysaccharidosis Immunodeficiency diseases Hydrocephalus

Table 27.1: Some causes of retarded growth in dogs and cats.

(Greco, 1995; Feldman and Nelson, 1996). Other abnormalities reflecting concurrent hypothyroidism or hypoadrenocorticism may be present (see Chapters 11 and 14). Histopathological examination of the skin demonstrates non-specific changes typical of endocrinopathies, and may reveal reduced numbers and size of dermal elastin fibres due to GH deficiency (Feldman and Nelson, 1996).

Assessment of pituitary function

Basal GH assay alone will not differentiate pituitary dwarfs from healthy animals. GH secretion in healthy animals is pulsatile, with trough values being similar to those seen in pituitary dwarfs (Feldman and Nelson, 1996; Rijnberk, 1996). The diagnosis of pituitary dwarfism is

Clonidine stimulation test

Dose:	10 µg/kg intravenously
Sampling times:	0, 15, 30, 45, 60, 120 minutes
Interpretation:	
Normal	Growth hormone (GH) >10 ng/ml (usually 10–15-fold increase) at 15–30 minutes followed by rapid decline
GH deficiency	Little or no increase in GH
Adverse reactions:	Sedation, bradycardia, hypotension, collapse, aggression, vomiting

Xylazine stimulation test

Dose:	100–300 µg/kg intravenously
Sampling times:	0, 15, 30, 45, 60, 120 minutes
Interpretation:	
Normal	GH >10 ng/ml (usually 10–20-fold increase) at 15–30 minutes followed by rapid decline
GH deficiency	Little or no increase in GH
Adverse reactions:	Sedation, bradycardia, hypotension, collapse, shock

Growth hormone releasing hormone (GHRH) stimulation test

Dose:	1 µg/kg intravenously (human GHRH)
Sampling times:	0, 15, 30, 45, 60, 120 minutes
Interpretation:	
Normal	2–4-fold increase in GH at 15–30 minutes followed by rapid decline*
GH deficiency	Little or no increase in GH
Adverse reactions:	None reported

* In some healthy animals a biphasic response may be seen (Abribat et al., 1989).

Table 27.2: Stimulation tests commonly used to detect hypopituitarism. Protocols for testing and sample handling may vary between laboratories; contact the laboratory concerned. At present GH assays are available at Department of Clinical Sciences of Companion Animals, Faculty of Veterinary Medicine, The University of Utrecht, PO Box 80.154, Utrecht 3508TD, The Netherlands.

Healthy adult dogs* and cats	200–800 ng/ml
Healthy dogs up to 1 year old	500–1000 ng/ml
Growth hormone deficiency, dogs and cats	<50 ng/ml
Acromegaly, dogs and cats	>1000 ng/ml

* Healthy toy breed dogs may have IGF-1 levels below this reference range.

Table 27.3: Interpretation of insulin-like growth factor-1 (IGF-1) assay results in dogs (medium to large breed) and cats. Validated by SCL Bioscience Services, 211 Cambridge Science Park, Milton Road, Cambridge CB4 4ZA.

confirmed by demonstrating inadequate release of GH following stimulation with either clonidine, xylazine, or GHRH (Feldman and Nelson, 1996). Test protocols commonly used are presented in Table 27.2. Age, nutritional state and concurrent disease, all affect pituitary responsiveness, and complicate interpretation of stimulation tests (Feldman and Nelson, 1996). GH assay is currently performed by species-specific radioimmunoassay, and is not widely available. Assessment of blood glucose concentrations during clonidine or high dose xylazine stimulation provides an alternative diagnostic marker. Glucose rises within 60 minutes in unaffected dogs, but fails to rise in pituitary dwarfs (Hampshire and Altszuler, 1981; Feldman and Nelson, 1996).

IGF-1 assay

IGF-1 assays are more readily available than GH assays. IGF-1 has a long half-life and its secretion is not episodic. A single basal sample can be used to assess pituitary function indirectly. Serum concentrations of IGF-1 are low in pituitary dwarfism but consideration of the breed is important because IGF-1 concentrations vary in proportion to size (Feldman and Nelson, 1996; Rijnberk, 1996) (Table 27.3).

Thyroid function

Assessment of thyroid function in pituitary dwarfs is necessary because of the similarities between congenital hypothyroidism and pituitary dwarfism, and the frequency with which the two disorders eventually co-exist in the latter disorder. Serum total T4 concentrations remain within the reference range in cases of isolated GH deficiency (Feldman and Nelson, 1996). Low serum total T4 concentrations in association with low–normal endogenous TSH concentrations support a diagnosis of hypothyroidism, and suggest the need for exogenous thyroid hormone replacement therapy in pituitary dwarfism. TSH, or thyrotropin releasing hormone (TRH), response tests (see Chapter 14) are rarely required. However, assessment of endogenous TSH concentrations before and after TRH administration is theoretically promising for confirmation of TSH deficiency.

Adrenal function

Adrenal function testing by ACTH stimulation is useful to detect those pituitary dwarfs requiring glucocorticoid supplementation because of secondary hypoadrenocorticism. A basal ACTH assay is also helpful (Feldman and Nelson, 1996) (see Chapter 11).

TREATMENT

Treatment of pituitary dwarfism is expensive and unrewarding. Canine or feline GH is not available but recombinant human GH can be given by subcutaneous injection at a dose of 0.1 IU/kg three times per week for 4–6 weeks (Feldman and Nelson, 1996). Porcine or bovine GH is not available in Europe, but is used at the same dose where it is available. Adverse reactions to GH therapy include hypersensitivity and diabetes mellitus, therefore daily urine glucose monitoring and weekly blood glucose determinations are recommended during GH therapy. Development of hyperglycaemia is an indication for early discontinuation (Feldman and Nelson, 1996). If indicated by thyroid or adrenal testing, T4 and/or glucocorticoid supplementation should be continued for life (see Chapters 11 and 14). Improvement of dermatological signs usually occurs within 6–8 weeks of beginning GH therapy, but most animals are presented too late for significant gain in size because of growth plate closure (Feldman and Nelson, 1996). Relapse of dermatological signs can be treated with GH at a dose of 0.1 IU/kg subcutaneously three times in one week (Feldman and Nelson, 1996). Response to GH therapy decreases in some cases; this may be due to development of antibodies to the injected GH (Feldman and Nelson, 1996; Rijnberk, 1996).

PROGNOSIS

The long-term prognosis of pituitary dwarfism is usually poor. Euthanasia of affected animals is often requested within 3–5 years because of mental dullness, alopecia, infections, degenerative diseases, and neurological signs (Feldman and Nelson, 1996; Rijnberk, 1996). More accurate documentation and early treatment of secondary endocrine deficiencies may improve the prognosis, even in animals where GH therapy is withheld.

REFERENCES

Abribat T, Regnier A and Morre M (1989) Growth hormone response induced by synthetic human growth hormone-releasing factor (1-44) in healthy dogs. *Journal of Veterinary Medicine, Berlin* **A36**, 367–373

Allan GS, Huxtable CRR, Howlett CR, Baxter RC, Duff B and Farrow BRH (1978) Pituitary dwarfism in German shepherd dogs. *Journal of Small Animal Practice* **19**, 711–727

Campbell KL (1988) Growth hormone-related disorders in dogs. *Compendium on Continuing Education for the Practicing Veterinarian* **10**, 477–481

Capen CC (1993) The endocrine glands. In: *Pathology of Domestic Animals, 4th edn*, ed KVF Jubb *et al.*, pp. 267–347. Academic Press, San Diego

Feldman EC and Nelson RW (1996) Disorders of growth hormone. In: *Canine and Feline Endocrinology and Reproduction, 2nd edn*, pp. 38–66. WB Saunders, Philadelphia

Greco DS (1995) Pediatric endocrinology. In: *Current Veterinary Therapy XII.*, ed JD Bonagura and RW Kirk, pp. 346–351. WB Saunders, Philadelphia

Hampshire J and Altszuler N (1981) Clonidine or xylazine as provocative tests for growth hormone secretion in the dog. *American Journal of Veterinary Research* **42**, 1073–1076

Nicholas F (1978) Pituitary dwarfism in German shepherd dogs: a genetic analysis of some Australian data. *Journal of Small Animal Practice* **19**, 167–174

Rijnberk A (1996) Hypothalamus–pituitary system. In: *Clinical Endocrinology of Dogs and Cats. An Illustrated Text*, ed. A Rijnberk, pp. 11–34. Kluwer, Netherlands

CHAPTER TWENTY EIGHT

Acromegaly

Mark E. Peterson

INTRODUCTION

Excess production of growth hormone (GH; somatotropin) causes overgrowth of bone, connective tissue, and viscera leading to giantism and acromegaly. In young patients, giantism develops when excess GH is secreted before closure of the epiphyses, whereas in adults acromegaly develops when excess GH is secreted after closure of the epiphyses. In patients with acromegaly, the increase in bone length is limited to the membranous bones such as the nose, mandible, and portions of the vertebrae, because the long bones cannot grow longitudinally once the epiphyses have fused. Acromegaly, but not giantism, has been documented in dogs and cats.

Growth hormone is normally synthesised by the somatotroph cells of the pars distalis of the pituitary gland. The secretion of GH is episodic and controlled by two hypothalamic hormones: GH-releasing hormone, which stimulates the production and secretion of GH, and somatostatin, which inhibits the secretion of GH. Growth hormone exerts its effects both directly and indirectly. The indirect actions of GH, mediated by insulin-like growth factor-1 (IGF-1) produced mainly by the liver, are anabolic and include increased protein synthesis and soft tissue and skeletal growth. In contrast, the direct effects of GH are predominantly catabolic, e.g. lipolysis and restricted cellular glucose transport.

Assays for plasma or serum GH concentrations permit confirmation of the diagnosis of acromegaly in both dogs and cats. Many of the clinical and laboratory findings in acromegalic dogs and cats are similar, but there are also some important differences between the two species.

PATHOGENESIS

The pathogenesis of GH excess is completely different in dogs and cats. In female dogs, acromegaly is most often caused by endogenous or exogenous progestogens that induce overproduction of GH (Eigenmann and Venker-van Haagen, 1981). Old, intact female dogs may spontaneously develop acromegaly because of the high progesterone concentrations characteristic of dioestrus. Attempts to suppress oestrus by administration of a long-acting progestogen such as medroxyprogesterone acetate, may also lead to acromegaly in dogs. This progestin-induced GH excess originates from foci of hypoplastic ductular epithelium in the mammary glands (Selman *et al.*, 1994a). Mammary GH is biochemically identical to pituitary GH.

In cats, as in humans, acromegaly is most often caused by a GH-secreting tumour of the pituitary gland (Heinrichs *et al.*, 1989; Peterson *et al.*, 1990). Progestogens do not stimulate excessive GH secretion in cats (Peterson, 1987).

CLINICAL FEATURES

Signalment

In humans, dogs, and cats, naturally occurring acromegaly is a disease of middle to old age. Unlike humans, in whom there is no sex predilection for acromegaly, more than 90% of acromegalic cats are male and all dogs with naturally occurring acromegaly are female. A bitch's predisposition for acromegaly is understandable, based on progesterone stimulation of GH production.

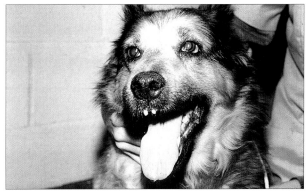

Figure 28.1: A 10 year old female intact dog with diabetes mellitus and acromegaly. Note the broad head, increase in interdental spaces, and inspiratory stridor (manifested by panting).

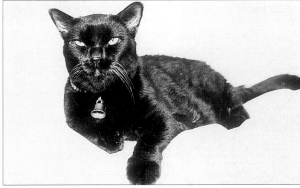

Figure 28.2: A 12 year old male castrated cat with severe insulin-resistant diabetes mellitus and acromegaly. The owners had noticed a gradual increase in the size of the cat's head and feet, and an increase in body weight. Note the broad face, prominent jowls, and increase in soft tissue over the eyes.

Finding	Dogs %	Cats %
Clinical signs:		
Polyuria/polydipsia	55	100
Inspiratory stridor	85	Rare
Renal failure	Rare	50
Cardiac failure	Rare	40
Arthropathy	Rare	40
Central nervous signs	0	15
Laboratory findings:		
Hyperglycaemia/glucosuria	30	100
Elevated serum alkaline phosphatase concentration	70	10
Azotaemia	Rare	50

Table 28.1: Manifestations of acromegaly in dogs and cats – similarities and contrasts.

General appearance

In humans, the earliest recognisable signs of acromegaly are soft tissue swelling and hypertrophy of the face and extremities. Facial alterations in humans include a large nose, thick lips, prominent skin folds, macroglossia, prognathism, and widened interdental spaces. Many of these same changes occur in acromegalic dogs and cats but, as in humans, the changes develop so insidiously that they are frequently overlooked. Both dogs and cats with acromegaly have been reported to show mandibular enlargement resulting in prognathism, widened interdental spaces, thickening of the bony ridges of the skull, large paws, and soft tissue swelling of the head and neck (Figures 28.1 and 28.2). Growth hormone-induced proliferation of connective tissue may cause the body to increase in size, most frequently manifested as marked weight gain and enlargement of the abdomen and face. Increases in body weight may occur despite the presence of the catabolic state of unregulated diabetes mellitus. The skin may become thickened and develop excessive folds, particularly around the head and neck. The growth and hypertrophy of all organs in the body, e.g. heart, liver, kidneys and tongue, is also a characteristic sign of acromegaly, especially in cats (Table 28.1).

Respiratory system

In acromegalic dogs, soft tissue proliferation in the oropharyngeal region may be so profound that panting, exercise intolerance, and inspiratory stridor due to compression of the upper airways occur (Figure 28.1). Inspiratory stridor due to narrowing of the upper airways is not seen in acromegalic cats; however, dyspnoea may develop as a result of pulmonary oedema or pleural effusion from GH-induced cardiac failure.

Diabetes mellitus

The most commonly recognised clinical manifestation of acromegaly in cats is insulin-resistant diabetes mellitus (Eigenmann *et al.*, 1984; Peterson *et al.*, 1990). Diabetes is also common in acromegalic dogs and, even in the absence of overt diabetes mellitus, many demonstrate carbohydrate intolerance (Eigenmann and Venker-van Haagen, 1981).

Growth hormone displays powerful diabetogenic activity, especially in carnivores (cats and dogs in particular), and seems to provoke hyperglycaemia, mainly by inducing peripheral insulin resistance. Excessive GH has been shown to reduce the number of insulin receptors and receptor binding affinity and induce a post-receptor insulin defect similar to that observed in patients with cortisol-induced insulin antagonism. This post-receptor defect in insulin action may lead to hyperinsulinaemia and subsequent downregulation of insulin receptors. These abnormalities in insulin binding and action result in hyperglycaemia and glucosuria and the accompanying clinical signs of polyuria, polydipsia, and polyphagia. Large doses of insulin are frequently needed to control the sustained hyperglycaemia.

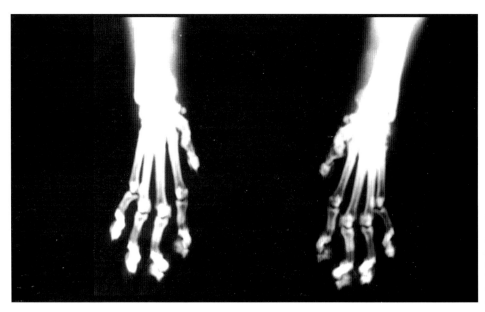

Figure 28.3: Dorsal palmar radiograph of the distal forelimb of a cat with acromegaly. Note the mild, diffuse soft tissue swelling, periarticular periosteal reaction, and collapse of the carpal joint spaces, consistent with degenerative joint disease.

Skeletal system

In some acromegalic cats, articular changes associated with degenerative arthritis may be severe and crippling. The articular changes initially result from fibrous thickening of the joint capsule and related ligaments, as well as overgrowth of bone and proliferation of articular cartilage. Later, as a result of the distorted joint architecture, features more typical of degenerative joint disease develop (Figure 28.3). Radiographic evidence of acromegalic arthropathy includes an increase in joint space secondary to thickening of the articular cartilage, cortical thickening, osteophyte proliferation, periarticular periosteal reaction, and collapse of the joint. Similar arthropathy has not been observed in acromegalic dogs.

Other bony changes that may occur in cats and dogs with acromegaly include enlargement of the mandible leading to prognathism and an overbite by the lower incisors. The spacing between the teeth may increase, as commonly occurs in acromegalic dogs. Finally, the bony ridges of the calvarium may be thickened, and marked spondylosis deformans of the spine may be evident in some patients.

Cardiovascular system

Cardiomyopathy occurs in some acromegalic cats (Peterson et al., 1990). Cardiovascular abnormalities that may be detected on physical examination include the presence of a systolic murmur, gallop rhythm, and, especially late in the course of disease, signs of congestive heart failure (e.g. dyspnoea, muffled heart sounds, and ascites). Radiographic findings may include mild to severe cardiomegaly, pleural effusion, and pulmonary oedema. Echocardiographic examination most frequently reveals left ventricular and septal hypertrophy; however, electrocardiographic findings are normal. Similar cardiac changes have not been observed in acromegalic dogs.

The cause of cardiac disease in acromegalic cats is not clear, but may be related to the general growth-promoting effect of excess GH on tissues. Hypertension, common in humans with acromegaly, may also contribute to the cardiac hypertrophy, but blood pressure determinations have not been reported consistently in acromegalic animals.

Nervous system

In acromegalic cats, central nervous system (CNS) signs can develop as a result of the extrasellar expansion of the pituitary tumour, but overt neurological signs are rare, even when a large pituitary tumour is compressing and invading the hypothalamus (Peterson et al., 1990). Acromegalic dogs do not have pituitary tumours so CNS signs are not expected.

Renal system

Polyuria and polydipsia are common signs of acromegaly in cats and dogs and seem to develop primarily because of the associated diabetic state. However, acromegaly also causes several other alterations in renal function. The kidneys become hypertrophied, leading to an increased glomerular filtration rate and renal blood flow.

In cats with longstanding acromegaly, azotaemia, proteinuria, and clinical signs of renal failure may develop (Peterson et al., 1990). Histologically, the kidneys of these cats are characterised by mesangial thickening of the glomeruli, changes similar to those described in humans with diabetic nephropathy. The mechanism of impairment of renal function in acromegalic cats is not clear, but may result from the glomerulosclerosis associated with unregulated diabetes mellitus or GH-mediated glomerular hyperfiltration. Renal failure has not been observed in acromegalic dogs.

Reproductive system

In dogs with progesterone-induced acromegaly, concomitant pyometra, mucometra, and mammary gland nodules may develop (Concannon et al., 1980). High circulating concentrations of progesterone alone could cause these conditions, however the high circulating GH concentrations superimposed on high progesterone concentrations may also play a role.

Hypoadrenocorticism

Low serum cortisol concentrations and atrophy of the adrenal cortex may develop in dogs in whom acromegaly is caused by chronic administration of progestogens. The intrinsic glucocorticoid-like activity of these progestogens suppresses adrenocorticotrophic hormone (ACTH) secretion, causing secondary hypoadrenocorticism (Selman et al., 1994b).

In contrast to dogs, in whom progestogen treatment or high circulating progesterone concentrations during dioestrus can stimulate excess GH production, progestogens do not stimulate GH secretion in cats (Peterson, 1987). However, administration of high doses of progestogens to cats also suppresses the pituitary–adrenal axis and leads to secondary hypoadrenocorticism (Peterson, 1987).

ROUTINE LABORATORY TESTS

Routine laboratory investigation of acromegaly often reveals hyperglycaemia and glycosuria, especially in affected cats. Less frequently there are increases in cholesterol, alanine aminotransferase, and serum alkaline phosphatase (ALP), which may be related to the diabetic state. However, even in many acromegalic dogs without diabetes, ALP activity is high; possible causes for this include production of steroid-induced or bone isoenzyme by progesterone, or hepatic lipidosis associated with GH-stimulated mobilisation of fat from adipose tissue.

DIAGNOSIS

Acromegaly should be suspected in bitches receiving progestogens, intact female dogs that develop diabetes mellitus or laryngeal stridor during metoestrus, and any cat that has severe insulin-resistant diabetes mellitus (i.e. persistent hyperglycaemia despite daily insulin doses greater than 20 IU/day), especially if other characteristic signs of acromegaly, such as arthropathy or cardiomyopathy, are also present.

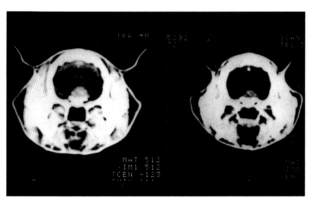

Figure 28.4: Computerised tomogram of the head of a cat with acromegaly, before and after external beam radiotherapy. (Left) Before radiotherapy: note the large mass in the region of the pituitary and hypothalamus following the intravenous administration of a positive contrast agent. (Right) Two months after radiotherapy: note the size of the pituitary tumor has decreased by approximately 50%.

Confirmation of the diagnosis requires demonstration of high circulating GH concentrations. Unfortunately, the availability of veterinary laboratories performing radioimmunoassays of GH in dogs and cats is limited. Instead, most acromegalic dogs are tentatively diagnosed on the basis of characteristic clinical and laboratory findings, exposure to a progesterone source, improvement in clinical signs after withdrawal of progesterone, and no evidence of spontaneous hyperadrenocorticism on adrenal testing. Similarly, in cats the presumptive diagnosis of acromegaly is made on the basis of characteristic clinical and laboratory features, normal results on thyroid and adrenal testing, and documentation of a pituitary mass with computerised tomography (Figure 28.4) or magnetic resonance imaging.

The determination of IGF-1 may also contribute to the diagnosis of acromegaly by indirectly evaluating the GH concentration. Dogs and cats with acromegaly have a high IGF-1 concentration.

TREATMENT

The treatment for progesterone-induced acromegaly in dogs is ovariohysterectomy or discontinuation of progestogen drugs (Eigenmann and Venker-van Haagen, 1981). The GH concentration will normalise (rapidly after ovariohysterectomy and more slowly after withdrawal of progestogen drugs) accompanied by resolution of the soft tissue proliferation and signs of respiratory stridor; however, skeletal changes may persist. The insulin requirement for GH-induced diabetes mellitus will also decline, but the reversibility of the diabetes depends on the insulin reserve of the pancreatic β islet cells.

In acromegalic cats, treatment should be directed at the pituitary tumour in one of three ways: drugs, irradiation, or hypophysectomy. Little has been published about any of these treatments. From the limited number of reported cases, it may be concluded that treatment with drugs such

as the dopamine agonist bromocriptine is not very effective in cats. The long-acting somatostatin analogue, octreotide, may lower circulating GH concentrations in some cats, but its use in clinical practice is questionable because it is expensive and needs to be injected several times a day. No reports have been published on the long-term use of octreotide. External beam radiotherapy has resulted in improvement in a few cats (see Figure 28.4). However, clinical improvement following radiotherapy is often slow in onset, and radiotherapy may not be effective in destroying large invasive pituitary tumours and is of limited availability. Finally, hypophysectomy may become the treatment of choice for small pituitary tumours, but surgical excision of GH-secreting tumours has not been evaluated in acromegalic cats.

PROGNOSIS

In dogs with progestogen-induced GH excess, the prognosis is good after removal of the progesterone source. Diabetes mellitus resulting from GH excess is sometimes reversible after removal of the GH source. Persistence of excess GH is accompanied by insulin resistance, which can be severe.

In cats, the short-term prognosis is relatively good, but although insulin-resistant diabetes mellitus can generally be managed satisfactorily, this requires large daily doses of insulin, at considerable expense. Complications such as congestive heart failure, renal failure, or an expanding pituitary tumour usually result in death within 1–2 years.

REFERENCES

Concannon P, Altszuler N, Hampshire J, Butler WR and Jansel W (1980) Growth hormone, prolactin, and cortisol in dogs developing mammary nodules and an acromegaly-like appearance during treatment with medroxyprogesterone acetate. *Endocrinology* **106**, 1173–1177

Eigenmann JE and Venker-van Haagen AJ (1981) Progestogen-induced and spontaneous canine acromegaly due to reversible growth hormone overproduction: Clinical picture and pathogenesis. *Journal of the American Animal Hospital Association* **17**, 813–822

Eigenmann JE, Wortman JA and Haskins ME (1984) Elevated growth hormone levels and diabetes mellitus in a cat with acromegalic features. *Journal of the American Animal Hospital Association* **20**, 747–752

Heinrichs M, Baumgartner W and Krug-Manntz S (1989) Immunocytochemical demonstration of growth hormone in an acidophilic adenoma of the adenohypophysis in a cat. *Veterinary Pathology* **26**, 179

Peterson ME (1987) Effects of megestrol acetate on glucose tolerance and growth hormone secretion in the cat. *Research in Veterinary Science* **42**, 354–357

Peterson ME, Taylor RS, Greco DS, Nelson RW, Randolph JF, Foodman MS, Moroff SD, Morrison SA and Lothrop CD (1990) Acromegaly in 14 cats. *Journal of Veterinary Internal Medicine* **4**, 192–201

Selman PJ, Mol JA, Rutteman GR, Van GE and Rijnberk A (1994a) Progestin-induced growth hormone excess in the dog originates in the mammary gland. *Endocrinology* **134**, 287–292

Selman PJ, Mol JA, Rutteman GR and Rijnberk A (1994b) Progestin treatment in the dog. II. Effects on the hypothalamic–pituitary–adrenocortical axis. *European Journal of Endocrinology* **131**, 422–430

CHAPTER TWENTY NINE

Feline Hyperadrenocorticism

Mark E. Peterson

INTRODUCTION

Hyperadrenocorticism (Cushing's syndrome) is caused by excessive production of glucocorticoids by either functional neoplasms of the adrenal cortex or bilateral adrenocortical hyperplasia. The latter results from over-production of adrenocorticotropic hormone (ACTH) by neoplastic or, less commonly, hyperplastic pituitary corticotrophs (pituitary-dependent hyperadrenocorticism). While hyperadrenocorticism seems to be rare, both pituitary-dependent hyperadrenocorticism and functional adrenal tumours (adenoma and carcinoma) have been identified in the cat (Peterson *et al.*, 1994; Duesberg and Peterson, 1997). Approximately 85% of cats with naturally occurring hyperadrenocorticism have the pituitary-dependent form of the disorder. In addition, although cats tend to be more resistant to the effects of exogenous glucocorticoid excess than dogs, iatrogenic hyperadrenocorticism is a well recognised disorder in cats.

CLINICAL FEATURES

Hyperadrenocorticism appears to be a disease of middle-aged and old cats. As with Cushing's disease in humans, there appears to be a strong female predilection in cats, unlike dogs in which there is no sex predilection (at least for pituitary-dependent hyperadrenocorticism).

The most common clinical signs associated with hyperadrenocorticism include polyuria, polydipsia, polyphagia, and a pendulous abdomen (Table 29.1). Despite the apparent similarity between cats and dogs with hyperadrenocorticism, there are major differences in clinical presentation.

Polyuria and polydipsia

Polyuria and polydipsia are usually the earliest signs of hyperadrenocorticism in dogs, and develop in over 80% of cases. In dogs, it seems that glucocorticoids inhibit the secretion or action of antidiuretic hormone, resulting in polyuria with secondary polydipsia. Although hyperglycaemic osmotic diuresis might also contribute to these signs, most dogs with hyperadrenocorticism have normal or only mild increases in blood glucose concentration. By contrast, the onset of polyuria and polydipsia in cats treated with large doses of glucocorticoids, or with naturally occurring hyperadrenocorticism, is often delayed and usually coincides with the development of moderate to severe hyperglycaemia and glucosuria, with subsequent osmotic

Abnormality	Number of cats (%)
Clinical signs:	
Polyuria/polydipsia	27 (90%)
Pot-bellied appearance	24 (80%)
Increased appetite	20 (67%)
Muscle wasting	19 (63%)
Hair loss	18 (60%)
Thin skin	17 (57%)
Lethargy	15 (50%)
Obesity/weight gain	11 (37%)
Fragile, tearing skin	11 (37%)
Infection	11 (37%)
Hepatomegaly	10 (33%)
Weight loss	10 (33%)
Seborrhoea (unkempt haircoat)	9 (30%)
Laboratory findings:	
Hyperglycaemia	28 (93%)
Glycosuria	28 (93%)
Lymphopenia	18 (62%)
Eosinopenia	15 (52%)
Hypercholesterolaemia	14 (47%)
Increased alanine amino-transferase	13 (43%)
Mature leucocytosis	13 (45%)
Monocytosis	7 (24%)
Increased alkaline phosphatase	6 (20%)
Ketonuria	4 (13%)

Table 29.1: *Clinical signs and abnormal laboratory findings in 30 cats*

diuresis. Therefore, it is likely that these signs would not be present during the less advanced stages of hyperadrenocorticism when glucose tolerance is still normal (i.e. before the development of diabetes mellitus).

Skin fragility

Extreme fragility of the skin, one of the major cutaneous manifestations of hyperadrenocorticism in cats, develops only rarely, if at all, in dogs with the disorder. Fragility of the skin, resembling that seen in cats with cutaneous asthenia (Ehlers–Danlos syndrome), developed in over a third of 30 cats reported with hyperadrenocorticism. In affected cats, the skin tends to tear with routine handling, leaving large denuded areas (Figure 29.1). Although many cutaneous features of hyperadrenocorticism in cats are similar to those reported in dogs (e.g. hair loss, atrophic

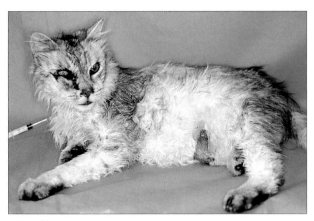

Figure 29.1: Cat with hyperadrenocorticism due to a unilateral adrenal adenoma. Note the unkempt haircoat, chronic eye infection, and open non-healing wound on the ventral abdomen. The non-healing would is secondary to severe thinning of the skin.

thin skin, and bruising of the skin), skin fragility seems to be a unique but serious manifestation of the disease in cats.

SCREENING LABORATORY TESTS

The abnormalities on routine laboratory testing of feline hyperadrenocorticism are variable. There may be a mature leucocytosis, eosinopenia, lymphopenia and monocytosis, but these findings are inconsistent (see Table 29.1).

By far the most striking serum biochemical abnormalities reported in feline hyperadrenocorticism are severe hyperglycaemia and glycosuria. Hypercholesterolaemia develops in about half of affected cats and is probably caused, at least in part, by a poorly controlled diabetic state. Elevated activity of serum alanine aminotransferase (ALT) also develops in about 40% of affected cats, probably related to the hepatic lipidosis associated with diabetes. In dogs with hyperadrenocorticism, steroid induction of a specific hepatic isoenzyme of alkaline phosphatase (ALP) causes increases in the serum activity of this enzyme in 85–90% of dogs, whereas only 20% of cats with hyperadrenocorticism have high serum ALP activity (see Table 29.1). The mild increase in serum ALP activity found in some cats probably results from the poorly regulated diabetic state rather than from a direct effect of glucocorticoid excess, since the serum ALP activity may normalise with insulin treatment alone, despite progression of the hyperadrenocorticism.

PITUITARY–ADRENAL FUNCTION TESTS

Basal serum cortisol determinations
Basal serum cortisol determinations are of little value in the diagnosis of feline hyperadrenocorticism. In a clinical setting, a large percentage of cats are likely to exhibit high–normal or high resting serum cortisol concentrations due to the effects of stress or non-adrenal disease. Conversely, a finding of a normal serum cortisol concentration should not be used to exclude a diagnosis of hyperadrenocorticism.

ACTH stimulation tests
The ACTH stimulation test is a valuable screening test for feline hyperadrenocorticism. One regimen commonly used for testing is to collect the blood for determination of serum (or plasma) cortisol concentration before and at 60–90 minutes after intravenous administration of 0.125 mg synthetic ACTH (tetracosactrin) (Peterson *et al.*, 1994); some authors recommend collecting two samples at 60 and 120 minutes (Sparkes *et al.*, 1990). Regardless of the basal cortisol value obtained, diagnosis of hyperadrenocorticism depends on the demonstration of a cortisol concentration after stimulation with ACTH that is significantly higher than the reference range.

Recent studies have reported that a variety of chronic illnesses not associated with hyperadrenocorticism can also influence ACTH-stimulated cortisol secretion in cats (Zerbe *et al.*, 1987). It is likely that the stress associated with chronic illness results in some degree of bilateral adrenocortical hyperplasia in ill cats, which could account for an exaggerated cortisol response to ACTH. Therefore, the diagnosis of hyperadrenocorticism should be based primarily on the cat's history, clinical signs, and routine laboratory findings, and not solely on the results of serum cortisol determination.

Dexamethasone suppression tests
Low- and high-dose dexamethasone suppression tests have proved useful in the diagnosis of hyperadrenocorticism in dogs and humans, but have not been well standardised in cats. Dexamethasone at a dose of 0.010–0.015 mg/kg intravenously is sufficient to suppress serum cortisol concentrations consistently to low or undetectable values for at least 8 hours in healthy cats (Peterson *et al.*, 1994; Duesberg and Peterson, 1997). However, further studies must be done before a low-dose dexamethasone suppression test can be considered a definitive diagnostic test for feline hyperadrenocorticism. As with the ACTH stimulation test, a variety of illnesses other than hyperadrenocorticism can influence the results of low-dose dexamethasone suppression tests. The high-dose dexamethasone suppression test (0.1 mg/kg intravenously) may be the preferred method of screening for hyperadrenocorticism, at least for now.

The ACTH stimulation test and the high-dose (0.1 mg/kg) dexamethasone suppression test — especially in the latter case when samples after dexamethasone administration are collected at 2–4 hours — appear to be useful screening tests for feline hyperadrenocorticism. Therefore, it may be reasonable to combine the two screening tests to help in the diagnosis, as only three or four blood samples need to be collected over a 3–4 hour period:

1 Collect a baseline blood sample for serum cortisol determination
2 Administer a high dose of dexamethasone (0.1 mg/kg, intravenously)
3 Collect a post-dexamethasone sample for serum cortisol determination at 2 hours
4 Immediately administer synthetic ACTH (0.125 mg, intravenously)

5   Collect post-ACTH sample for cortisol determination at 3 hours (1 hour after ACTH administration).

Most cats with hyperadrenocorticism do not show serum cortisol suppression after dexamethasone administration, and have markedly exaggerated responses to ACTH stimulation. By contrast, normal cats and diabetic cats without hyperadrenocorticism show marked serum cortisol suppression after dexamethasone administration and have normal cortisol responses after ACTH stimulation.

Endogenous ACTH determinations

The determination of basal endogenous ACTH concentration appears to be a valuable test for differentiating the origin of hyperadrenocorticism in cats with clinical signs and screening test results diagnostic for hyperadrenocorticism (Peterson *et al.*, 1994; Duesberg and Peterson, 1997). Endogenous ACTH concentrations are high in cats with pituitary-dependent hyperadrenocorticism, but low to undetectable in cats with functional adrenocortical tumours. It is important to remember that blood samples for determination of endogenous ACTH concentration need to be handled carefully, in accordance with the instructions of the laboratory performing the assay. Mishandling of samples could result in a falsely decreased value, erroneously suggesting an adrenal tumour.

TREATMENT

There is limited experience with the treatment of feline hyperadrenocorticism, but effective treatment is not easily accomplished. Potential options for treatment include the use of the adrenocorticolytic agent mitotane (o,p'-DDD), drugs that block cortisol synthesis (e.g. ketoconazole and metyrapone), unilateral adrenalectomy for adrenocortical tumour, bilateral adrenalectomy for pituitary-dependent hyperadrenocorticism, or radiotherapy for pituitary adenoma. In general, adrenalectomy seems to be the most successful method of treatment for most cats with hyperadrenocorticism, whereas medical management and the use of pituitary radiotherapy have yielded mixed results (Peterson *et al.*, 1994; Duesberg and Peterson, 1997).

Mitotane

A number of different protocols for the medical treatment of cats with hyperadrenocorticism have been used with varying levels of short-term success; however, long-term results have generally been discouraging. Mitotane has been used extensively in dogs but its use in cats has often been discouraged because of potential sensitivity to chlorinated hydrocarbons. Additionally, in a small number of cats treated orally with 50 mg/kg mitotane (divided twice daily), the drug did not effectively suppress adrenocortical function or alleviate clinical signs of the disease (Peterson *et al.*, 1994; Duesberg and Peterson, 1997).

Ketoconazole

Ketoconazole, an imidazole derivative primarily used in the treatment of deep fungal infections, has been used in canine hyperadrenocorticism with some success. By contrast, the drug does not seem to suppress adrenocortical function reliably in either normal cats or cats with hyperadrenocorticism, and therefore cannot be recommended.

Metyrapone

Metyrapone inhibits the action of 11-β-hydroxylase, the enzyme that converts 11-desoxycortisol to cortisol, and has been used with mixed results in cats. Dosages ranging from 250–500 mg/cat/day have been used (Daley *et al.*, 1993); although most cats appeared to tolerate these doses, drug-induced vomiting and inappetence necessitated discontinuation of treatment in some cats. If metyrapone is effective, there should be a reduction in baseline and ACTH-stimulated cortisol concentrations and the amelioration of clinical signs of the disease. Overall, the use of metyrapone in cats with hyperadrenocorticism does offer some promise, at least for short-term use in preparation for surgical adrenalectomy.

Radiotherapy

Radiotherapy has been used with partial success to treat a few cats with pituitary-dependent hyperadrenocorticism. Although radiotherapy seems a promising method for treating cats with pituitary-dependent hyperadrenocorticism, especially pituitary macroadenomas, its effectiveness remains to be determined. However, the limited availability and expense of radiotherapy might prevent it from becoming a common treatment in cats.

Adrenalectomy

Adrenalectomy seems to be the most successful method of treating cats with hyperadrenocorticism (Duesberg *et al.*, 1995). Unilateral adrenalectomy should be performed in cats with functional unilateral adrenocortical tumours, whereas bilateral adrenalectomy must be performed in cats with bilateral adrenocortical hyperplasia resulting from pituitary-dependent hyperadrenocorticism. Cats undergoing unilateral adrenalectomy generally require glucocorticoid supplementation for approximately 2 months postoperatively, until the glucocorticoid secretory function of the atrophied contralateral gland recovers. By contrast, cats undergoing bilateral adrenalectomy require consistent, lifelong replacement of both mineralocorticoid and glucocorticoid hormones.

Affected cats that are successfully treated by adrenalectomy typically, within 2–4 months postoperatively, have resolution of the clinical signs of polyuria, polydipsia, polyphagia and lethargy, and resolution of the physical abnormalities of pot belly, muscle wasting, alopecia, thin skin, hepatomegaly, and infections. Additionally, many cats have decreased requirements for exogenous insulin therapy. Unfortunately, cats debilitated by chronic hypersecretion of glucocorticoids have an increased risk of infection and delayed wound healing postoperatively. Presurgical medical stabilisation (e.g. metyrapone) of cats with severe clinical signs may improve postsurgical outcome.

Without treatment, most cats will succumb to

complications attributable to hyperadrenocorticism. The immunosuppressive effects of glucocorticoid excess predispose cats to infection, and chronic hypercortisolism may adversely affect the cardiovascular system leading to hypertension, pulmonary thromboembolism, or congestive heart failure. Thus, the deleterious consequences of chronic cortisol excess on metabolic, immune, and cardiovascular function are frequently responsible for the death of untreated cats with hyperadrenocorticism.

REFERENCES

Daley CA, Zerbe CA, Schick RO and Powers RD (1993) Use of metyrapone to treat pituitary-dependent hyperadrenocorticism in a cat with large cutaneous wounds. *Journal of the American Veterinary Medical Association* **202**, 956–960

Duesberg CA, Nelson RW, Feldman EC, Vaden SL and Scott-Moncrieff JCR (1995) Adrenalectomy for treatment of hyperadrenocorticism in cats: 10 cases (1988–1992). *Journal of the American Veterinary Medical Association* **207**, 1066–1070

Duesberg C and Peterson ME (1997) Adrenal disorders in cats. *Veterinary Clinics of North America: Small Animal Practice* **27**, 321–347

Peterson ME, Randolph JF and Mooney CT (1994) Endocrine diseases. In: *The Cat: Diagnosis and Clinical Management, 2nd edn,* ed. RG Sherding, pp. 1404–1506. Churchill Livingstone, New York

Sparkes AH, Adams DT, Douthwaite JA and Gruffydd-Jones TJ (1990) Assessment of adrenal function in cats: Response to intravenous synthetic ACTH. *Journal of Small Animal Practice* **31**, 2–5

Zerbe CA, Refsal KR, Peterson ME, Armstrong PJ, Nachreiner RF and Schall WD (1987) Effect of nonadrenal illness on adrenal function in the cat. *American Journal of Veterinary Research* **48**, 451–454

CHAPTER THIRTY

Canine Thyroid Tumours and Hyperthyroidism

Carmel T. Mooney

INTRODUCTION

Thyroid tumours account for 1.2–3.75% of all tumours and approximately 10–15% of all head and neck neoplasms in the dog (Brodey and Kelly, 1968; Mitchell *et al.*, 1979; Birchard and Rousel, 1981; Harari *et al.* 1986). Thyroid tumours in the dog are usually non-functional, invasive, carcinomatous masses whereas in the cat, they are generally functional, non-invasive, relatively small adenomatous masses. The prognosis is therefore guarded but treatment may be possible by surgery, chemotherapy or radiotherapy, either alone or in combination.

TUMOUR CLASSIFICATION

In pathological studies, benign adenomas account for approximately 30–50% of all thyroid tumours (Brodey and Kelly, 1968; Leav *et al.*, 1976). However, benign thyroid tumours are usually small focal lesions which are not commonly detected during life. Occasionally, these tumours, particularly if cystic, may be obvious by palpation as mobile ovoid masses within the cervical area. Rarely, clinical signs referable to compression of surrounding organs may be apparent. In most cases only one thyroid lobe is affected, although bilateral involvement is possible.

Carcinomas, while responsible for approximately 50–70% of all thyroid tumours diagnosed post mortem, account for up to 90% of those tumours detected antemortem and therefore all thyroid masses are usually presumed malignant until proven otherwise. Carcinomas are usually larger than adenomas, coarsely multinodular, non-mobile, and often have necrotic or haemorrhagic centres or, occasionally, focal areas of mineralisation or bone formation. Unilateral involvement is twice as common as bilateral involvement, and when the latter occurs the neoplastic process is usually extensive. It is therefore difficult to determine if the tumour arose in both thyroid lobes or if metastases occurred from one lobe to the other. Occasionally ectopic thyroid tissue located in the media-stinum becomes neoplastic and thyroid tumours must therefore be included in the differential diagnosis of heart-base tumours.

Carcinomas are poorly encapsulated and commonly extend into or around the trachea, cervical muscles, oesophagus, larynx, nerves and blood vessels although invasion into the oesophageal or tracheal lumen is unusual. The major lymphatic drainage of the thyroid gland is in the cranial direction and metastatic spread to the retro-pharyngeal and cervical lymph nodes is common. However, early invasion into the cranial and caudal thyroid veins with the formation of tumour cell thrombi leads to multiple pulmonary metastases, often before involvement of regional lymph nodes. Other reported, but rare, sites of metastatic lesions include kidney, adrenal gland, liver, spleen, spinal cord and bone.

Histopathologically, thyroid carcinomas are usually well differentiated and classified as follicular, compact, mixed or papillary. In humans, papillary carcinoma is the most common type; it has a low grade of malignancy and therefore a more favourable prognosis. This type of tumour is rare in the dog where the majority are mixed, follicular or, less commonly, compact. The correlation between the histopathological classification and ultimate prognosis is unclear. However, the probability of metastases increases in proportion to the size of the tumour. Dogs with small thyroid tumours (<20 cm^3) have a less than 20% incidence of metastatic disease, whereas nearly all dogs with large tumours (>100 cm^3) have metastases. Undifferentiated (anaplastic) thyroid tumours appear to be highly malignant but are rare. Medullary (parafollicular, C-cell) carcinoma is also considered rare. However, medullary carcinoma may be difficult to distinguish from other thyroid carcinomas by light microscopy alone. When specific immunocytochemical stains are used, the incidence of medullary thyroid carcinoma is much higher (Carver *et al.*, 1995). These tumours may have a more favourable prognosis as distant metastatic spread is uncommon. They also appear to be well encapsulated and easily resectable at the time of surgical thyroidectomy.

THYROID FUNCTION

In general, canine thyroid tumours are non-functional and euthyroidism is maintained throughout the course of the disease. It has been suggested that up to 30% of dogs with detectable thyroid tumours are hypothyroid (Feldman and Nelson, 1996). Hypothyroidism may arise because of destruction of all normal thyroid tissue by aggressive bilateral carcinomas. Alternatively, large tumours could potentially produce excessive inactive thyroid hormones capable of pituitary TSH suppression and eventual atrophy of normal thyroid tissue (Branam *et al.*, 1982). However, in the author's experience, hypothyroidism is rare and may be coincidental occurring before the development of the thyroid tumour. Hyperthyroidism occurs in approximately 10–20% of thyroid carcinomas. Functional tumours tend to be unilateral, small to medium in size, and mobile with less compressive effects on adjacent structures than non-functional tumours. Hyperthyroidism is a rare consequence of thyroid adenoma in the dog (Lawrence *et al.*, 1991).

MULTIPLE ENDOCRINE NEOPLASIA (MEN)

In humans, neoplasms may develop in several different endocrine organs simultaneously. Certain of these multiple endocrine neoplasms have emerged as distinct clinical entities which can occur in related individuals. Medullary thyroid carcinoma is occasionally associated with phaeochromocytoma and parathyroid hyperplasia/ neoplasia (MEN type IIa) or phaeochromocytoma (MEN type IIb). Although rare, MEN does occur in dogs (Feldman and Nelson, 1996). The possibility of MEN should always be suspected in dogs presenting with thyroid carcinoma and clinical signs referable to dysfunction of other endocrine glands.

SIGNALMENT

Thyroid tumours occur in middle-aged and older dogs with an average age at onset of 10 years. Almost all dogs are greater than 4 years old at the time of diagnosis. There is no sex predilection unlike the situation in humans where women are twice as commonly affected as men. Beagles and Golden Retrievers appear predisposed to the development of thyroid carcinomas and Boxers to the development of both adenomas and carcinomas.

CLINICAL SIGNS

Most dogs are presented because of a visible mass in the neck and/or its associated consequences (Table 30.1 and Figure 30.1). The duration of these signs varies from weeks to months. The mass is usually felt in the region of the thyroid gland, below the larynx, but occasionally larger tumours may descend towards the thoracic inlet. Clinical signs referable to regional (enlarged lymph nodes or cording of local lymphatic and blood vessels) or distant (dyspnoea from pulmonary metastases) metastatic spread may be apparent. A few dogs may present with the additional clinical signs of hypothyroidism (see Chapter 14) or hyperthyroidism. Dogs with hyperthyroidism exhibit similar clinical signs to those in cats (weight loss, polyphagia, polyuria/polydipsia, restlessness, tachycardia) but tend to be less symptomatic.

DIAGNOSIS

The differential diagnosis for large cervical swellings includes abscess, granuloma, thyroid tumour, other

Clinical feature	% of dogs
Visible mass in neck	84
Coughing	37
Dyspnoea	31
Dysphagia	28
Dysphonia	18
Weight loss	15
Vomiting/regurgitation	13
Polydipsia/polyuria	10
Depression	8
Anorexia	6
Hyperactivity	6
Diarrhoea	4
Increased appetite	4
Facial oedema	3

Table 30.1: *Common presenting signs in a series of 146 dogs with thyroid tumours. (Adapted from Feldman and Nelson, 1996.)*

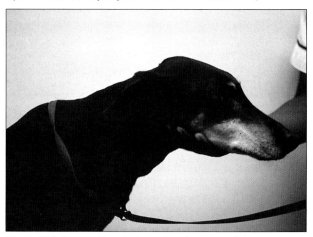

Figure 30.1: *Large midcervical mass in a hyperthyroid dog.*

tumours, and salivary mucocoele. Fine needle (21 to 23 gauge) aspiration is helpful in distinguishing thyroid tumours from abscesses, salivary mucocoeles and enlarged lymph nodes. Unfortunately, because of the vascular nature of thyroid tissue, samples are frequently heavily contaminated with blood and exfoliation of neoplastic cells can be poor (Thompson *et al.*, 1980). Cytological examination, or total T4 estimation of any fluid removed, helps confirm the thyroidal origin of the sample but a definitive diagnosis of malignancy is not often possible. Evaluation of wide bore needle biopsies, while of greater diagnostic yield, significantly increases the risk of haemorrhage and should only be carried out under ultrasound guidance. Even with these needle biopsies, there may still be difficulty in distinguishing benign from malignant tumours and the latter is often only confirmed by demonstration of vascular or capsular invasion in biopsies taken at the time of surgical thyroidectomy.

Results of post-mortem studies show that up to 80% of dogs have evidence of distant metastatic spread, although this decreases to 30–50% in clinical cases. Thus, it is imperative that once a mass is identified as

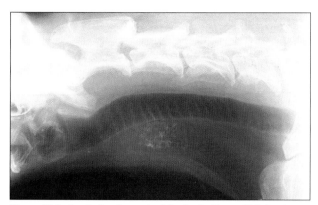

Figure 30.2: *Cervical radiograph of the dog in Figure 30.1 showing dorsal displacement of the trachea by a large calcified soft tissue swelling.*

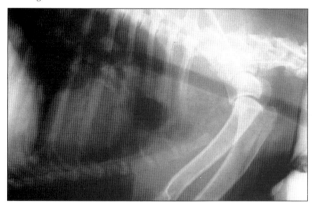

Figure 30.3: *Pulmonary metastases in a dog with thyroid carcinoma. Treatment is rarely attempted as the prognosis is so poor.*

thyroid, a systematic search for metastatic spread is instigated. Routine haematological and biochemical examinations may be helpful in identifying possible organs containing metastases or concurrent problems which may ultimately affect the prognosis. Local lymph nodes should be carefully examined and biopsied as necessary. Radiography of the cervical area may help to assess the size of the mass and the extent of local invasion (Figure 30.2). Thoracic radiographs should always be evaluated for evidence of pulmonary spread (Figure 30.3). Abdominal radiography and ultrasonography may also be useful in cases where hepatic metastasis is suspected.

As in cats, thyroid scintigraphy using pertechnetate may be useful. Pertechnetate scans do not provide any information with regard to thyroid function but are helpful in depicting location of the tumour and regional meta-stases (Marks *et al.*, 1994). Some thyroid tumours fail to concentrate pertechnetate adequately and it has been suggested that these are less likely to respond to radio-active iodine administration (Feldman and Nelson, 1996). Compared with thoracic radiography, thoracic scintigraphy is not considered useful to depict pulmonary metastases.

Measurement of serum total T4 concentration is necessary in dogs with appropriate clinical signs of thyrotoxicosis. Elevations are generally moderate, compared with the marked elevations often seen in hyperthyroid cats.

TREATMENT

Surgical thyroidectomy remains the cornerstone of treatment of thyroid tumours, provided there is no evidence of distant metastatic spread. Surgical thyroidectomy allows gross examination for local invasion and submission of adequate tissue for histopathological examination which is helpful in differentiating adenoma from carcinoma. The functional status of the thyroid tumour does not alter this treatment choice. However, as in cats, carbimazole therapy (5 mg three times daily initially and subsequently adjusted for effect) is recommended for thyrotoxic animals prior to surgery.

The surgical technique is similar to that described for cats. However, in dogs most tumours are unilateral and therefore, it is not necessary to preserve parathyroid glands on the affected side. Adenomas and relatively small, mobile carcinomas are easy to remove and surgery alone results in long-term survival (Klein *et al.*, 1995). However, in many cases extensive tumour invasion precludes complete removal and aggressive surgical attempts significantly increase the risk of extensive haemorrhage and damage to the recurrent laryngeal nerves and parathyroid glands. In these cases, surgical debulking followed by chemotherapy is usually preferable. Patients with large tumours, even without evidence of metastatic spread, may also benefit from subsequent chemotherapy because the probability of metastases is so high.

Various chemotherapeutic protocols have been recommended following surgical thyroidectomy. These usually involve doxorubicin either alone or in combination with cyclophosphamide and/or vincristine. The reader is referred to relevant oncology textbooks for further information regarding these regimens.

Other treatment modalities include administration of high doses of radioactive iodine or cobalt irradiation but facilities offering these forms of therapy are rare (Peterson *et al.*, 1989; Adams *et al.*, 1995; Feldman and Nelson, 1996).

Standard dose thyroxine supplementation is necessary following bilateral thyroidectomy. In addition, thyroxine therapy is usually recommended after unilateral thyroidectomy. Receptor affinity and concentration, and functional response to TSH are similar in healthy and carcinomatous thyroids (Verschueren *et al.*, 1992). Although it is unclear whether TSH has any growth-stimulating properties in thyroid neoplasia *in vivo*, thyroxine therapy seems a wise precaution.

REFERENCES AND FURTHER READING

Adams WH, Walker MA, Daniel GB, Petersen MG and Legendre AM (1995) Treatment of differentiated thyroid carcinoma in 7 dogs utilizing 131I. *Veterinary Radiology and Ultrasound* **36**, 417–424

Birchard SJ and Rousel OF (1981) Neoplasia of the thyroid gland in the dog: a retrospective study of 16 cases. *Journal of the American Animal Hospital Association* **17**, 369–372

Branam JE, Leighton RL and Hornof WJ (1982) Radioisotope imaging for the evaluation of thyroid neoplasia and hypothyroidism in a dog.

Journal of the American Veterinary Medical Association **180**, 1077–1079

Brodey RS and Kelly DF (1968) Thyroid neoplasms in the dog. A clinicopathologic study of fifty-seven cases. *Cancer* **22**, 406–416

Carver JR, Kapatkin A and Patnaik AK (1995) A comparison of medullary thyroid carcinoma and thyroid adenocarcinoma in dogs: a retrospective study of 38 cases. *Veterinary Surgery* **24**, 315–319

Feldman EC and Nelson RW (1996) Canine thyroid tumors and hyperthyroidism. In: *Canine and Feline Endocrinology and Reproduction, 2nd edn*, pp. 166–185 WB Saunders, Philadelphia

Harari J, Patterson JS and Rosenthal RC (1986) Clinical and pathologic features of thyroid tumours in 26 dogs. *Journal of the American Veterinary Medical Association* **188**, 1160–1164

Klein MK, Powers BE, Withrow SJ, Curtis CR, Straw RC, Ogilivie GK, Dickinson KL, Cooper MF and Baier M (1995) Treatment of thyroid carcinoma in dogs by surgical resection alone: 20 cases (1981-1989). *Journal of the American Veterinary Medical Association* **206**, 1007–1009

Lawrence D, Thompson J, Layton AW, Calderwood-Mays M, Ellison G and Mannella C (1991) Hyperthyroidism associated with a thyroid adenoma in a dog. *Journal of the American Veterinary Medical Association* **199**, 81–83

Leav I, Schiller AL, Rijnberk A, Legg MA and der Kinderen PJ (1976) Adenomas and carcinomas of the canine and feline thyroid. *American Journal of Pathology* **83**, 61–93

Marks SL, Koblik PD, Hornof WJ and Feldman EC (1994) [99]mTc-pertechnetate imaging of thyroid tumors in dogs: 29 cases (1980–1992). *Journal of the American Veterinary Medical Association* **204**, 756–760

Mitchell M, Hurov LI and Troy GC (1979) Canine thyroid carcinomas: clinical occurrence, staging by means of scintiscans, and therapy of 15 cases. *Veterinary Surgery* **8**, 112–118

Peterson ME, Kintzer PP, Hurley JR and Becker DV (1989) Radioactive iodine treatment of a functional thyroid carcinoma producing hyperthyroidism in a dog. *Journal of Veterinary Internal Medicine* **3**, 20–25

Thompson EJ, Stirtzinger T, Lumsden JH and Little PB (1980) Fine needle aspiration cytology in the diagnosis of canine thyroid carcinoma. *Canadian Veterinary Journal* **21**, 186–188

Verschueren CP, Rutteman GR, Vos JH, Van Dijk JE and de Bruin TWA (1992) Thyrotrophin receptors in normal and neoplastic (primary and metastatic) canine thyroid tissue. *Journal of Endocrinology* **132**, 461–468

PART FIVE

Therapeutics and Endocrine Tests

CHAPTER THIRTY ONE

Monitoring Thyroid Replacement

Kent R. Refsal and Ray F. Nachreiner

INTRODUCTION

Making an accurate diagnosis of canine hypothyroidism continues to pose a challenge to clinicians, compounded by recognition of an ever widening array of clinical mani-festations of the disorder. Diagnostic testing of canine hypothyroidism has expanded from the measurement of iodothyronines, to the addition of antithyroid autoantibodies and, most recently, canine thyrotropin (thyroid stimulating hormone, TSH). The integration of clinical signs with laboratory results, especially when these are at variance, often results in uncertainty in the diagnosis. Thyroid hormone supplementation may thus be initiated from the perspective of a type of clinical trial, using the dog's response to establish or refute the diagnosis. After initiation of thyroid supplementation, the clinician must then assess the clinical response and consider changing the dose accordingly. Thyroid supplementation and its evaluation have received relatively little attention in terms of clinical or experimental studies, when compared with the literature defining clinical manifestations of hypothyroidism or endocrine testing for diagnosis of hypothyroidism. This chapter outlines the treatment of hypothyroidism with L-thyroxine (T4).

ASSESSMENT OF CLINICAL RESPONSE

T4 supplementation results in dramatic and often complete resolution of clinical signs of canine hypothyroidism when there has been an accurate diagnosis. Usually the first indicator of improvement is increased activity, with weight loss evident in the first month; neurological signs may take longer to resolve. A useful review on treatment of hypothyroidism provides further insight into the interpretation of the clinical response (Panciera, 1997). In our experience, overt iatrogenic thyrotoxicosis is an infrequent complication, presumably because of the comparatively short half-life of T4 in the dog. It has not been determined whether subclinical hyperthyroidism is of clinical relevance in the dog.

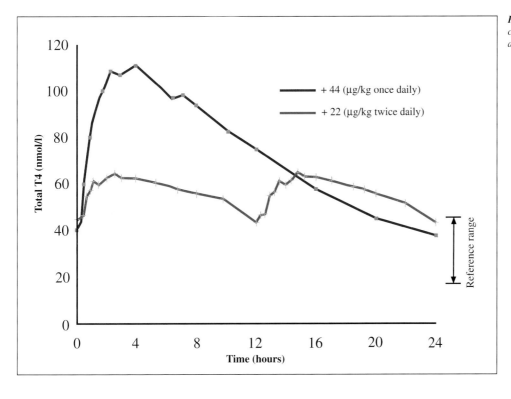

Figure 31.1: Serum total T4 concentration after administration of L-thyroxine.

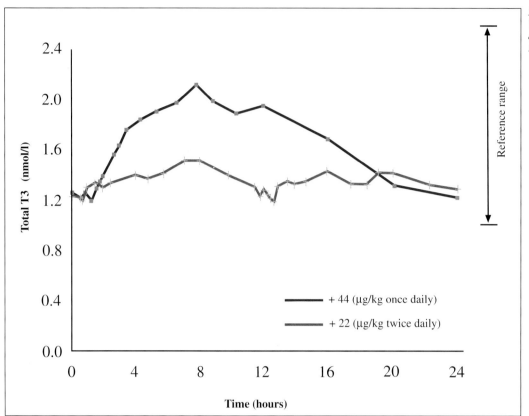

Figure 31.2: *Serum total T3 concentration after administration of L-thyroxine.*

ENDOCRINE ASSESSMENT OF T4 SUPPLEMENTATION

Assays for canine TSH have been available for clinical application for approximately 2 years, and reports on their diagnostic usefulness are starting to appear (Dixon *et al.*, 1997; Graham *et al.*, 1997; Peterson *et al.*, 1997). The available data indicate that the majority of hypothyroid dogs have the combination of low iodothyronine concentrations and elevation of TSH. Oral administration of T4 produces an increase in circulating concentrations, and subsequent increase in circulating triiodothyronine (T3), from the peripheral deiodination of exogenous T4. Pharmacokinetic studies on oral T4 supplementation in experimentally induced hypothyroid dogs have helped to define relations between the dose of T4 and serial changes in circulating T4 and T3 concentrations, with recognition of the variation in efficiency of absorption of T4 among dogs (Nachreiner *et al.*, 1993). Figure 31.1 shows the average concentrations of serum T4 in 12 dogs receiving 44 µg/kg/day of T4 given as a single or divided daily dose. While T4 supplementation may produce circulating concentrations of T4 above the normal range for a considerable part of the day, serum T3 usually remains within the reference range (Figure 31.2).

Current recommendations to monitor T4 supplementation are based on the collection of serum between 3 and 8 hours after treatment, the time at which serum T4 is best correlated with the area under the curve. Where treatment is given twice daily to a dog, a serum T4 concentration between 30 and 65 nmol/l provides evidence for good absorption of T4. A serum concentration of T4 above 70 nmol/l at this time is not necessarily excessive for the dog, but allows the option of decreasing or changing the schedule from twice to once daily. In our experience, evidence for adequate absorption of T4 is usually accompanied by normalisation of TSH in a hypothyroid dog with elevated TSH at the time of initial diagnosis. A daily dose of T4 of ≥20 µg/kg was sufficient to maintain normal TSH concentrations in hypothyroid dogs (Ferguson and Hoenig, 1997). Studies are needed to determine whether normalisation of canine TSH equates with clinical euthyroidism irrespective of the therapeutic concentration of T4 Current assays for canine TSH cannot distinguish clinically low results from normal and thus do not help identify dogs at risk of thyrotoxicosis. To date, there has been a relative lack of clinical studies devoted to evaluation of thyroid supplementation in the dog. We should not disregard the possibility that measurement of T3 or free T4 by equilibrium dialysis may further refine laboratory monitoring of T4 supplementation.

DECISION-MAKING IN MONITORING THYROID SUPPLEMENTATION

The following factors should be considered when evaluating the clinical response to T4 supplementation in light of therapeutic concentrations of iodothyronines and canine TSH. Decisions to continue, change, or stop T4 supplementation rely on confidence in the initial diagnosis of hypothyroidism.

Clinical response satisfactory

If the clinical response is satisfactory but the concentrations of thyroid hormones are below the desired therapeutic range, then consider:

• Owner compliance: the sample was collected ≥1 day

before treatment and the laboratory results do not reflect absorption of T4

- Other medications or supplements: other treatments interacting and affecting solubility and/or absorption of T4 are recognised in people; this topic has not been studied in the dog
- The clinical response has been partial to date and an increase in the dose of T4 would be of further benefit: this is especially pertinent if TSH is elevated in the therapeutic monitoring sample
- Whether or not the response was due to thyroid supplementation, especially if TSH is not elevated in the therapeutic monitoring sample.

If the clinical response is satisfactory and the concentrations of thyroid hormones are in the desired therapeutic range, then consider:

- Continuing with the dose and schedule of treatment: there is a possibility that the dose could be changed in the future, especially if there is further weight loss
- The initial confidence in the diagnosis of hypothyroidism: if treatment was initiated as a therapeutic trial (without low T4 or elevated TSH concentrations in the diagnostic sample), you may question whether or not the clinical improvement was due to thyroid supplementation. In primary hypothyroidism, T4 supplementation is lifelong; it may be of merit to stop T4 supplementation and see if clinical signs return.

If the clinical response is satisfactory but the concentrations of thyroid hormones are above the therapeutic range (recall that the therapeutic range extends above the reference range), then:

- Look for evidence of thyrotoxicosis
- Decrease the daily dose of T4 or change the dose to once rather than twice daily
- The following may also be applicable: assess the initial confidence in the diagnosis of hypothyroidism; if treatment was initiated as a therapeutic trial (without low T4 or elevated TSH concentrations in the diagnostic sample), you may question whether or not the clinical improvement was due to thyroid supplementation. It may be of merit to stop T4 supplementation and see if clinical signs return.

Inadequate clinical response

If a dog is not showing an adequate clinical response and the concentrations of thyroid hormones are below the therapeutic range, then:

- Increase the dose of T4, especially if TSH is elevated; bear in mind that the magnitude of the change of serum T4 is usually below, or at best similar to, the incremental increase of the dose of T4. The reasons for inadequate absorption of T4 in some dogs are unknown — assess client compliance with the treatment
- Change the T4 product and continue with the same

dose: questions arise about the consistency of potency or bioavailability among different products
- Consider other medications or supplements: other treatments interacting and affecting solubility and, or, absorption of T4 is recognised in people; this topic has not been studied in the dog.

If the dog is not showing an adequate clinical response but the concentrations of thyroid hormones are in the desired therapeutic range, then:

- Reconsider the diagnosis of hypothyroidism
- Consider whether the response is as good as can be expected; the dog may have multiple problems that would not completely resolve with thyroid supplementation alone.

If the dog is not showing an adequate clinical response and the concentrations of thyroid hormones are excessive, then:

- Reconsider the diagnosis of hypothyroidism
- Thyrotoxicosis may be contributing to the unsatisfactory response; for example, catabolic effects of excess T4 may impair regrowth of hair.

REASSESSING THE DIAGNOSIS OF HYPOTHYROIDISM IN THYROXINE-TREATED DOGS

If a dog is on treatment but the clinician concludes the dog is not hypothyroid, then the treatment should be withdrawn. It is likely that the thyroid glands will have undergone some atrophy from the negative feedback of administration of exogenous T4. Abrupt discontinuation of T4 supplementation could leave the dog with low concentrations of iodothyronines for several weeks, until its pituitary–thyroid axis has had time to recover. The possibility of critical complications arising from abrupt discontinuation of thyroid supplementation is assumed to be very low. After stopping T4 supplementation, a minimum of one month should be allowed to identify return of thyroid function in a euthyroid dog (Panciera et al., 1990).

REFERENCES

Dixon RM, Graham PA, Harvie J and Mooney CT (1997) Comparison of endogenous serum thyrotropin (cTSH) concentrations with bovine TSH response test results in euthyroid and hypothyroid dogs. *Journal of Veterinary Internal Medicine* **11**, 121

Ferguson DC and Hoenig M (1997) Re-examination of dosage regimens for l-thyroxine (T4) in the dog: bioavailability and persistence of TSH suppression. *Journal of Veterinary Internal Medicine* **11**, 121

Graham PA, Nachreiner RF, Refsal KR, Hauptman J and Watson GL (1997) Heterogeneity of thyroid function in beagles with lymphocytic thyroiditis. *Journal of Veterinary Internal Medicine* **11**, 120

Nachreiner RF, Refsal KR, Ravis WR, Hauptman J, Rosser EJ and Pedersoli WM (1993) Pharmacokinetics of l-thyroxine after its oral administration in dogs. *American Journal of Veterinary Research* **54**, 2091–2098

Panciera DL (1997) Treating hypothyroidism. *Veterinary Medicine* **92**, 58–68

Panciera DL, MacEwen EG, Atkins CE, Bosu WTK, Refsal KR and Nachreiner RF (1990) Thyroid function tests in euthyroid dogs treated with l-thyroxine. *American Journal of Veterinary Research* **51**, 22–26

Peterson ME, Melian C and Nichols R (1997) Measurement of serum total thyroxine, triiodothyronine, free thyroxine, and thyrotropin concentrations for diagnosis of hypothyroidism in dogs. *Journal of American Veterinary Medical Association* **211**, 1396–1402

CHAPTER THIRTY TWO

Management of Glucocorticoid Therapy

Jonathan Elliott

INTRODUCTION

Glucocorticoid drugs consist of a number of analogues of the natural glucocorticoid hormone, cortisol. They are used in the therapy of diverse conditions in veterinary medicine and, if applied in a rational manner, are a most valuable and important part of our therapeutic armoury. When using glucocorticoid drugs it is most important to:

- Make a specific diagnosis before instituting therapy
- Recognise those conditions where glucocorticoid therapy is inappropriate
- Understand potential adverse effects and how to avoid them
- Remember that the underlying cause of the disease is not being treated in most cases.

ACTIONS OF GLUCOCORTICOIDS

Steroid hormones affect cells by altering protein synthesis, either by inducing or inhibiting the transcription of cellular proteins which mediate their effects. They achieve this effect by binding to a receptor in the nucleus of their target cells which then undergoes a conformational change, enabling it to bind to a steroid responsive element in DNA. There are believed to be 10–100 steroid responsive genes in each cell, some examples of which are considered below. For this reason, the actions of glucocorticoid drugs, which are summarised in Table 32.1, occur throughout the body and their biological half lives exceed their pharmacological half lives.

System affected	Effect of glucocorticoids
Metabolism:	
Carbohydrate	Insulin antagonism:
	• Inhibition of glucose uptake into cells
	• Increased formation of glucose from amino acids
	• Stimulation of glycogen synthesis by the liver, possibly as a result of increased insulin secretion in response to hyperglycaemia
Protein synthesis	General decrease in tissue protein synthesis and increase in protein catabolism
Lipid	Permissive effect on lipolysis stimulated by catecholamines, redistribution of body fat
Mineral homeostasis	Negative calcium balance and hypercalciuria as a result of:
	• Decreased Ca^{2+} absorption from the intestine
	• Increased Ca^{2+} excretion (reduced renal tubular absorption)
	• Increased secretion of parathyroid hormone
	• Inhibition of osteoblast and stimulation of osteoclast activities, mobilising Ca^{2+} and PO_4^{2-} from bone
	• Blockade of the vitamin D_3-induced synthesis of osteocalcin
Water and electrolyte balance	Affect renal concentrating mechanisms by inhibiting the secretion of ADH and reducing the responsiveness of the kidney to the effects of ADH
	Most of the synthetic glucocorticoids do have some affinity for mineralocorticoid receptors and thus enhance K^+ and reduce Na^+ excretion by the kidney to a degree
Inflammation and immune system:	
Humoral mediators (inhibit the production of the enzymes phospho-lipase A_2 and cyclo-oxygenase 2)	Inhibit the production of:
	• Prostaglandins
	• Leukotrienes
	• Platelet-activating factor
	• Cytokines (e.g. interleukins)
	• Complement components
Inflammatory cells	Reduce:
	• Migration of polymorphonuclear lymphocytes and macrophages and their ability to generate oxygen free radicals
	• Ability of macrophages to kill organisms they phagocytose
	• Clonal expansion of T and B lymphocytes
	• Activity of fibroblasts, thus fibrosis and wound healing
Hypothalamic–pituitary–adrenocortical axis (HPA)	Inhibit CRH and ACTH secretion (immediate effect) which if persistently inhibited for several weeks will lead to adrenal gland atrophy

Table 32.1: *Actions and effects of glucocorticoids. (ACTH, adrenocorticotropic hormone; ADH, antidiuretic hormone; CRH, corticotropin releasing hormone.)*

Separation of the actions of glucocorticoids

So far, the production of synthetic analogues of cortisol has not resulted in drugs which possess the anti-inflammatory actions of glucocorticoids but lack their metabolic hypothalamic–pituitary–adrenocortical (HPA) axis suppressant effects. Indeed, the anti-inflammatory potencies of glucocorticoid drugs closely follow their metabolic effects. The only separable property is Na$^+$ retention, which is mediated via the mineralocorticoid receptor. Thus, the prospect of potent broad spectrum anti-inflammatory and immunosuppressive drugs without the attendant metabolic and other side effects does not appear to be realistic.

CLINICAL APPLICATIONS OF GLUCOCORTICOIDS

Indications for glucocorticoid therapy

Glucocorticoid drugs are indicated for the following problems in small animal veterinary medicine:

- Treatment of circulatory shock (endotoxaemic shock in particular)
- Treatment of central nervous system (CNS) oedema (neoplasia and trauma)
- As part of a cytotoxic drug therapy protocol for malignant lymphoma, multiple myeloma and mast cell tumours

- Treatment of hypercalcaemia once the underlying cause has been identified
- Management of immune-mediated disease
- Suppression of acute or chronic inflammatory disease where the underlying cause cannot be addressed or ascertained
- Diagnostic testing for hyperadrenocorticism
- Replacement therapy in hypoadrenocorticism.

Although in many of the above situations glucocorticoids are being used as palliative rather than curative therapy, their use is of great value in the control of these diseases and in some cases they can be life-saving. The indications have been listed in approximate decreasing order of the dose of glucocorticoid generally required in each case, which may vary from one individual animal to the next.

Choice of glucocorticoid preparation, formulation and route of administration

Available drugs and formulations

There are five main glucocorticoid drugs available as authorised veterinary products in various formulations, with a further two preparations available as human authorised products. The properties which should be considered when deciding which of these drugs to use are detailed in Table 32.2.

Compound	Relative glucocorticoid activity	Relative mineralocorticoid activity	Duration of biological effect (hours)	Additional comments and availability of products for veterinary use
Hydrocortisone	1	1	8–12	Identical to natural hormone (cortisol) Parenteral and oral preparations are all human products
Cortisone	0.8	0.8	8–12	Metabolised to cortisol to be activated. No authorised veterinary products
Prednisolone	5	0.8	12–36	Oral forms authorised for veterinary use, parenteral forms are human products
Prednisone	4	0.8	12–36	Metabolised to prednisolone. No authorised veterinary products
Methylprednisolone	5	minimal	12–36	Both oral and parenteral preparations are authorised for veterinary use
Triamcinolone	5*	none	24–48	Only long-acting parenteral preparation is authorised for veterinary use. Oral forms are human products
Dexamethasone	30	minimal	36–72	Both oral and parenteral preparations are authorised for veterinary use
Betamethasone	30	negligible	36–72	Both oral and parenteral preparations are authorised for veterinary use

Table 32.2: *Properties of available glucocorticoid drugs.*
* Some authors suggest triamcinolone is 30 times more potent than hydrocortisone

The duration of biological effect is an important consideration when deciding which drug to choose. The figures quoted in Table 32.1 apply to formulations of the drugs that are rapidly absorbed from their site of administration. This would include formulations given by the oral route, where the drug is rapidly and effectively absorbed from the gastrointestinal tract, and water-soluble injectable formulations which are suitable for intravenous administration. There are a number of water-insoluble preparations which are suitable for intramuscular, sub-cutaneous or intralesional (including intra-articular) injection. These esters of the glucocorticoids are slowly absorbed into the systemic circulation, the ester being hydrolysed to release the free steroid. Their duration of effect therefore is more dependent on the speed of absorption from the site of administration rather than the rate of clearance of the drug from the body. The different formulations of glucocorticoid preparations and their duration of action are detailed in Table 32.3.

There are many topical eye, ear and skin preparations that contain glucocorticoids, usually as the acetate, acetonide, benzoate, butyrate and valerate esters. Acetonides are well absorbed into the dermis where they are bound, thus limiting their access to the general circulation. For topical eye preparations, penetration into the anterior chamber is necessary in the treatment of anterior uveitis, and prednisolone acetate appears to be the preparation of choice. Prednisone and cortisone require activation by the liver and so are not suitable for local administration.

Which drug and which formulation is appropriate for the required use?

In deciding which drug and which formulation should be used it is necessary to consider the following:

- Is the duration of therapy likely to be short or long term?
- Is an immediate onset of action necessary?
- Is additional mineralocorticoid action desirable or undesirable?
- What is the most practical route of administration for the animal concerned?

Short-term therapy: Acute conditions which benefit from short-term glucocorticoid treatment may only require one dose. The most appropriate choice in these situations would be drugs with a long duration of action (betamethasone and dexamethasone) administered in a formulation which gives a rapid onset of action (soluble esters or the free steroid), usually by intravenous injection as most of the indications for short-term therapy require an immediate onset of effect. Orally administered drugs will be rapidly absorbed and should produce their effects as rapidly as intramuscular or subcutaneous injections of soluble formulations. Indications for short-term therapy include:

- Anaphylactic reactions
- Circulatory shock (particularly endotoxaemic shock)
- CNS trauma or oedema of other causes (e.g. neoplasia)
- Severe asthmatic attacks (cats)
- Prevention of post-surgical oedema (e.g. following airway surgery)

Preparation	Duration of action following intramuscular injection*	Examples (authorised veterinary products unless stated)

Short acting
Free steroid alcohols solubilised in a suitable vehicle (polyethylene glycol)
Soluble esters:
    Sodium succinate
    Sodium phosphate
	12–72 hours (rapid onset of action)
	
	12–72 hours (onset of action within minutes)
		Dexamethasone
		
		Betamethasone
		Dexamethasone
		Hydrocortisone†
		Methylprednisolone

Intermediate acting
Insoluble esters:
    Acetate
    Diproprionate
    Isonicotinate
    Phenylproprionate
    Undecanoate
	2–4 weeks (slow onset of action)
	Some products are co-formulated with soluble esters to give rapid onset of action
		Betamethasone
		Dexamethasone
		Methylprednisolone
		Triamcinolone

Long acting
Very insoluble esters
    Acetonide
    Pivalate
	>4 weeks (very slow onset of action)	Triamcinolone
		Dexamethasone

Table 32.3: Formulations of glucocorticoid preparations for injection.

* Approximate guide only; also depends on the vehicle in which the drug is formulated and dose given.

† Only available in human authorised products

- Emergency management of severe hypercalcaemia
- Management of acute moist dermatitis (hot spots).

In general, with short-term usage of glucocorticoids, the adverse effects discussed below are not considered to be a problem.

Long-term therapy: With long-term therapy, adverse effects of glucocorticoids are a major consideration. These can be predicted from the actions of glucocorticoids discussed above, and in the choice of agent and its formulation for long-term therapy the primary concern is limiting adverse effects. The practicalities of long-term dosing mean that either the oral route or topical administration are chosen. Cats which are impossible to dose by mouth are the exception to this rule and in such cases long acting injectable preparations are often used (e.g. methylprednisolone acetate).

Principles which are followed in situations where long-term glucocorticoid therapy is necessary are:

- Once the condition you are treating is brought under control, find the lowest possible effective dose of glucocorticoid
- Administer this dose with the longest possible interdosing interval
- Consider other additional treatments which may lower the dose of glucocorticoid necessary
- Re-evaluate the animal on a regular basis to detect complications of therapy or concomitant disease which may lead to failure of therapy.

The most suitable glucocorticoid drugs for long-term therapy are those with an intermediate duration of biological effect (e.g. prednisolone). If these drugs can be used on an every other day basis, the long-term complications which can occur with glucocorticoid therapy tend to be much less severe. In theory, dosing every 48 hours with a drug whose biological effect lasts a maximum of 36 hours leaves the body at least 12 hours between each dose to recover from the effects of the drug. This is particularly true of the effects of HPA axis suppression which can lead to severe adrenal cortical atrophy with long-term continuous glucocorticoid dosing. HPA axis suppression has been documented with administration of topical preparations containing glucocorticoids.

Time of dosing of glucocorticoids is often recommended such that it coincides with the peak of cortisol and ACTH secretion. In man there is a definite diurnal rhythm for cortisol secretion, and glucocorticoids are recommended to be given in the morning to minimise HPA axis suppression. In the dog and cat, the natural diurnal rhythm has been less well studied and is less obvious.

Additional mineralocorticoid effects: Synthetic glucocorticoid preparations have been produced to reduce the mineralocorticoid effects when compared with cortisol (hydrocortisone). In man, Na^+ retention can be a major problem with glucocorticoid therapy. Salt and water retention does not appear to occur to the same extent in dogs and cats treated with compounds which still have significant residual mineralocorticoid effects (e.g. prednisolone) and in many instances this factor is not very important in the decision as to which glucocorticoid should be used. It should perhaps be considered in patients with concomitant diseases which would make them more susceptible to the additional mineralocorticoid effects (i.e. less able to compensate for them) (see Table 32.5).

In the emergency management of adrenocortical insufficiency, use of a glucocorticoid preparation which also has significant mineralocorticoid effects could be considered to be advantageous. The preparation of choice in this regard would be hydrocortisone sodium succinate (human preparation) given by the intravenous route. Unfortunately, administration of hydrocortisone interferes with the interpretation of the ACTH stimulation test and must only be used after this test has been completed. It is more common, therefore, to treat these patients with dexamethasone (soluble preparation) immediately, which does not cross react with cortisol in assays commonly used. Glucocorticoids are important as an adjunct to shock doses of fluid therapy (0.9% saline) to facilitate survival of the acute crisis. Oral fludrocortisone acetate can then be administered on a longer term basis to maintain such a patient (see Chapters 11 and 19). No suitable injectable mineralocorticoid preparation is readily available in the UK.

Dose rates and dosing regimens

The dose of glucocorticoid required to treat a particular problem will depend on the nature of the problem. In most inflammatory and immune-mediated diseases, where long-term treatment is necessary, an induction dose will be required for a variable period of time to bring the disease under control, followed by a reduction in dose in an attempt to find the dose rate which keeps the disease under control without giving unacceptable adverse effects (see below).

Initial (induction) dose rates

Each animal should be treated as an individual and dose rates given in Table 32.4 should be treated as guidelines only.

Any animal that has received glucocorticoid therapy for more than 24 hours should have the dose of glucocorticoid it is receiving gradually reduced rather than abruptly stopped, to prevent glucocorticoid withdrawal syndrome due to HPA axis suppression. The severity of HPA axis suppression increases with the duration of therapy and the dose used. Recommendations for dose reduction in inflammatory and immune-mediated diseases are discussed below.

Maintenance therapy for inflammatory and immune-mediated disease

As discussed above, in order that the adverse effects of glucocorticoids are avoided or minimised with chronic therapy, the lowest dose of oral prednisolone that will control the disease process should be established as soon as possible. Again, only guidelines can be suggested and individual patients should be managed according to their response.

Therapeutic aim	Examples of disease states*	Preferred preparation and initial dose†	Additional comments
Glucocorticoid replacement therapy	Addison's disease Glucocorticoid withdrawal syndrome	Prednisolone (oral) 0.1 mg/kg–0.25 mg/kg every 12 h depending on degree of stress As above	Used in maintenance phase of the disease, particularly if animal is to encounter stress. In emergency, crisis dose as for shock
Anti-inflammatory therapy	Atopic / flea allergic dermatitis Chronic / allergic bronchitis	Prednisolone (oral) 0.25–0.5 mg/kg every 12 h (dog) 1.0 mg/kg every 12 h (cat) As above (If methylprednisolone acetate has to be used in cats, 2 mg/kg is injected every 2 weeks initially)	These are standard anti-inflammatory doses; cats requiring higher doses than dogs. Reduce dose after 5–7 days (see text) Inflammatory bowel disease in dog and cat are generally treated with immuno-suppressive doses
Immunosuppression	Immune-mediated: Anaemia Thrombocytopenia Polyarthritis Skin disease	Prednisolone (oral) 1–2 mg/kg every 12 h (dog) 2–4 mg/kg every 12 h (cat)	These are standard immunosuppressive doses Reduce dose after 10–28 days according to response (see text)
Cancer chemotherapy	Malignant lymphoma Multiple myeloma Mast cell tumour	Consult individual chemotherapy protocols	Use as part of a chemotherapy protocol – if used alone, glucocorticoids can induce multiple drug resistance in cancer cells
CNS oedema	Brain trauma or neoplasia leading to acute problems Spinal cord trauma	Dexamethasone (soluble preparation intravenously) 2 mg/kg every 6 h Methylprednisolone sodium succinate – 30 mg/kg intravenously every 6 h	Use for 24 hours then reduce dose and switch to oral prednisolone if still required Use for 24 hours and then stop
Management of shock	Acute trauma and haemorrhage Endotoxaemic shock	Dexamethasone (soluble preparation) 5 mg/kg intravenously once Prednisolone sodium succinate 15 mg/kg intravenously once	Use of glucocorticoids in shock is controversial. Experimentally, the beneficial effects come from pre-treatment of animals, particularly in endotoxaemic models of shock

Table 32.4: Recommendations for dose rates of glucocorticoids.
* These examples are illustrative and not meant to be an exhaustive list – consult texts on individual disease states for more detailed information
† In the cases where dosing with prednisolone every 12 h is suggested, equal success can often be achieved by dosing on a once daily basis

Anti-inflammatory therapy: In general terms, most inflammatory diseases can be brought under control after 5–7 days of treatment but this may depend on the chronicity of the disease. With anti-inflammatory doses, the first stage is to reduce the frequency of dosing without reducing the total dose given until the drug is administered on an every other day basis. So, for example, if the dose is 0.5 mg/kg once daily, the every other day dose should be 1 mg/kg. The dose can then be gradually reduced on an every other day basis. Prednisolone is the drug best suited to every other day dosing for the reasons discussed above. If control is not achieved with prednisolone, it may be worth trying another glucocorticoid provided the animal has been fully evaluated for any factors which would complicate the response to steroid therapy. It should be appreciated that every other day therapy with dexamethasone, betamethasone or triamcinolone will still produce significant HPA axis suppression and other adverse effects with long-term administration. Moving to every third day therapy with these drugs is not usually possible without losing control of the problem.

Immunosuppressive therapy: When using prednisolone for immunosuppressive therapy, the same principles as discussed for anti-inflammatory therapy should be followed. The time scale over which the dose can be reduced is usually longer, however, with 10–28 days of dosing at the induction dose rate being required to bring the disease under control. It may be necessary to use other immunosuppressive drugs at this stage to help control refractory cases and reduce the dose of glucocorticoid required. Frequent monitoring for signs of recurrence of the disease under treatment should be undertaken as the dose is reduced.

ADVERSE EFFECTS OF GLUCOCORTICOIDS

The adverse effects of glucocorticoids can be predicted from the actions of glucocorticoids and from the clinical manifestations of hyperadrenocorticism. They are best avoided by:

- Using the lowest dose of glucocorticoid that is necessary, dosing on an every other day basis with oral prednisolone if possible

- Monitoring animals on glucocorticoids carefully, not merely increasing the dose when the owner reports that signs of the disease have reappeared, but examining the animal carefully for new problems which may require different therapy
- Recognising concomitant diseases which will be exacerbated by glucocorticoids and deciding on the risk–benefit of glucocorticoid therapy
- Managing withdrawal of glucocorticoid therapy carefully to avoid iatrogenic hypoadrenocorticism.

The adverse effects of glucocorticoids that are most commonly seen with chronic glucocorticoid therapy are:

Organ/System	Adverse effect	Comments
Cardiovascular	Hypertension (Na+ and water retention and vascular effects)	Tendency to cause Na+ retention varies with the preparation chosen Should avoid glucocorticoids in states where this may contribute to the disease process e.g.: • Cardiac disease where salt and water retention may precipitate signs of congestion • Chronic renal disease – animals are unable to excrete excess salt and water and tend to be hypertensive and hypokalaemic (especially cats) • Some forms of liver disease where hyperaldosteronism is already a complicating factor in the disease, leading to oedema formation and hypokalaemia
Endocrine	Insulin antagonism Thyroid hormone testing	Glucocorticoids antagonise the effects of insulin on peripheral tissues – subclinical diabetics may become overtly diabetic and clinical diabetics will require more insulin for control Glucocorticoids affect pituitary–thyroid function – cause confusion in the interpretation of total plasma thyroxine concentration
Eyes	Raise intraocular pressure Delay corneal healing	Glucocorticoids do raise intraocular pressure with long-term use but may be helpful in the acute phase of some forms of glaucoma where there is also an anterior uveitis present Glucocorticoids are contraindicated in ulcerative keratitis as they delay corneal healing and potentiate infectious agents
Gastrointestinal	Ulceration Perforation Pancreatitis Hepatopathy	Slow the rate of turnover of enterocytes and therefore may potentiate the ulcerogenic effects of non-steroidal anti-inflammatory drugs Trauma to the spinal cord may predispose to gastrointestinal tract ulceration severe enough to cause colonic perforation. Dogs undergoing spinal surgery are particularly susceptible to this problem Although controversial, it has been suggested that glucocorticoids can be one of the trigger factors for acute pancreatitis and as such should be avoided in dogs with a history of this problem Glucocorticoids cause accumulation of glycogen in hepatocytes and also lead to organelle damage with prolonged high-dose therapy. Some forms of liver disease with active inflammatory pathology will respond to glucocorticoids, in others glucocorticoid will be detrimental, particularly where there is hepatic encephalopathy (catabolic effects) or ascites (Na+ retaining effects)
Musculoskeletal	Arthropathy Osteoporosis	There are clear indications for steroid use in inflammatory arthritides but in degenerative joint disease their use is controversial. They inhibit cartilage synthesis, may accelerate its destruction and reduce its proteoglycan content, particularly after multiple intra-articular injections. Their use in degenerative joint disease is reserved for refractory cases to provide symptomatic relief after other treatment has failed Osteoporosis and vertebral compression fractures occur in man. Less of a problem in dogs and cats but would expect bone healing to be slow and metabolic bone disease to be potentiated in conditions such as renal failure
Nervous system	Behaviour changes	These are not well documented in veterinary medicine. High-dose glucocorticoid therapy can cause increased anxiety and aggression in some human patients. Anecdotal reports would suggest the same is true of dogs
Reproductive system	Infertility, birth defects and abortion	Glucocorticoids are not recommended for use during pregnancy because of these potential adverse effects

Table 32.5: Some adverse effects of glucocorticoids leading to specific concerns over their use.

- Polyphagia
- Polyuria and polydipsia
- Atrophy of the skin
- Redistribution of fat and hepatomegaly giving a pot-bellied appearance
- Increased susceptibility to infection by micro-organisms – viral infections in particular may worsen following glucocorticoid therapy
- Slow wound healing and tissue repair
- Iatrogenic hypoadrenocorticism on glucocorticoid withdrawal.

Other potential adverse effects that give rise to specific contraindications or concerns for the use of glucocorticoids are summarised in Table 32.5.

FURTHER READING

Behrend EN and Greco DS (1995) Clinical applications of glucocorticoid therapy in nonendocrine disease. In: *Current Veterinary Therapy XII*, ed. JD Bonagura, pp. 406–413. WB Saunders, Philadelphia

Ferguson EA (1993) Glucocorticoids – use and abuse. In: *Manual of Small Animal Dermatology*, ed. PH Locke *et al.*, pp. 233–243. BSAVA, Cheltenham

Keen PM (1984) Uses and abuses of corticosteroids. In: *Veterinary Annual 27th edn*, ed. CGS Grunsell *et al.*, pp. 45–62. Scientechnica, Bristol

Moore GE, Mahaffey EA and Hoenig M (1992) Hematologic and serum biochemical effects of long term administration of anti-inflammatory doses of prednisone to dogs. *American Journal of Veterinary Research* **53**, 1033–1037

Roberts SM, Lavach JD, Macy DW and Severin GA (1984) Effect of ophthalmic prednisolone acetate on the canine adrenal gland and hepatic function. *American Journal of Veterinary Research* **45**, 1711–1714

Rutgers HC, Batt RM, Valliant C and Riley JE (1995) Subcellular pathologic features of glucocorticoid induced hepatopathy in dogs. *American Journal of Veterinary Research* **56**, 898–907

Scott DW (1995) Rational use of glucocorticoids in dermatology. In: *Current Veterinary Therapy XII*, ed. JD Bonagura, pp. 573–581. WB Saunders, Philadelphia

Sera DA (1991) Glucocorticoid therapy. In: *Consultations in Feline Internal Medicine*, ed. JR August, pp. 271–277. WB Saunders, Philadelphia

van den Broek AHM and Stafford WL (1992) Epidermal and hepatic glucocorticoid receptors in dogs and cats. *Research in Veterinary Science* **52**, 312–315

Zenoble RD and Kemppainen RJ (1987) Adrenocortical suppression by topically applied corticosteroids in healthy dogs. *Journal of the American Veterinary Medical Association* **191**, 685–688

CHAPTER THIRTY THREE

Collection, Storage and Transport of Samples for Hormone Assay

Ray F. Nachreiner and Kent R. Refsal

INTRODUCTION

Hormone testing continues to assume a prominent role in small animal practice, and clinical studies provide new insight into the interpretation of the results. There are continuous efforts to evaluate new hormone assays for diagnostic application, and laboratories now face the challenge of changing from the long-established techniques of radioimmunoassay (RIA) to immunoassays, methods that do not rely on radioactivity. It is important that as changes in hormone testing occur, there is continuous evaluation of sample quality and sample handling so that the best results can be achieved. This chapter outlines factors to consider when collecting, storing, and handling samples for hormone assay.

SERUM OR PLASMA

Most hormones can be accurately and validly assayed in serum samples; the exceptions are adrenocorticotropic hormone (ACTH), which requires EDTA as anticoagulant, and antidiuretic hormone (ADH), which has special requirements for collection. Cortisol is often assayed in EDTA plasma samples because, in some animals, it adheres to red blood cells after extended contact. However, when samples are centrifuged within 30 minutes of collection, the results are comparable in both serum and plasma. Laboratories do not tend to use heparin as an anticoagulant for cortisol and other hormones, as fibrin often forms, and precipitates from heparinised plasma can collect at pipette tips and invalidate results. The measurement of progesterone from cattle samples poses a problem, as a red blood cell enzyme metabolises the progesterone, thus falsely lowering the result. However, dogs and cats do not have such an enzyme and therefore special handling (cooling or rapid sample processing) is not required. Centrifuging samples shortly after the blood has clotted is always the best approach. Separating the serum from the clot will assure a valid sample and avoid haemolysis if, for example, the sample was inadvertently frozen.

PROTEOLYSIS

Hormones such as ACTH, parathormone, insulin and ADH are often affected by proteolytic enzymes present in serum and plasma, and special sample handling is required. Generally, cooling will retard the activity of proteolytic enzymes. Other compounds can inhibit proteolytic activity, such as aprotinin; unfortunately, this preservative is not readily available to practitioners. If protease inhibitors do become available in the future they would be a tremendous advantage in the transportation of protein and peptide hormones. Of the protein hormones, thyrotropin seems to be an exception as it is quite stable in both serum and plasma, even at 37°C; hence, special sample handling is not required.

HAEMOLYSIS

Many laboratories use RIA procedures for hormone assays. These procedures are quite robust and unaffected by slight haemolysis. However, severe haemolysis, which occurs when a whole blood sample is frozen, causes questionable results. As more laboratories change to enzyme immunoassays and other procedures with colorimetric end points, haemolysis will become a significant factor.

LIPAEMIA

Excess lipids in blood, or lipaemia, is not a problem for many RIA procedures because they tend to be reliable in their ability to detect hormones; however, at least one commercially available direct assay for free triiodothyronine is an exception, as the concentrations are falsely elevated when samples are lipaemic. Some ACTH assays are known to be affected by lipaemia as well. Lipaemia can also be a problem in hormone assays that use a colorimetric indicator.

SERUM SEPARATOR TUBES

Serum separator tubes contain a chemical that has a density between that of red blood cells and serum, and forms a gelatinous barrier between the two. This enables serum to be easily poured from the tube into the container used for sample transportation. A number of studies have been performed to test the effect of serum separator tubes on assay results. In our laboratory, we found that there were no important differences in the results of RIA using serum

Hormone	Temperature (^{0}C)	Number of days	Percentage hormone remaining	Temperature (^{0}C)	Number of days	Percentage hormone remaining
Adrenoncorticotropin	22	1	80	22	3	65
Aldosterone	22	7	95	37	7	12
Antidiuretic hormone	4	1	59	22	1	1
Cortisol	22	7	95	37	3	35
Insulin	24	3	90	37	3	52
Insulin-like growth factor	22	7	105	37	7	103
Parathormone	6	7	65	24	7	19
Parathormone related protein	4	4	97	37	4	82
Total thyroxine (T4)	22	7	95	37	7	75
Total triiodothyronine (T3)	22	7	75	37	4	48
Free T4 direct	22	7	105	37	7	77
Free T3	22	7	85	37	7	30
Free T4 by dialysis	4	7	105	37	7	160
Canine thyrotropin	20	4	110	37	4	98
Vitamin D (1,25-dihydroxycholecalciferol)	4	6	105	22	6	95

Table 33.1: Percentage of hormone remaining after incubation at various temperatures and for varying numbers of days.

separator tubes; some procedures, however, have been reported to be affected and this appears to be especially important when some of the new non-RIA procedures are used. The manufacturer's instructions and laboratory protocol should always be followed.

GLASS TUBES

ACTH is a relatively small molecule which will adsorb to glass; silicone additives can prevent this, although plastic tubes seem to overcome the problem. Hence, an EDTA glass tube may be used to collect a blood sample, but the blood should be transferred to a plastic tube before centrifugation or transportation.

TEMPERATURE

A number of studies have been performed in our laboratory over the past 10 years to determine the effects of time and temperature on the stability of hormones in canine serum samples; the times and temperatures studied represent those to which samples are subjected during transportation. The times varied, but the usual incubation period was 4–7 days and the incubation temperatures usually 4ºC, 20–22ºC and 37ºC. Hormone concentrations were determined using validated RIA techniques (Table 33.1).

While some hormones degrade because of conditions during transportation, it is interesting to note that measured concentrations of free thyroxine (T4) by dialysis increase. The binding globulins either seem to lose some of their affinity for T4 or some of the binding proteins

degrade and the free fraction becomes greater.

CONTAINERS

We have tested a number of commercially available containers used for sample transportation. One suitable container is a polystyrene box measuring 20 cm × 16 cm × 13 cm with walls 2.4 cm thick. The box contains two 450 g gel packs: when these gel packs are frozen at –24ºC, a 2 ml sample can remain below 7ºC for 24 hours when the entire package is incubated at 22ºC, and below 10ºC for 8 hours when the entire package is incubated at 37ºC. Hence, samples to be assayed for plasma renin activity and ADH would need to be transported on dry ice, but samples to be assayed for most other hormones would be valid after overnight delivery. Results indicate that most hormone samples can be transported to laboratories at some distance provided specific conditions for the samples are met (Table 33.2).

EPISODIC HORMONE SECRETION

A number of hormones are released episodically by the pituitary because of pulsatile secretion of their respective releasing hormones from the hypothalamus. Many species possess such cycles, which appear to last for about 1–2 hours. Hence, a sample collected at the end of a cycle could give low results compared with a sample collected from the same animal at the peak of a cycle. A misconception in adrenal function testing is that dogs follow a diurnal hormone release pattern similar to that of humans (lowest at bedtime and highest upon waking). In fact, cortisol release in dogs follows a random episodic pattern which cannot be predicted using sleep–wake infor-mation. Hence, there is nothing unique about obtaining a sample at 8 a.m. or at any other time of the day; adrenal function testing can be accomplished at any time.

Hormone	Sample	Transportation requirements
Adrenocorticotropin	EDTA[†], plasma	Plastic tube, frozen to <4°C for 24 hours
Aldosterone	EDTA[†], plasma	Transport on 1 kg frozen gel packs (<72 hours)
Ionised calcium	Serum	Overnight delivery on 1 kg frozen gel packs, and adjust result for pH change
Cortisol	EDTA[†], plasma	Transport on 1 kg frozen gel packs (<72 hours)
Gastrin	Serum	Transport on 1 kg frozen gel packs (<72 hours)
Insulin	Serum	Transport on 1 kg frozen gel packs (<72 hours)
Insulin-like growth factor	Serum	Transport on 1 kg frozen gel packs (<72 hours)
Parathormone	Serum	Overnight delivery on 1 kg frozen gel packs
Plasma renin activity	EDTA[†], plasma	Collect in chilled tube, centrifuge in cold centrifuge, freeze plasma, transport on dry ice
Progesterone	Serum	Transport on 1 kg frozen gel packs (<72 hours)
Testosterone	Serum	Transport on 1 kg frozen gel packs (<72 hours)
Thyroid function testing:		
Total thyroxine (T4)*	Serum	Room temperature (<7 days)
Total triiodothyronine	Serum	Room temperature (<7 days)
Direct free T4	Serum	Room temperature (<7 days)
Direct free T3	Serum	Room temperature (<7 days)
Reverse T3	Serum	Room temperature (<7 days)
Canine thyrotropin*	Serum	Room temperature (<7 days)
Free T4 by dialysis	Serum	Room temperature for 24 hours or <15°C for 48 hours
Vitamin D (1,25-dihydroxycholecalciferol)	Serum	Overnight delivery on 1 kg frozen gel packs
Urine cortisol	Urine	Transport on 1 kg frozen gel packs (<72 hours)

[†] EDTA samples are not recommended for hormone assays by chemiluminescent methods.
* Known to give false results when serum separator tubes are used to harvest serum if chemiluminescent or enzyme immunoassays are performed in the laboratory.

Table 33.2: Sample handling and shipping suggestions for transportation.

CHAPTER THIRTY FOUR

Reference Ranges and Test Protocols

Carmel T Mooney and Andrew G. Torrance

INTRODUCTION

This chapter is intended as a quick reference guide to laboratory tests, indications and interpretation. All of the ranges quoted are for guidance only and each individual laboratory should furnish its own reference ranges. In addition, it is advisable to follow the exact protocol recommended by the laboratory for dynamic function tests. Where applicable, cross-referencing to other chapters for further information is included.

ROUTINE LABORATORY SCREENING TESTS

Guideline reference ranges for screening laboratory tests are outlined in Tables 34.1, 34.2 and 34.3.

Haematology	Dog	Cat
PCV (l/l)	0.35–0.55	0.26–0.46
Hb (g/l)	120–180	80–150
RBC ($\times 10^{12}$/l)	5.4–8	5–11
MCV (fl)	65–75	37–49
MCH (pg)	22–25	12–17
MCHC (g/l)	340–370	320–350
Reticulocytes (%)	0–1	0–1
Reticulocytes ($\times 10^9$/l)	20–80	20–60
Platelets ($\times 10^9$/l)	150–400	150–400
WBC ($\times 10^9$/l)	6–18	5.5–19.5
Neutrophils (band)	0–0.3	0–0.3
Neutrophils (mature)	3–12	2.5–12.5
Lymphocytes	0.8–3.8	1.5–7
Monocytes	0.1–1.8	0–0.85
Eosinophils	0.1–1.9	0.1–1.5
Basophils	0–0.2	0–0.2
BMT (minutes)	<5	<2.5
OSPT (seconds)	7–12	7–12
APTT (seconds)	12 – 15	12–22

Table 34.1: *Routine haematological and haemostatic values for dogs and cats. In young dogs up to 6 months old, lymphocyte number may be increased by as much as 50%.*
MCV (fl) = (PCV × 1000) ÷ RBC; MCHC (g/l) = (Hb concentration) ÷ PCV; BMT, buccal mucosal, bleeding time; OSPT, one stage partial thromboplastin time; APTT, activated partial thromboplastin time.

Serum biochemistry	Dog	Cat
Total protein (g/l)	50–78	60–82
Albumin (g/l)	22–35	25–39
Alanine aminotransferase (ALT) (IU/l)	<100	<75
Aspartate aminotransferase (AST) (IU/l)	7–50	7–60
Alkaline phosphatase (ALP) (IU/l)	<200	<100
Lactate dehydrogenase (LDH) (IU/l)	50–350	50 – 350
γ-Glutamyl transferase (γ-GT) (IU/l)	0–8	0–8
Bilirubin (μmol/l)	0–6.8	0–6.8
Urea (mmol/l)	3–9	5–10
Creatinine (μmol/l)	20–110	40–150
Calcium (mmol/l)	2.2–2.9	2.1–2.9
Ionised calcium (mmol/l)	1.2–1.4	1.2–1.4
Phosphate (mmol/l)	0.5–2.6	1.1–2.8
Potassium (mmol/l)	3.8–5.8	3.6–5.8
Sodium (mmol/l)	140–158	145–165
Sodium:potassium ratio	>23:1	>23:1
Chloride (mmol/l)	105–122	112–129
Creatine kinase (CK) (IU/l)	0–500	0–600
Cholesterol (mmol/l)	2.7–9.5	1.5–6.0
Triglycerides (mmol/l)	<1	<1
Glucose (mmol/l)	3.5–5.5	3.5–6.5
Bile acids (fasting and post-prandial) (μmol/l)	<15	<15
Ammonia (μmol/l)	0–60	0–60
Amylase (IU/l)	400–2000	400–2000
Lipase (IU/l)	0–500	0–700
Glycosylated haemoglobin (%)	<5	<2
Fructosamine (μmol/l)	160–350	175–400
Fair control of diabetes mellitus	<450	<550
Poor control of diabetes mellitus	>450	>550
Trypsin-like immuno-reactivity (TLI) (ng/ml)	>5	>5
Bicarbonate (mmol/l)	21–23	15–23
pH	7.31–7.53	7.32–7.44
Osmolality (mOsmol/kg)	275 – 305	299–327

Table 34.2: *Routine serum biochemical values in dogs and cats. Alkaline phosphatase concentrations may be higher in young animals.*

Urinalysis		Dog	Cat
Specific gravity		1.015–1.045 (1.005 (min) – 1.050 (max))	1.015–1.060 (1.005 (min) – 1.060 (max))
pH		5.5–7.5	5.5–7.5
Volume (ml/kg/24 hours)		20–40	22–30
Osmolality (mOsmol/kg)		500–1200 (161(min)–2830(max))	50–3000
Bilirubin		0–trace	0
Glucose/ketones		0	0
Protein semiquantitative		0–trace/1+	0–trace/1+
Protein:creatinine ratio		<0.6	<0.6
	Equivocal	0.6–1.0	0.6–1.0
	Abnormal	>1.0	>1.0
Sediment	Leucocytes (/hpf)	0–5	0–5
	Erythrocytes (/hpf)	0–5	0–5
	Casts (/hpf)	0	0

Table 34.3: Routine urinalysis results in dogs and cats. hpf = high power field.

HORMONE ANALYSES

Conversion of hormones to SI units is outlined in Table 34.4 and guideline reference ranges for the more commonly used hormones are given in Table 34.5.

Measurement	SI unit	Common unit	Common to SI*	SI to Common*
Aldosterone	pmol/l	ng/dl	27.7	0.036
Adrenaline	pmol/l	pg/ml	5.46	0.183
Adrenocorticotropin (ACTH)	pmol/l	pg/ml	0.22	4.51
Cortisol	nmol/l	µg/dl	27.59	0.036
β-Endorphin	pmol/l	pg/ml	0.292	3.43
Gastrin	ng/l	pg/ml	1.00	1.00
Gastrointestinal polypeptide	pmol/l	pg/ml	0.201	4.98
Glucagon	ng/l	pg/ml	1.00	1.00
Growth hormone	µg/l	ng/ml	1.00	1.00
Insulin	pmol/l	µIU/ml	7.18	0.139
Insulin-like growth factor-1	µg/ml	ng/ml	1.00	1.00
α Melanocyte stimulating hormone (αMSH)	pmol/l	pg/ml	0.601	1.66
Noradrenaline	nmol/l	pg/ml	0.006	169.00
Oestrogen (Oestradiol)	pmol/l	pg/ml	3.67	0.273
Pancreatic polypeptide	mmol/l	mg/dl	0.239	4.18
Progesterone	nmol/l	ng/ml	3.18	0.315
Prolactin	µg/l	ng/ml	1.00	1.00
Renin	ng/l/s	ng/ml/h	0.278	3.60
Somatostatin	pmol/l	pg/ml	0.611	1.64
Testosterone	nmol/l	ng/ml	3.47	0.288
Total thyroxine (T4)	nmol/l	µg/dl	12.87	0.078
Free T4	pmol/l	ng/dl	12.87	0.078
Total triiodothyronine (T3)	nmol/l	ng/dl	0.0154	64.90
Vasoactive intestinal polypeptide	pmol/l	pg/ml	0.301	3.33

Table 34.4: Conversion to SI (système internationale) units for hormone assays.
* Factor to multiply by to convert one unit to another

Hormone	Guideline ranges	
	Dog	**Cat**
Total thyroxine (T4) (nmol/l)	15–50	15–60
Free T4 (pmol/l)*	10–45	10–45
Total triiodothyronine (T3) (nmol/l)	0.5–2.5	0.5–2.5
Canine thryotropin (cTSH) (ng/ml)	<0.6	
Cortisol (nmol/l)	20–250	20–250
Urine cortisol:creatinine ratio	$<10 \times 10^{-6}$	$<10 \times 10^{-6}$
Adrenocorticotropic hormone (ACTH)* (pg/ml)	20–80	20–80
Parathormone* (pg/ml)	10–60	3–25
Insulin (μIU/ml)*	5–20	5–20
Growth hormone (GH) (μg/l)	2–5	2–5
Insulin-like growth factor-1 (IGF-1) (ng/ml)	200–800	200–800
Healthy dogs up to 1 year	500–1000	
Progesterone (nmol/l)		Dependent on oestrus cycle
Pro-oestrus	5.4±0.95	
Oestrus	<5.4	
Dioestrus	57±20	
Metoestrus	76±10	
Anoestrus	1.9±0.3	
Oestradiol (pmol/l)		
Pro-oestrus	213±26	
Oestrus	253±40	
Dioestrus	84±26	
Metoestrus	66±11	
Anoestrus	121±55	
Males	50–200	

Table 34.5: *Guideline reference ranges for the commonly requested hormones.*

Total thyroxine (T4)
- Widely available
- Indications:
  Screening test for hypothyroidism (Chapter 14 and 25)
  Diagnosis of canine hypothyroidism when combined with cTSH (Chapter 14)
  Diagnosis of hyperthyroidism (Chapter 15 and 30)
  Monitoring thyroid hormone supplementation (Chapter 31)
  Monitoring antithyroid medication (Chapter 15)
  Prognostic indicator (Chapter 5)
- Use in dynamic function tests:
  TSH stimulation test
  TRH stimulation test
  T3 suppression test

Free thyroxine (T4)
- Specialised laboratory
  Equilibrium dialysis recommended
- Indications:
  More sensitive but less specific than total T4 for feline hyperthyroidism (Chapter 15)
  More specific than total T4 for diagnosing canine hypothyroidism (Chapter 14)

Total triiodothyronine (T3)
- Widely available
- Indications:
  No advantage over total T4
- Use in dynamic function tests:
  Monitoring tablet administration in the T3 suppression test

Canine thyroid stimulating hormone (cTSH)
- Widely available
- Indications:
  Diagnosis of canine hypothyroidism when combined with total or free T4 (Chapter 14)
  Monitoring T4 supplementation.
- Use in dynamic function tests
  TRH stimulation test (usefulness in diagnosing hypothyroidism not yet evaluated)

Cortisol
- Widely available
- Indications:
  Basal cortisol concentrations not diagnostically valuable
  Urinary cortisol:creatinine ratio may be valuable as a screening test for hyperadrenocorticism (Chapter 10)

- Use in dynamic function tests
  ACTH stimulation test
  Low dose dexamethasone suppression test

Adrenocorticotropin

- Specialised laboratory
- Indications:
  Differentiation of pituitary-dependent from adrenal-dependent hyperadrenocorticism. Values >45 pg/ml are consistent with the former and values <10 pg/ml with the latter (Chapter 10)
  Investigation of primary or secondary hypoadreno-corticism (Chapter 11)

Insulin

- Specialised laboratory
- Indications:
  Assessment of pancreatic function in diabetes mellitus (Chapter 12)
  Diagnosis of insulinoma (Chapter 17). Blood glucose concentrations must be assessed simultaneously. Values >10 μIU/ml in the face of hypoglycaemia are consistent with a diagnosis of insulinoma. Values <5 μIU/ml are inconsistent with such a diagnosis. In equivocal cases the insulin:glucose ratio (IGR) or amended insulin:glucose ratio (AIGR) can be used.
  IGR = insulin (μIU/ml) ÷ glucose (mmol/l). Values ≥ 4.2 IU/mol consistent with insulinoma.
  AIGR = (plasma insulin (μIU/ml) × 100) ÷ (plasma glucose (mg/dl)–30). Values ≥ 30 consistent with insulinoma

Growth hormone (GH)

- Specialised laboratory outside UK
- Indications:
  Diagnosis of acromegaly. Values >6 μg/l consistent with this diagnosis (Chapter 28)
- Use in dynamic function tests:
  As part of clonidine, xylazine or growth hormone releasing hormone stimulation tests for the diagnosis of pituitary dwarfism (Chapter 27)

Insulin-like growth factor-1 (IGF-1)

- Specialised laboratory
- Indications:
  Diagnosis of pituitary dwarfism. Values <50 ng/ml consistent with such a diagnosis (Chapter 27)
  Diagnosis of acromegaly (Chapter 28). Values >1000 ng/ml are consistent with such a diagnosis

Parathormone (PTH)

- Specialised laboratory
- Indications:
  Investigation of hypercalcaemia (Chapter 16). High or high-normal values in association with hypercalcaemia are highly suggestive of primary hyperparathyroidism. Extremely elevated concentrations may be found with renal disease. Low to low-normal values in association with hypercalcaemia are highly suggestive of malignancy associated hypercalcaemia

Diagnosis of hypoparathyroidism (Chapter 16)
Values are low to low-normal in association with hypocalcaemia

Progesterone

- Widely available
- Indications:
  Assessment of timing of mating (Chapter 8)
  Mating/insemination is recommended within 4–6 days of the plasma progesterone concentration exceeding 6.5 nmol/l or the day after values exceed 25.0–32.0 nmol/l
  Establishing stage of oestrous cycle together with vaginal cytology in mismated bitches (Chapter 9)

Oestradiol

- Widely available
- Indications:
  Diagnosing Sertoli cell tumours in dogs (Chapter 3)
  High values are highly suggestive of this diagnosis but normal values do not exclude it
  Investigation of bitches for ovarian remnants
  Evaluating the stage of the oestrous cycle (in conjunction with progesterone)

DYNAMIC FUNCTION TESTS

Dynamic function tests are indicated to confirm a diagnosis particularly where results of basal hormone analyses overlap between healthy, sick and affected animals. In addition, dynamic function tests may be used to predict the site of malfunction when more than one abnormality is capable of producing the same end result.

TSH stimulation test

- Indications:
  Confirmation of hypothyroidism in dogs (Chapter 14)
  Confirmation of hypothyroidism in cats (Chapter 25)
- Method:
  Measurement of total T4 before and 6 hours after the intravenous administration of 0.1 IU/kg (dogs) or 0.5 IU/kg (cats) bovine TSH
- Interpretation:
  Post-TSH total T4 concentrations increase over 1.5 times basal and exceed 30 nmol/l in healthy dogs
  Post-TSH total T4 concentrations do not exceed 20 nmol/l in hypothyroid dogs. Values between these ranges are equivocal and may be the result of hypothyroidism, non-thyroidal illness or concurrent drug therapy
  Total T4 concentrations usually double after TSH administration in healthy cats but do not significantly increase in hypothyroidism.

TRH stimulation test

- Indications:
  Confirming euthyroidism in dogs suspected of hypothyroidism (Chapter 14)
  Diagnosis of feline hyperthyroidism in equivocal

cases (Chapter 15)

Diagnosis of feline hypothyroidism (Chapter 25)

- Method:

  Measurement of serum total T4 concentrations before and 4 hours after the intravenous administration of 500 μg (dogs) or 100 μg/kg (cats) TRH. Side effects are common

- Interpretation:

  Post-TRH total T4 concentrations increase over 1.5 times basal concentrations representing an increment >6 nmol/l in healthy dogs. Values below this are consistent with hypothyroidism, non-thyroidal illness or drug therapy but occasionally occur in healthy dogs

  Post-TRH total T4 concentrations are usually 60–100% higher than basal concentrations in healthy cats. Increases below 50% are consistent with hyperthyroidism in cats with high basal concentrations and with hypothyroidism in cats with low basal total T4 concentrations

T3 suppression test

- Indications:

  Diagnosis of feline hyperthyroidism in equivocal cases (Chapter 15)

- Method:

  Measurement of serum total T4 concentrations before and 2–4 hours after 7 consecutive 8 hourly oral doses of 20 μg tertroxin. Simultaneous measurement of serum total T3 concentrations ensures adequate compliance in administering the drug

- Interpretation:

  Serum total T4 concentrations decrease to <20 nmol/l with >50% suppression of basal values in healthy cats. Serum total T4 concentrations remain >20 nmol/l with less than 50% suppression in hyperthyroid cats. In both cases, serum total T3 concentrations increase

ACTH stimulation test

- Indications:

  Diagnosis of canine hyperadrenocorticism and canine and feline hypoadrenocorticism (Chapter 10 and 11)

  Combined with dexamethasone suppression for the diagnosis of feline hyperadrenocorticism (Chapter 29)

- Method:

  Measurement of circulating cortisol concentrations before and one hour after the intravenous or intramuscular injection of 0.25 mg synthetic ACTH (tetracosactrin). In cats, synthetic ACTH is injected

intravenously at a dose of 0.125 mg

- Interpretation:

  Post-ACTH cortisol concentrations usually are below 450 nmol/l in healthy dogs. Post-ACTH cortisol concentrations that exceed 600 nmol/l are consistent with a diagnosis of hyperadrenocorticism. Reference range values do not exclude the diagnosis

  In both dogs and cats with hypoadrenocorticism, basal cortisol concentrations are low and show little or no increase following ACTH administration

  Similar results are seen after therapy with glucocorticoids or progestogens

Low-dose dexamethasone suppression test (LDDS)

- Indications:

  Diagnosis of canine hyperadrenocorticism (Chapter 10)

  Differentiation of adrenal tumour from pituitary-dependent hyperadrenocorticism (Chapter 10)

- Method:

  Measurement of circulating cortisol concentrations before and 3 and 8 hours after the intravenous administration of 0.01–0.015 mg/kg dexamethasone.

- Interpretation:

  Post-dexamethasone cortisol concentrations that exceed 40 nmol/l at 8 hours are consistent with a diagnosis of hyperadrenocorticism. Suppression at 3 hours followed by escape is consistent with pituitary-dependent hyperadrenocorticism

Combined high-dose dexamethasone suppression and ACTH stimulation test

- Indications:

  Diagnosis of feline hyperadrenocorticism (Chapter 29)

- Method:

  Measurement of circulating cortisol concentrations before and 2 hours after the intravenous administration of 0.1 mg/kg dexamethasone followed by the immediate intravenous administration of 0.125 mg ACTH and measurement of cortisol concentrations 1 hour later

- Interpretation:

  Failure to suppress cortisol concentrations after dexamethasone with an exaggerated response to ACTH is consistent with a diagnosis of feline hyperadrenocorticism

Index

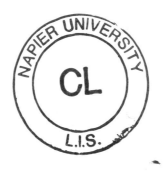
256